P9-CFP-293

Language Disorders

A Functional Approach to Assessment and Intervention

Robert E. Owens, Jr.

State University of New York at Geneseo

Merrill, an imprint of
Macmillan Publishing Company
New York

Collier Macmillan Canada, Inc.
Toronto

Maxwell Macmillan International Publishing Group
New York   Oxford   Singapore   Sydney

For information about the Macmillan Catalog write: Macmillan Publishing Company, 445 Hutchinson Ave., Columbus, OH 43235

Editor: Ann Castel
Production Editor: Constantina Geldis
Photo Editor: Gail Meese
Cover Designer: Brian Deep

Copyright © 1991 by Macmillan Publishing Company.
Merrill is an imprint of Macmillan Publishing Company.

Printed in the United States of America

All rights reserved. No part of this book may be reproduced
or transmitted in any form or by any means, electronic or mechanical,
including photocopy, recording, or any information storage and retrieval system,
without permission in writing from the Publisher.

Macmillan Publishing Company
866 Third Avenue, New York, New York 10022

Collier Macmillan Canada, Inc.

Library of Congress Cataloguing-in-Publication Data
Owens, Robert E.
    Language disorders : a functional approach to assessment and
    intervention / Robert E. Owens, Jr.
        p.   cm.
    Includes bibliographical references and indexes.
    ISBN 0-675-20773-8
    1.   Language disorders in children.   I.   Title.
RJ496.L35094   1990
618.92'855—dc20   90-6525
                                                                    CIP

Photo credits: p. 2, Merrill Publishing; p. 24, Tim Cairns/Merrill Publishing; pp. 60 and 198, Lloyd Lemmerman/Merrill Publishing; p. 84, Gail Meese/Merrill Publishing; p. 122, Jean Greenwald/Merrill Publishing; p. 150, Michael Siluk; p. 172, Nancy P. Alexander; p. 214, David Napravnik/Merrill Publishing; p. 260, Paul Conklin; p. 282, Randall D. Williams; p. 306, David Strickler

Printing: 1 2 3 4 5 6 7 8 9   Year: 1 2 3 4

To my parents,
who have freely given of their love
and
asked for nothing in return.

Preface

Language Disorders: A Functional Approach to Assessment and Intervention is the culmination of several years of work in speech-language pathology with both presymbolic and symbolic children and adults. In this book, I concentrate on children because of the special problems they exhibit in learning language. Adults who are acquiring language, or who have lost language and are attempting to regain it, represent a much more diverse group and would be difficult to address in one text. This does not mean that children are a homogeneous group or that intervention with this group is easy. Any school speech-language pathologist will attest otherwise.

I call the model of assessment and intervention presented in this text *functional language.* The approach goes by other names, such as environmental or conversational, and includes elements of several other models. Where I have borrowed someone's model, ideas, or techniques, full credit is given to that person. I find assessment and intervention an adaptation of a little of this and a little of that within an overall theoretical framework. Readers should approach this text with this in mind. Some ideas presented are very practical and easy to implement, whereas others may not apply to particular intervention settings. Readers should use what they can, keeping in mind the goal of trying to use the natural environment and natural conversations as the context for training language. I am the first to acknowledge that I do not have a monopoly on assessment and intervention methods.

Within *Language Disorders,* I have made some content decisions that should be explained. First, I have used the feminine pronoun when referring to the speech-language pathologist in recognition of the fact that most speech-language pathologists are women. I apologize to male speech-language pathologists, who should take comfort in the fact that the much overworked masculine pronoun has been given a deserved rest. Second, I group all children with language problems, both delays and disorders, under the general rubric of *language-impaired*. This expedient decision was made recognizing that this text would not be addressing specific disorder populations except in a tangential manner. Third, I address two special cases in Chapter 10, which discusses classroom applications of the functional model, and in Chapters 11 and 12, which discuss presymbolic and minimally symbolic children. Chapter 10 recognizes the large numbers of speech-language pathologists who work within the public schools and the revolution in service delivery that is occurring there. Chapters 11 and 12 address a population close to my heart and to my initial clinical experiences.

No text is written without the aid of other people. I acknowledge the advice and counsel of Brenda Rogerson, director, Central Ohio Speech and Hearing Center, a colleague, confidant, and dear friend of long standing; and Dr. Addie Haas, chair, Department of Communication, State University of New York at New Paltz, a constant inspiration and breath of freshness. In addition, special thanks and love to Tom Menzel for his patience, support, and understanding. Other contributors include Dr. Linda House, chair, Department of Speech Pathology and Audiology, State University of New York at Geneseo; Dr. Kathy Jones, Department of Speech Pathology and Audiology, Nazareth College; and Donna Cooperman, Department of Speech Pathology and Audiology, College of St. Rose.

Additionally, I appreciate the comments and suggestions made by the following reviewers: Lynne E. Rowan, University of Illinois—Urbana-Champaign; Lynn S. Bliss, Wayne State University; Thomas Klee, Vanderbilt University; Darlene Gould Davies, San Diego State University; Diana L. Hughes, Central Michigan University; Nan Bernstein Ratner, University of Maryland; A. Lynn Williams, California State University—Fullerton; Karen Steckol, St. Louis University; Jim Halle, University of Illinois—Urbana-Champaign; Linda McCormick, University of Hawaii—Manoa; Lauren Nelson, The Ohio State University; and Joe Reichle, University of Minnesota.

Finally, my deepest gratitude to Dr. James MacDonald, Department of Speech Pathology and Audiology, The Ohio State University, for introducing me to the potential of the environment in communication intervention.

Robert E. Owens, Jr.

Contents

ONE
Introduction

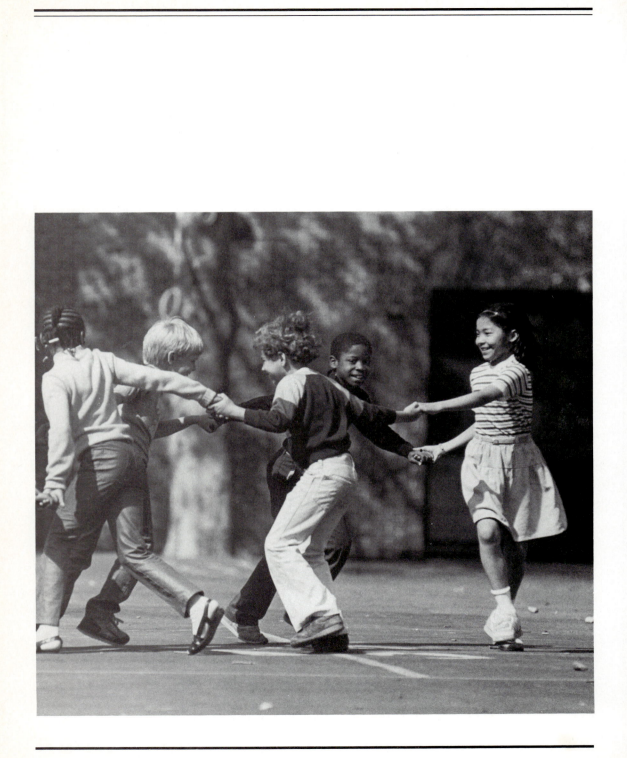

1
A Functional Language Approach

L anguage is a vehicle for communication or participation in conversations (Loban, 1979). In other words, ''language is a social tool'' used in communication interactions (McLean & Snyder-McLean, 1978, p. 47). Implicit in the use of language is the assumption that the user is communicating meanings with someone else. Thus, language can be viewed as a dynamic force or process rather than as a product (Muma, 1978). The goal of speech-language intervention, therefore, should extend beyond language itself to include better communication. Newly trained language skills should be evaluated to the extent that these skills enhance overall communication. This is the goal of a functional language approach.

A functional language approach to assessment and intervention, as described in this text, targets language as it is used or as it works for the language user as a vehicle for communication. In clinical intervention, a functional approach to language impairment is a communication-first approach. The focus is the overall communication of the language-impaired child and of those who communicate with the child. The goal is better communication that works in the client's natural communicative contexts. Thus, ''if the therapeutic strategy does not result in the child's acquiring a generalized communicative repertoire, we have failed (or at least have not succeeded)'' (Warren & Rogers-Warren, 1985, p. 5). The speech-language pathologist needs to ensure that the language skills that are targeted and trained generalize to the actual everyday environment of the child. This concern for language use necessitates a new primacy for pragmatics in intervention protocols.

In short, in a functional language approach, conversation between children and their communication partners becomes the vehicle for change. By manipulating the linguistic and nonlinguistic contexts within which a child's utterances occur, the partner facilitates the use of certain structures and provides evaluative feedback while maintaining the conversational flow. From the early data collection stages, through target selection, to the intervention process, the speech-language pathologist and other communication partners are concerned with the enhancement of overall communication. The functional approach, therefore, is a holistic one that uses as much of the child's natural environment as possible.

Traditionally, language-training programs have focused more or less on language form and content with little consideration given to pragmatics or language use (Spinelli & Terrell, 1984). The typical approach to teaching language forms has been a highly structured, behavioral one emphasizing the teaching of specific behaviors within a stimulus-response-reinforcement paradigm (Fey, 1986). Thus, language is a product or response elicited by a stimulus or produced in anticipation of reinforcement.

Many speech-language pathologists prefer structured approaches because the clinician can predict accurately the language-impaired child's response to the training stimuli. In addition, structured behavioral approaches increase the probability that the client will make the appropriate, desired response. Language lessons are usually scripted as drills and, therefore, are repetitive and predictable for the clinician.

The child becomes a passive learner, and active processing by the child is disregarded. Cognitive processes and the child's individual cognitive style, motivation, and communication intent are often minimized.

The clinician manipulates structured stimuli in order to elicit responses and dispenses reinforcement. In other words, clinical procedures are unidirectional and clinician directed (Fey, 1986; Snow, Midkiff-Borunda, Small, & Proctor, 1984). The clinician's overall style is highly directive (Ripich & Panagos, 1985; Ripich & Spinelli, 1985). Fey (1986) labels these approaches "trainer-oriented" and finds them deficient in the area of developing meaningful uses for the newly acquired form or content.

Structured behavioral or trainer-oriented approaches that exhibit intensity, consistency, and organization have been successful in teaching some language skills to the mentally retarded (Guess, Sailor, & Baer, 1974) and to other language-impaired populations, such as language learning disabled (LLD) children. Such approaches work, and the results are easily measured because the objectives are specific and discernible.

A major problem with present clinical approaches, however, is generalization from clinical to more natural contexts. Such generalization usually is not automatic (Spinelli & Terrell, 1984). This lack of generalization may be a function of the material selected for training, the learning characteristics of the child, or the training paradigm.

Stimuli present in the clinical setting, which directly or indirectly affect the behavior being trained, may not be found in other settings (Costello, 1983). For example, the child may learn to respond only in the presence of certain specific stimuli found in the clinical setting. Some of these stimuli may be intentional, such as training cues, whereas others, such as the clinician, may be unintentional. In addition, clinical cues or consequences used for teaching may be very different from those encountered in everyday situations. This lack of natural consequences may also remove the motivation to use the behavior elsewhere.

In contrast, functional approaches give more control to the language-impaired child and decrease the amount of structure in intervention activities. Indices of improvement are an increase in successful communication rather than the number of correct responses (Marion, 1983). Procedures used by the speech-language pathologist and communication partners more closely resemble those in the language learning environment of nonimpaired children. In addition, the everyday environment of the language-impaired child is also included in training.

Children who are inactive or passive communicators seem to achieve especially well within the supportive, responsive, accepting atmosphere of functional intervention (Fey, 1987). Children who possess a well-established active communication style may benefit less.

The effectiveness of any language-teaching strategy will vary with the characteristics of the language-impaired child (Connell, 1987a; Friedman & Friedman, 1980). For example, children with language learning disabilities seem to benefit more from specific language training than do other language-impaired children (Nye, Foster, & Seaman, 1987). Likewise, more severely language-impaired children initially benefit more from a structured imitative approach.

Although this text advocates a functional approach, it is recognized that exclusive use of any one strategy is too inflexible. It is probably more efficient to merge functional interactive models with more direct behavioral instruction. To rely exclusively on a functional interactive approach does not allow for the needs of individual language-impaired children.

Direct instruction might be used initially to introduce a new language structure that can then be generalized through use of more interactive techniques. Syntactic disorders seem to respond best to direct teaching, whereas pragmatic disorders improve very little (Nye et al., 1987).

Functional language approaches have been used to increase mean length of utterance and multiword utterance production; the overall quantity of communication; pragmatic skills, such as requesting, responsiveness, and initiation; vocabulary growth; language complexity; receptive labeling; intelligibility and the use of trained forms in novel utterances in children with mental retardation, autism, specific language impairment, language learning disability, and multiple handicaps (Alpert & Rogers-Warren, 1984; Friedman & Friedman, 1980; Girolametto, 1988; Halle, Baer, & Spradlin, 1981; Hart & Risley, 1974, 1975, 1980; McGee, Krantz, Mason, & McClannahan, 1983; Nye et al., 1987; Scherer & Olswang, 1989; Schwartz, Chapman, Terrell, Prelock, & Rowan, 1985; Warren, McQuarter, & Rogers-Warren, 1984). Even minimally symbolic children who require a more structured approach benefit from a conversational milieu (Hart & Rogers-Warren, 1978; MacDonald & Gillette, 1982; Owens, McNerney, Bigler-

Burke, & Lepre-Clark, 1987). In addition, functional interactive approaches may result in improved generalization even when the immediate results differ little from more direct instructional methods (Alpert & Rogers-Warren, 1984; Cole & Dale, 1986; Halle et al., 1981; Hart & Risley, 1968; Rogers-Warren & Warren, 1980; Warren & Kaiser, 1986a).

In this chapter, we explore a rationale for a functional language approach. This rationale is based on the primacy of pragmatics in language and on the generalization of language intervention.

PRAGMATICS

Pragmatics is the relationship between communicative partners and the form and meaning of the language being used. In short, pragmatics consists of the intentions or communication goals of each speaker and of the linguistic adjustments made by each speaker for the listener in order to accomplish these goals. Most features of language are affected by pragmatic aspects of the conversational context. For example, the selection of pronouns, verb tenses, articles, and adverbs or adverbial phrases of time involves more than syntactic and semantic considerations. The conversational partners must be aware of the preceding linguistic information and of each other's point of reference.

Pragmatics and accompanying issues of context have raised concerns about the number and type of features that speech-language pathologists should assess and train (Duchan, 1983b). An earlier interest by speech-language pathologists in psycholinguistics has led to the present therapeutic emphasis on increasing utterance length by increasing syntactic complexity. The speech-language pathologist's role has been to discover each child's individual learning strategies and to use these within a unidirectional, clinician-directed approach (Snow et al., 1984). Intervention goals have usually been based on language form with use frequently ignored. In short, the child's communicative intentions have been considered irrelevant. More pragmatic intervention goals might include communication functions, turn taking, discourse structures, and registers or styles of language.

With the therapeutic shift in interest to semantics or meaning in the early 1970s, there was a new recognition of the importance of cognitive or intellectual readiness but little understanding of the importance of the social environment. Most intervention approaches maintained structural behavioral teaching techniques.

The influence of sociolinguistics and pragmatics in the late 1970s and 1980s has led to interest in conversational rules and contextual factors. Everyday contexts have provided a backdrop for explanations of linguistic performance (Duchan, 1984). Of specific interest is the way individuals negotiate interactions and meanings with one another.

In working with special populations, the focus is shifting to a continuation of the communication process rather than to treating specific symptoms of disorder (Duchan, 1982a, 1984; Frankel, 1982). Previously, for example, children's behaviors were considered either appropriate or inappropriate to the stimulus-reinforcement situation rather than as a part of the interaction. Echolalia and unusual language patterns of autistic, psychotic, and retarded children were considered inappropriate and, therefore, were extinguished (Schreibman & Carr, 1978) or punished (Lovaas, 1977) in order to decrease their frequency of occurrence. When emphasis shifts to pragmatics and to the processes that underlie behavior, however, the child's language can be considered on its own terms (Tager-Flusberg, 1981). Echolalia and delayed echolalia are said to occur when the child does not understand or when the child expresses certain intentions (Curcio & Paccia-Cooper, 1982; Duchan, 1983a; Paccia-Cooper & Curcio, 1982; Prizant & Duchan, 1981; Prizant, 1983a).

The sociolinguistic model acknowledges not only individual differences across children but also stylistic differences within children as they interact with varying communicative partners. ''The natural outgrowth of such [sociolinguistic] procedures is to involve families and teachers in training programs in which they create environments and interactive modes that are finely tuned and responsive to the communicative attempts and language competencies of [language-impaired] . . . children'' (Duchan, 1984, p. 67).

The traditional or formalist view of language as a composite of various rule systems, consisting of syntax, morphology, phonology, semantics, and pragmatics (Figure 1.1), may be inadequate (Prutting, 1982). This multileveled formalist approach has given way to a functional intervention model and to a more holistic approach to intervention. Language is a social tool, and, as such, considerations of language use are paramount. The formalist model is being replaced for many

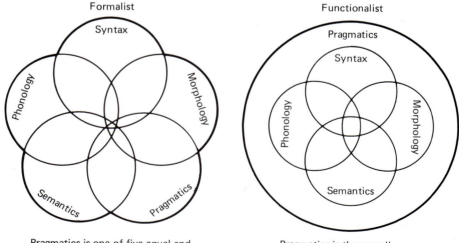

Pragmatics is one of five equal and interrelated aspects of language.

Pragmatics is the overall organizing aspect of language.

FIGURE 1.1
Relationship of the aspects of language

speech-language pathologists by one in which pragmatics is the overall organizing framework. Increasingly, speech-language pathologists are recognizing that structure and content are heavily influenced by the conversational constraints of the communication context.

This view of language has necessitated a very different approach to language intervention (Prutting, 1983). In effect, intervention has moved from an *entity approach,* which targets discrete isolated bits of language, to a *systems approach,* which targets language within the overall communication process. Therapy has become process rather than product oriented (Snow et al., 1984).

The major implication of a systems approach is a change in both the targets and the methods of training (Craig, 1983; Muma, Pierce, & Muma, 1983). If, as formalists contend, pragmatics is just one of five equal aspects of language, then it offers yet another set of rules for training. Thus, there will be additional training goals, but the methodology need not change. The training can still emphasize the *what* with little change in the *how,* which can continue in a structured behavioral paradigm.

In contrast, an approach in which pragmatics is the organizing aspect of language necessitates a more interactive conversational training approach, one that mirrors the transfer environment in which the language will be used. Therapy becomes bidirectional and child oriented, and conversation is viewed as a language-learning context (Cook-Gumperz & Gumperz, 1978; Snow et al., 1984; Waterson & Snow, 1978; Wells, 1981). Such an approach has been demonstrated to be effective (Friedman & Friedman, 1980). Thus, the conversational context becomes the teaching *and* transfer environment.

Dimensions of Communication Context

Language is more than just uttering words in linear sequence (Steinmann, 1982). Language is purposeful and takes place within a dynamic context. "We do not experience language in isolation . . . [but] in relation to a scenario, some background of persons and actions and events from which the things are said to derive their meaning" (Halliday, 1974, p. 28).

In other words, context affects form and content and may in turn be affected by them. Context consists of a complex interaction of the following six factors (Dudley-Marling & Rhodes, 1987):

> *Purpose.* Language users begin with a purpose that affects what to say and how to say it (Knoblauch, 1980).
> *Content.* We use language to communicate about something. The topic of discourse will affect the form and the style.
> *Type of discourse.* Certain types of discourse, such as a debate or speech, use a characteristic type of structure related to the purpose.
> *Participant characteristics.* Participant characteristics that affect context are background knowledge, roles, life experiences, moods, willingness to take risks, relative age, status, familiarity, and relationship in time and space (Graves, 1981).
> *Setting.* Setting includes the circumstances under which the language occurs.

Activity. The activity in which the language users are engaged will affect language, especially the choice of vocabulary.

Speech community. The speech community is that group with whom we share certain rules of language. It may be as large as the speakers of a language, such as English, or as small as two people who share a secret language of their own.

Mode of discourse. The purpose and the relations of language users in time and space are usually determined by the mode of discourse. Speech and writing are modes that require very different types of interaction from the participants.

Within a discourse, participants must continually assess these factors and their changing relationships.

The context imposes certain responsibilities on language users in the form of an implicit contract. These responsibilities include the following six conversational and politeness maxims (Grice, 1975; Lakoff, 1973):

Be relevant. Speakers are expected to stay on topic unless they signal a topic change.

Be truthful. The amount of truthfulness varies with the context, but each participant believes the other to be speaking the truth.

Be orderly. Discourse must be orderly and cohesive.

Avoid ambiguity. Speakers are expected to be as clear as possible. In turn, listeners are expected to signal when they do not understand the information transmitted.

Be brief. Speakers are expected to know their audiences and to provide no more information than is needed.

Be polite. Speakers do not impose on their listeners. Instead, they observe the rules of turn-taking, select the appropriate mode of address, and so on.

The actual rules observed in a conversation will depend on the contract between the participants and on the context (Dudley-Marling & Rhodes, 1987).

The speech-language pathologist should be a master of the conversational context. Unfortunately, it is too easy to rely on overworked verbal cues, such as ''Tell me about this picture'' or ''What do you want?'' to elicit certain language structures. As simple a behavior as waiting can be an effective intervention tool when appropriate (Hart, 1985). Similarly, a seemingly nonclinical utterance, such as ''Boy, that's a beautiful red sweater,'' can easily elicit negative constructions when directed at a child's green socks. Speech-language pathologists who know the dimensions of communication context understand these dimensions more effectively and manipulate them more efficiently.

At least five dimensions to the communication context must be considered by the speech-language pathologist (Prutting, 1982). They are the *cognitive context*, the *social context*, the *physical context*, the *linguistic context*, and the *nonlinguistic context*.

The cognitive context includes the communication partners' shared knowledge about the physical world. Obviously, two individuals cannot share the same exact knowledge base. A toddler and her mother, for example, have very different knowledge bases, and yet, they can communicate.

Parents adapt their behavior to the assumed knowledge level of their child. In part, parental behavior is constrained by parents' limited shared knowledge with the child. If the parents want the child to understand, they must adhere to topics that are known by the child or that differ only slightly (Hunt, 1961). The child provides feedback that is used in turn by the parents in structuring the conversation.

In the clinical setting, pathologists know much more than the client about the behavior being taught and must modify their behavior accordingly. Thus, for example, pathologists should ensure that the child understands the concepts of temporal order and reversibility before attempting to teach linguistic marking of these concepts.

The social context includes each communication partner's knowledge of the social world. Such knowledge encompasses the communication setting, the partner, and the interactional rules used by each partner. In the clinic, the speech-language pathologist should consider each child's social skills. For example, severely delayed clients or those with affective disorders often function as if they do not understand the concept of communication. These clients may seem asocial, and yet their behavior may be used in several atypical ways to communicate a great deal. Preschoolers who seem unaware of the need to self-monitor and to repair their production may not have social knowledge of listener needs. The speech-language pathologist must be aware of the child's social knowledge to understand the child's behavior.

In the physical context are each partner's perceptions of the people, places, and objects that form that context. For example, pictures are very concrete for adults but may be very abstract for young preschoolers. I worked with an emotionally disturbed adolescent who perceived the therapy room as very threatening despite my best efforts to dispel any fears. The speech-language pathologist can manipulate the variables within this context to resemble more closely the transfer environment. Better still, intervention can occur in settings in which the training targets are likely to occur.

The linguistic context consists of the verbal features that precede, accompany, and follow a verbalization and that are used by each partner for processing. For example, a question is usually followed by an answer; there is an obligation to reply. Earlier in this chapter we discussed the speech-language pathologist's skilled manipulation of the linguistic content in order to facilitate generalization.

Finally, the nonlinguistic context contains the nonlinguistic and paralinguistic events that surround a verbal production, that is, the activity in which the conversational partners are engaged. Some activities, such as group projects, encourage conversation, whereas others, such as silent reading, do not. The importance of this context as a facilitator of verbal production cannot be overlooked in the clinical setting. Speech-language pathologists who focus exclusively on the linguistic context produce conversations consisting of a series of didactic exchanges.

Summary

"We are in an exciting era in our attempts to understand the relationships among linguistic, pragmatic, social and cognitive aspects of language behavior" (Prutting, 1982, p. 132). In the clinical setting, speech pathologists are becoming more aware of the effects of context on communication. How well language-impaired children regulate their relationships with other people depends on their ability to monitor context (Prutting, 1982). Given the dynamic nature of conversational contexts, it is essential that intervention also address generalization to the child's everyday communication contexts.

GENERALIZATION

One of the most difficult aspects of therapeutic intervention in speech-language pathology is generalization or carry-over to nontraining situations (Fey, 1988; Halle, 1987; Warren, 1988; Warren, Rogers-Warren, Baer, & Guess, 1980). For our purposes, let us consider generalization to be the ongoing interactive process of clients and of their newly acquired language feature with the communication environment. For example, if I am trying to teach a child the new word *doggie*, I might repeat the word several times in the presence of the family dog and then cue the child with "Say doggie." If the child repeats the word only in this situation, he has not learned to use the word. If he says the word spontaneously and in the presence of other dogs, however, then I can reasonably assume that the child can produce the word without a model and thus has learned the word.

The degree to which generalization is a factor in language acquisition depends on the level of language rule learning involved (Johnston, 1988). For example, quantitative changes, such as the gradually more successful use of a target structure, may involve less generalization than qualitative changes, such as the broadening of linguistic categories or rules.

The factors that affect generalization may lie within the training content, the learner, or the teaching program but will vary as particular aspects of the teaching situation change. The training content, the trainer, and the teaching environment are salient components of any learning situation. If a response is to occur in a nontraining situation, then some aspects of that situation must be present in the training situation in order to signal that the response should occur. In other words, the speech-language pathologist concerned with language use must consider the effects of the various teaching contexts on generalization to everyday contexts.

Time and again, we speech-language pathologists bemoan the fact that although Johnny performed correctly 100% of the time in therapy, he could not transfer this performance to the playground. When language features taught in one setting are not generalized to other content and contexts, "the mutual goal of communicative competence is not realized" (Rieke & Lewis, 1984, p. 41).

Failure of speech and language intervention to affect the child's everyday usage causes concern for the ethics of providing intervention services (Fey, 1988). This state of affairs has led some professionals to conclude that "the traditional therapeutic model characterized by an adult working with a child a few minutes a day in an isolated context can never result in acceptable generalization" (Warren & Rogers-Warren, 1985, p. 5). Even though this conclusion may be overstated, it does pose the general problem: How can we get the language features trained in the therapy session to generalize to the client's other use environments?

In part, the difficulty experienced with generalization of trained features reflects a failure to manipulate the variables that affect generalization. Instead, we may use a "train and hope" strategy (Stokes & Baer, 1977), in which we have faith that the training will generalize but little influence over that possibility. Language training may not generalize because it is taught out of context, does not represent either the child's communicative functions or linguistic knowledge or experiences, and/or presents few communicative opportunities. To some extent, generalization is also a result of the procedures used and of the variables manipulated in language training. Finally, the very targets chosen for remediation may contribute to a lack of carryover. In each case, the speech-language pathologist needs to ask, Will this procedure (or target) work in the child's everyday environment? Is there a need within the everyday communication of the client for the feature that is being trained, and do the methods used in its teaching reflect that everyday context?

In a recent meeting with a student clinician, the answer to these questions was no. As a result, we decided to forego auxiliary verb training with a middle-aged retarded adult in favor of communication features more likely to be used within the client's everyday communication environment, such as ordering at a fast food restaurant, asking directions, and using the telephone.

Variables that Affect Generalization

Generalization or the "flexible use of knowledge" (Brown, Kane, & Echols, 1986) is an essential part of learning. Even the young child using her first word must learn to generalize its use to novel content, as mentioned previously. The word *doggie* may be used with other four-legged animals. Eventually, the child abstracts those cases in which the word *doggie* is correct and those in which it is not. A Doberman, a poodle, and a stuffed animal are doggies, but a deer and a sheep are not. In short, the child is learning those contexts that obligate the use of doggie and those that preclude its use. Such contextual learning contributes to the underlying meaning of the word. In similar fashion, formation of sentences is controlled by the context in which each sentence occurs. Contexts regulate application of learned language rules (Connell, 1982).

Likewise, the young child who can say "May I have a cookie, please?" has not learned this new utterance until it is used in the appropriate contexts. For example, it is inappropriate to use the utterance in a hardware store unless someone present has cookies. The child cannot learn all possible contexts; rather, the child learns the appropriate contextual cues, such as the presence of cookies, that govern use of the utterance.

The contexts in which training takes place influence what the child actually learns. In fact, correctness is not inherent in the child's response itself but is found in the response in context, as illustrated in the "May I have a cookie, please?" example. The relationship of context to learning is not a simple one, and the stimuli controlling a response may be multiple combinations of complex stimulus conditions (Goldstein, 1984).

Generalization is an integral part of the language intervention process. Thoughts on generalization should not be left until after the intervention program is designed. Generalization is not a single-line entry at the end of the lesson plan, nor is it homework.

To facilitate the acquisition of truly functional language—language that works for the child—it is essential that speech-language pathologists manipulate the variables related to generalization throughout the therapeutic process. Table 1.1 includes a list of the major generalization variables.

There are two broad types of generalization, *content generalization* and *context generalization*. Content is the *what* of training. Content generalization occurs when the language-impaired child induces a language rule from examples and from actual use. Thus, the new feature (e.g., plural *s*) may be used with content not previously trained, such as words not used in the therapy situation. Content generalization is affected by the *targets* chosen for training, such as use of negatives, and by the specific choice of *training items,* such as the words and sentences used to train negation.

Overall, the content selected for training reflects a clinician's theoretical concept of language and of the strategies for language learning. More and more, speech-language pathologists are selecting targets that reflect use rather than grammatical units. When grammatical units are targeted, different uses or functions for those units are essential to training.

Context is the *how* of training. Context generalization occurs when the client uses the new feature, such as the use of auxiliary verbs in questions, within everyday communication, such as in the classroom, at home, or in play. In each of these contexts, there are differences in persons present and in the location, as well as in the linguistic events that precede and follow the newly learned behavior. Only recently has the literature recognized the importance of context as an intervention variable (Gallagher, 1983). Yet, we know from child development research that context is often crucial in determining meaning. In short, generalization can be facilitated when the communication contexts of the training environment and of the natural environment are similar (Spinelli & Terrell, 1984).

Context includes an intrapersonal component unique to each individual and an interpersonal component shared by all persons in the communication set-

---

TABLE 1.1
Variables that affect generalization

Content Variables	Context Variables
Training Targets	Method of Training
Training Items	Trainers Involved
	Training Cues
	Training Contingencies
	Training Location

ting (Spinelli & Terrell, 1984). Intrapersonal variables would include each partner's cognitive and social knowledge or context, variables that may differ greatly across special populations. These variables, discussed previously, influence the selection of content and the individualization of program design.

Interpersonal intervention variables include situational factors (e.g., method of training, personnel involved, training cues, reinforcement method, and location and time of training and objects present) and participant factors (e.g., conversational roles of the participants). The effects of some of these variables on generalization are discussed in detail in the following sections.

Training Targets

The very complexity of language probably makes it impossible for the speech-language pathologist to teach everything that a language-impaired child needs to become a competent communicator. Obviously, some language features must be ignored. Target selection, therefore, is a conscious process with far-reaching implications. Training target selection should be based on the actual needs and interests of each child within his or her communication environments.

The focus of instruction should be on increasing the effectiveness of child-initiated communication. Both the frequency and sophistication of this communication can be increased through intervention (McCormick, 1986).

Language is a dynamic process that is heavily influenced by context. Thus, language features selected for training should be functional or useful for the child in the communication environment. Forms acquire real meaning only when they are used to accomplish some intention. In clinical intervention, we should remember that forms are best learned when they are needed to fulfill some intention of the client. The optimum moment for training "Want cookie" is when the child desires one. Only when the utterance works does it generalize to the child's use repertoire.

Generalization is also a function of the scope of the training target and of the child's characteristics and linguistic experience with the target. Language knowledge exists along a continuum from restricted or specific rules with a narrow application to broad, unrestricted rules with wide application. The scope of a training target will affect generalization. In general, language rules with broad scope generalize more easily than do those with more restricted scope (Kamhi, 1988).

Because an individual's conceptual knowledge and view of reality naturally consist of theories and principles with wide application, it is almost impossible to impede generalization of this broad-based type of knowledge. Even language-impaired children are capable of generalizing this type of knowledge, although the process appears to take a little longer (Kamhi, Gentry, & Mauer, 1987).

The scope of rule application can be a function of the way it is taught. Language-impaired children may not recognize the analogous relationships within language (Kamhi, 1988). For example, the language-impaired child may not recognize the similarity in use of auxiliary verbs with both negatives and interrogatives. In part, restricted teaching may reflect a behaviorist bias in the methods of speech-language pathologists that reduces training targets to easily identifiable and observable units. The clinically perceived need to have children perform to some acceptable criterion level forces clinicians to address narrow, restricted targets. Rules interpreted by the child as applying to a limited set of lexical items combined in a very specific manner will involve little generalization (Johnston, 1988).

The language-impaired child's prior knowledge of language also influences generalization. The failure of training to generalize may reflect training targets that are inappropriate for the knowledge level of the child. For example, it would be inappropriate to train indirect commands prior to the child's understanding and using yes/no questions and direct commands.

In conclusion, training targets should be selected based on each child's actual communication needs and abilities rather than on some preconceived agenda. The targets selected for training should be functional or useful in the client's everyday communication environment. We can expect optimum generalization only when the content logically flows from one training level to the next and when the client has a need and a use for this content in communication. More broad-based language rules generalize better than do rules with limited scope and application.

Training Items

The actual items selected for intervention, such as the specific verbs to be used in training past tense or the sentences to be used in training negation, and the linguistic complexity of these intervention items can also influence generalization. In general, it is best if these items come from the natural communication environment of the language-impaired child. Structured observation of this environment can aid intervention programming. For example, the active child may use the verbs *walk, jump,* and *hop* frequently. It is more likely that use of the past tense *-ed* will generalize if these frequently occurring words are used in the training.

Individualization is important because of the many different use environments across language-impaired children. The institutionalized child may have very different content to discuss than does the child residing at home. The interests of younger children are also very different from those of adolescents.

Targeted linguistic forms, whether word classes or larger linguistic structures, should be trained across several functions. For example, negatives used with auxiliary verbs can occur in declaratives (''That doesn't fit''), imperatives (''Don't touch that''), and interrogatives (''Don't you want to go?'') and in functions, such as denying (''I didn't do it'') or requesting information (''Why didn't you go?'').

For optimum generalization, then, it is necessary to select training items from the child's everyday environment. In addition, these items should be trained across linguistic forms and/or functions and across linguistic and non-linguistic contexts.

Method of Training

The training of discrete bits of language devoid of the communication context may actually retard learning and growth (Cazden, 1972; Damico, 1988). The prevailing construct of language as separate and autonomous components, however, assumes little or no interaction among the linguistic units. Such fragmentation allows minute analysis units to eclipse the essential language qualities of intentionality and synergy (Damico, 1988). In other words, language use in communication is lost. Language should be viewed holistically. In the past, intervention that focused on specific, discrete, structural entities fostered drills and didactic training. These adversely affect the flow, intentionality, and meaningfulness of language (Oller, 1983).

The training of language involves much more than just the training of words and structures. Clients should be learning strategies for comprehending language directed at them and for generating novel utterances within several conversational contexts.

Training should occur in actual use within a conversational context. Prutting (1983) states that language intervention should meet the *Bubba* criterion. *Bubba* is Yiddish for *grandmother.* If we were to explain our intervention approach to our Jewish grandmother, she would reply: "Oh, I could have told you that. It just makes sense to use conversations to train. Why didn't you ask me?" In other words, the training regimen should make sense. Our intervention methodology should flow logically from our concept of language.

If language is a social tool and if the goal is to train for generalized use, then it follows that language should be trained in conditions similar to the ultimate use environment. Thus, the speech-language pathologist should modify the interactional context within which language is trained so that it closely resembles, or actually takes place within, the child's ongoing everyday communication environment. It is important, therefore, to view context not as a backdrop but as an ongoing process (Cook-Gumperz & Corsaro, 1976; Cook-Gumperz & Gumperz, 1978).

Often called *incidental teaching,* training that occurs in everyday contexts can closely resemble the language development environment of nonimpaired children. This approach attempts to ensure that children learn and have ample opportunity to use language within naturally occurring activities (McCormick, 1986). Generalization increases with the similarity of the original learning situation to the transfer situation (Brown & Campione, 1984).

As intervention agents, speech-language pathologists can systematically modify the number of trainers, the training cues, and the consequences that constitute this context to resemble more closely the real world in which the language is to be used. Through the use of multiple trainers and multiple cues and consequences, the speech-language pathologist can facilitate generalization by weakening irrelevant stimulus cues that can influence the trained feature.

A few years ago, I worked with a nonspeaking brain-injured adolescent who, after considerable effort, learned to communicate with a few simple pictures but would not use them with anyone except me. In this case, I had become what behaviorists call a *discriminative stimulus* (S^D) for communication with the pictures. In other words, the client had learned that the pictures were to be used only in my presence. This condition was not a training goal, but rather an uncontrolled result of the training situation. If multiple trainers had been employed, my personal characteristics, which were irrelevant to his picture use, would have been negated. Similarly, a young child may exhibit one type of language in the clinical setting and quite another at home. In this case, the clinic room and the home are S^Ds for certain language features. In another example, the client who learns to say single words only in response to ''What's that?'' is unlikely to generalize this behavior to spontaneous expressive use. Thus, truly functional language training requires that the goal of conversational use within the client's everyday environment be an essential aspect of training from the onset.

Discussion of the method of training leads naturally to consideration of the other contextual variables. For optimum generalization, training should occur within a conversational context with varying numbers of trainers, cues, consequences, and locations.

Language Trainers

''To ensure that the language trained is functional and, therefore, most likely to be generalized, language training should be conducted by those who spend the most time communicating with the child'' (Warren & Rogers-Warren, 1985, p. 7). This conclusion suggests that parents, teachers, aides, and unit personnel, in addition to the speech-language pathologist, should be language trainers because of their relationship with and the amount of time each spends with the client.

Interactional partners form communication environments for each other (McDermott, Gospodinoff, & Aram, 1976), and it is essential that the client experience newly learned language in a number of everyday communication environments. Because language is contexually variable, it will differ within the context created by the child with each communication partner. Thus, generalization depends on the number of different communication partners we can involve in the intervention process (Craig, 1983).

Because most nonimpaired children learn language through interaction with several individuals, it is highly unlikely that the work of one caregiver, such as the speech-language pathologist, constitutes the most effective method by which a child can develop language (Lieven, 1984). In fact, the number of different individuals the child sees during the week is positively correlated with the rate of language development (Nelson, 1973).

Language facilitators are ''adults who increase the child's potential for communication success'' (Craig, 1983, p. 110). Through training, these adults could maximize their teaching potential. Of particular importance is the use of informal incidental techniques within the everyday activities of the child (Owens, 1982; Warren & Rogers-Warren, 1985).

A wealth of data indicates that programs that involve the child's communication partners, especially parents, produce greater gains for children than do programs that do not (Baker, Murphy, Heifetz, & Brightman, 1975; Fredricks, Baldwin, & Grove, 1974; Watson & Bassinger, 1974). Despite the acknowledged importance of parent training, it is the exception rather than the rule in most speech-language intervention settings (McDade & Varnedoe, 1987). Usually, parents assume the role of uninformed spectators (Baker, 1976).

With parent or caregiver training, parents or teachers can function on a continuum from paraprofessionals to general language facilitators (Adler, 1983; King, 1976; McDade & Varnedoe, 1987; Owens, 1982). Each speech-language pathologist must establish the caregiver role that best suits her model of intervention.

Parents offer a channel for generalizing intervention into the natural environment of the home (Tiegerman & Siperstein, 1984). This can be accomplished within everyday events in the home. With these additional language facilitators, the traditional role of the speech-language pathologist changes. The pathologist has the skill to train other people to grab the communication moment that happens in naturally occurring conversation or is created by the clinician and to turn it into a conversational learning moment (Craig, 1983). In essence, the speech-language pathologist becomes a programmer of the child's environment, manipulating the variables to ensure successful communication and generalization.

To be effective, the speech-language pathologist must recognize that the language-impaired child is not the only client. Another goal of therapy is to modify the communication environment of the child and to make it more facilitating. Thus, the child's communication partners are also clients as well as agents of change (MacDonald, 1985).

In part, the success of parent or teacher training rests on recognition of two facts. First, these individuals are capable of training language in children. Second, their use within the intervention program increases the amount of training the child receives, even if there is a decrease in direct clinician-child interaction (McDade & Varnedoe, 1987).

In addition to training the client and the client's communication partners, the speech-language pathologist acts as a consultant, helping each interactive dyad fine-tune its conversational behaviors. For example, the speech-language pathologist might help the teacher to follow the child's conversational lead or might demonstrate for a parent a more conversational consequence than the commonly used ''Good talking.''

Training Cues

Too often children are trained solely to respond to trainer cues. Goals for the child should include both initiating and responding behaviors and the situations in which each is appropriate.

It is highly unlikely that the child will initiate spontaneous use of content that has been trained in a response mode. Therefore, the speech-language pathologist must consider training language through a great variety of both linguistic and nonlinguistic cues reflected in the style of interaction.

Parents of nonimpaired children use at least two interactive styles, the nurturant and the directive. The nurturant style is child directed or child centered with the adult responding to child initiations. The adult encourages child utterances by subtle manipulation of the context and responds to the child in a conversational manner. In contrast, the directive style consists of didactic exchanges: the adult initiates the exchange, usually with a question, awaits the child's reply, and then provides evaluative feedback.

Research has demonstrated the beneficial effects of the nurturant style on children's language acquisition (Barnes, Gutfreund, Satterly, & Wells, 1983; Cross, 1978, 1984). A functional language approach adapts these techniques as naturally as possible to intervention. Clinicians use conversational techniques to facilitate child utterances or use familiar routines and activities that will encourage verbal initiations by the child. The nonlinguistic context can be manipulated along a continuum from highly structured routines that can promote interactions with noninteractive children to more open-ended, less structured conversations (Duchan & Weitzner-Lin, 1987).

Contingencies

The nature of the reinforcement used in training is also a strong determiner of generalization. Edibles or social reinforcement used in training may have little relationship to the language feature being trained. For best generalization to the natural use environment, "consequences that are related directly to the language utterance and communication function made by the student should be provided" (Stremel-Campbell & Campbell, 1985, p. 266). Everyday, natural consequences are best. If the child requests a paintbrush, he should be given one, unless, of course, there is a good reason not to give it. If that is the case, then the child should not have been required to learn the request.

Weaning the child away from edible reinforcers in favor of social ones is commendable as long as the social reinforcer is likely to be found in the natural communication environment. Such verbal or social training consequences as "Good talking" may be encountered only rarely by the child in the course of everyday conversations. Although such consequences may be helpful in initial training, they should be discontinued as soon as possible in favor of more natural responses.

Functional approaches offer a variety of response modes that demonstrate acceptance or rejection and redirection of the child's utterance while maintaining the conversational flow. Consequences such as "Good talking" end social interaction by commenting on the correctness of the child's utterance only and leaving little that the child can say in return ("Yes, I do talk well, don't I?"). Verbal responses that combine feedback about correctness/incorrectness with additional information can be both a language-learning opportunity and a communicative turn (Rieke & Lewis, 1984).

Not every utterance is reinforced in the natural environment. In some situations, such as residential institutions, clients are rarely reinforced for initiating communication, and the speech-language pathologist must train communication partners to provide more reinforcement. Even in the course of everyday conversations, many utterances are not reinforced. Meanwhile, in typical language intervention, every utterance by the child may be reinforced. Behaviors continuously reinforced are easy to extinguish. Intermittently reinforced responses are much more resistant. In addition, intermittent schedules more closely resemble the reinforcement patterns found in the real world.

Location

The location of training involves not only places but also events. For maximum generalization, language should be trained in the locations, such as the home, clinic, school, or unit, and in activities where it is used, such as play or household chores. Children removed from familiar contexts ''may be unable to exhibit their most creative uses of language'' (Lieven, 1984, p. 22).

Language should be trained within the daily activities of the client (Hart & Rogers-Warren, 1978). Daily routines can provide a familiar framework within which conversation can occur (Lieven, 1982, 1984; Snow & Goldfield, 1983). The familiar situation provides a frame that allows for a degree of automatization important in the acquisition of such skills as language (Reason & Mycielska, 1982). More important, the conditions for training and use are the same, alleviating the need for contrived generalization strategies.

Activity heavily influences language (Levinson, 1978), so the forms used to some extent depend on these activities. The ideal training situation is one in which the language-impaired child is engaged in some meaningful activity with a conversational partner who models appropriate language forms and functions (Staab, 1983). In this way, the child learns language in the conversational context in which it is likely to occur. It is within these everyday events that language is naturally acquired and to these events that the newly trained language is to generalize.

Within these daily events are naturally occurring communication sequences (Craig, 1983), such as the following:

#1. Hello.
#2. Hello, is John home?
#1. No, I'm sorry. He went to the store. He should be back in a minute. Can I take a message?
#2. No, That's fine. I'll call back later if that's okay.
#1. Fine. Bye.
#2. Bye.

The second sequence is very different.

#1. I just got back from Nantucket.
#2. So that's where you got that tan. I've never been there.
#1. Oh, you'd love it. I really love to ride my bike to some deserted beach to swim.
#2. I'd love a deserted beach, but we go to Atlantic City, and it's just too crowded.

Each sequence has its own content and its own style. The first sequence is more formal, more scripted, whereas the second is more casual, more familiar. Daily events, such as phone calls, friendly meetings, dinner preparation, and even dressing, can provide a framework for language and for language training. The frame provides a guide to help the participants organize their language and their language learning. Routines and ''familiar situations may provide the child with support for the next step'' (Lieven, 1984, p. 22). The speech-language pathologist can plan conversational roles and language training through the use of such daily events. Natural communication sequences are not so much the *where* of language training as the *how*.

Summary

Language training should be a dynamic process of exchange that occurs during natural events in different environments and with different conversational partners (Snow et al., 1984). Reinforcement should be the intrinsic conversational success of the child. The variables relative to content and context can, if manipulated carefully, facilitate generalization of newly learned language features.

Unfortunately, in practice, generalization is too often the final step in planning client training. Instead, ''communication goals and effects should be preserved and considered the first, pervasive, and most basic step in intervention planning and not some final set of generalization rules'' (Craig, 1983, p. 110).

CONCLUSION

The functional approach emphasizes nurturant and naturalistic approaches (Duchan & Weitzner-Lin, 1987). The nurturant aspect requires the clinician to relinquish control to the child and to respond to the child's communication initiations. The naturalistic aspect emphasizes everyday events and contexts. Language is trained as it is actually used. Thus, functional language training works in everyday contexts. The training generalizes.

It is easy to deride functional approaches as offering no framework for learning, allowing the child total freedom. Yet, the approach outlined in this chapter is not one in which the speech-language pathologist and child converse briefly with little intervention. Under such conditions, there is little development on the part of the child and little generalization.

Professionals often cast a wary eye on implementation of conversational and communication-based approaches to language intervention (as recommended in this text). There is a fear that intervention will deteriorate into a ''Hey, man, what's happenin'?'' approach, too open-ended to be effective in changing client behavior. Although this danger does exist, it is not inherent in functional approaches. As this text progresses, we discuss assessment and training procedures that enable speech-language pathologists to maintain a teaching momentum within the more natural context of conversation.

Beginning with assessment, we explore the collection and analysis of conversational and narrative data. In following chapters, an intervention paradigm and various techniques are presented along with discussion of two special applications, one to an environment (the classroom) and one with a population (presymbolic and minimally symbolic children).

Learning and generalization are the result of good planning based on a knowledge of the variables that affect generalization and the individual needs of each child. The content selected for training and the context within which this training takes place are both important aspects of the generalization process. The speech-language pathologist must determine the best response for the child's initiations and the best contexts for facilitating intervention targets.

Although the role of the speech-language pathologist within the functional language paradigm will change from primary direct service provider to language facilitator and consultant, the primary responsibilities will still be planning and intervention. Recognizing the need to meet these responsibilities more effectively, many professionals have proposed more functional intervention goals and procedures.

Language makes sense only when used within a communication context. Thus, the speech-language pathologist must become a master in the manipulation of that context in order to facilitate communication and generalization.

TWO
Communication Assessment

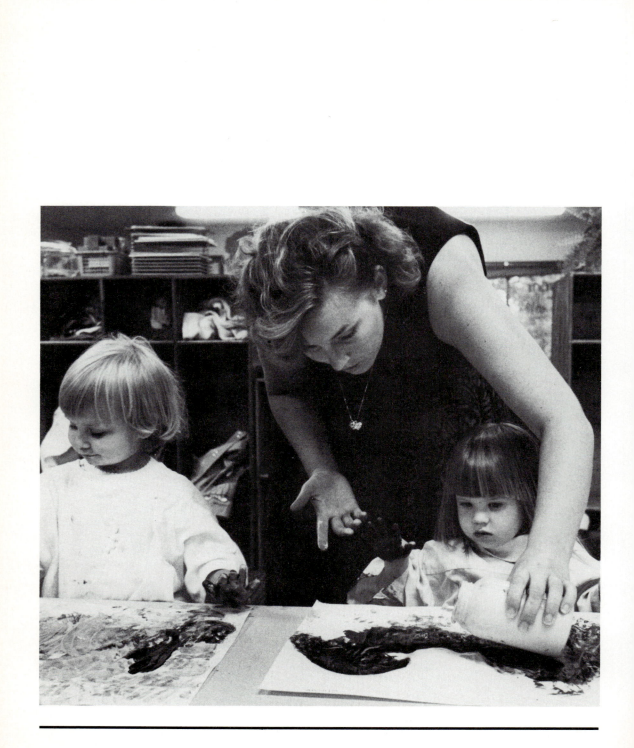

2
Communication Assessment of Children Using Symbols

There is no clear line between assessment and intervention. Both are part of the intervention process, and portions of each are found in the other. Ideally, assessment and measurement are ongoing throughout intervention. "In this way diagnosis becomes an ongoing process rather than a one-time occurrence at the initial evaluation" (Kamhi, 1984, p. 227). No clinical goal should be determined or modified without first attaining data on the communication performance of the affected child. This chapter explores the differences between psychometric and descriptive assessment paradigms and describes a combined or integrative approach that attempts systematically to address the shortcomings of both approaches while describing the child's use of language in context.

PSYCHOMETRIC VERSUS DESCRIPTIVE PROCEDURES

The goals of communication assessment are to identify and describe the unique pattern of communication behaviors exhibited by the language-impaired child. Through this process, the speech-language pathologist determines (a) whether there is a problem, (b) the causal-related factors, and (c) the overall intervention plan. There are two major philosophical approaches to this task. The normalist philosophy is based on a norm or average performance level—usually a score—that society considers typical of normal functioning and that is reflected in more

traditional language assessment procedures. In contrast, the neutralist or criterion-referenced approach compares the child's present performance to past performance and/or is descriptive in manner.

Traditional language assessment procedures heavily emphasize the use of
standardized psychometric or norm-referenced tests (Craig, 1983; Muma, 1983).
This situation is reflected in the fact that there are more than 100 commercially
available norm-referenced language assessment tools. Ideally, a standardized
test has been given to a large number of children from various populations, has
demonstrated reliability and validity, and has normative data that provide either
scale-score, age equivalent, or numerical score comparisons (Miller, 1978).

Reliability is the repeatability of measurement. More precisely, reliability is
the accuracy or precision with which a sample at one time represents performance based on either a different but similar sample, or the same sample at a
different time. Factors that might affect reliability include individual change over
time, sample differences, or the limited nature of the sample. Very limited samples usually result in unstable or undependable scores. Thus, the test must include a sample large enough to be reliable yet not unwieldy.

Test makers and users are concerned with both internal consistency and
various measures of reliability. *Internal consistency* is the degree of relationship
among items and the overall test. If a test has high internal consistency, children
who score well overall should tend to get the same items correct, whereas those
who score low should tend to perform similarly among themselves. Measures of
internal consistency are usually stated as item-test or subtest-test correlations or
as the correlation of passing/failing an item or subtest with passing/failing the
test.

Measures of reliability include test-retest reliability, alternate form reliability, and split-half reliability. In test-retest reliability, the child is administered the
same test with a time interval between each administration. With alternate forms,
the child is administered equivalent or parallel forms of a measure. Finally, a test
may be divided into equivalent halves. In each case, the two test scores are compared and the consistency of scores measured. This value is expressed as a reliability or correlational coefficient or as a standard error of measure. The closer the
reliability coefficient to a value of one and the lower the standard error or standard deviation of the error scores, the more reliable is the measure.

In addition, the speech-language pathologist is concerned with the probability of two judges' scoring the same behavior in the same manner, thus describing the child's behavior more accurately. As a group, scoring procedures that use
a definite criterion for correct-incorrect determination, such as accepting only
specific responses as correct, are more reliable than are those that use scaled scoring, such as grading responses by their degree of correctness. The latter can have
increased reliability if each score has definite criteria or if the tester has received
specific training.

Validity is the effectiveness of a test in representing, describing, or predicting an attribute of interest to the tester. In short, it is a measure of the test's ability
to assess what it purports to assess. The tester is interested in measuring all of the

attribute but nothing other than the attribute. For example, some tests of receptive language abilities require the child to respond verbally. Clearly, this requirement goes beyond the stated domain of the attribute being tested.

Tests are not presentations of the overall attribute or behavior but are merely samples of that attribute or behavior. From the samples, testers make inferences about the overall attribute or behavior. If the samples are not valid measures, the inferences will be incorrect. Validity is not self-evident and must be proven. Three types of proof or evidence are criterion validity, content validity, and construct validity.

Criterion validity is the effectiveness or accuracy with which a measure predicts success. This is usually calculated as the degree to which a measure correlates with some other suitable measures of success. Finding other suitable measures can be difficult.

Content validity is the faithfulness with which the sample or measure represents some attribute or behavior. In other words, the sum of the tasks involved should define or constitute the attribute or behavior being measured. For example, a test maker or user must decide what constitutes correct and effective use of language. A valid test would assess the use or process as well as the content of language. Measures should reflect the professional literature, research, and expert opinion on the constitution of the attribute or behavior. If there is a good correspondence, then the test has some content validity.

Finally, *construct validity* is the accuracy with which or the extent to which a measure describes or measures some trait or construct. Professionals are interested in the accuracy and significance of results and in how precisely the measure notes individual or group differences. Construct validity is usually determined by comparing the measure with other acceptable measures of the attribute or behavior in question. This procedure is also based on the assumption that the first test is valid.

Tests or measures help the speech-language pathologist determine how the child's performance, in the form of a score, compares to children who supposedly possess the same characteristics (McCauley & Swisher, 1984a; 1984b). Most frequently, tests are used to determine average and less-than-average performance for decisions about the need for intervention services (Lund & Duchan, 1988).

Unfortunately, many traditional assessment procedures do not reflect current definitions of the nature of language (Craig, 1983; Ray, 1989). Although normative tests may be good for measuring isolated skills, they provide very little information on overall language use. Thus, important linguistic processes needed in conversational exchange may not be measured.

More descriptive approaches, such as language sampling, highlight the individualistic nature of the child's communicative functioning noted in language development studies. In contrast, psychometric normative testing imposes group criteria on an individual, thereby obviating an assessment of the individual (Muma & Pierce, 1981). Each method of assessment has its strengths and weaknesses as well as possible applications within the clinical setting. These are described in the following sections.

PSYCHOMETRIC ASSESSMENT PROTOCOLS

Ideally, a test elicits a standard and representative sample of a behavior. Tests are standardized by administration to a sample from a specific population using specified explicit procedures. As such, tests enable the clinician to compare individual performance to that of a larger population. In general, norm-referenced assessment tools have the advantages of objectivity, replicability, and elimination of unwanted or uncontrolled variation (Weiner & Hoock, 1973). Tests help to focus and sharpen observational skills and are particularly helpful when deciding whether a problem exists (Longhurst, 1984).

Although standardized tests are potentially valid, reliable, and precise in measurement, it is difficult to find a language test that is acceptable in all three areas (Darley, 1979). In addition, standardized tests do not easily accommodate cultural and individual variation, nor do they begin to provide a true picture of the richness and complexity of the child's communication behavior (Leonard, Prutting, Perozzi, & Berkley, 1978; Newhoff & Leonard, 1983).

Tests are less complex than is the language being assessed (Ray, 1989). Language is multidimensional, and its use individualistic, making it difficult to measure (Dale, 1980; Damico, 1988; Fillmore, Kempler, & Wang, 1979). ''Attempts to assess the ability to use language on the basis of responses to items on a formal test,'' declared one expert, ''are probably a waste of time and money for the practitioner faced with real children'' (Dever, 1978, p. 19).

Test Differences

Language assessment instruments differ widely even when purported to measure the same entity. For example, the Bankson Language Screening Test (Bankson, 1977), a rambling, multidimensional tool, and the Fluharty Preschool Speech and Language Screening Test (Fluharty, 1978) purport to identify young children with language impairments. The Bankson correlates well with ratings from Developmental Sentence Scoring (DSS) (Lee, 1974) of a spontaneous language sample. In contrast, the Fluharty fails to identify many children who would be classified as language-disordered based on their DSS ratings (Blaxley, Clinker, & Warr-Leeper, 1983).

Even tests that seem to be significantly correlated, suggesting an interrelationship of criterion validity, may seem less so when subtests or various portions of tests are compared. For example, the Peabody Picture Vocabulary Test-Revised (PPVT-R) (Dunn & Dunn, 1981), the Test of Early Language Development (TELD) (Hresko, Reid, & Hammill, 1981), and the Preschool Language Scale (PLS) (Zimmerman, Steiner, & Pond, 1979) are significantly correlated, although the expressive and receptive portions of the TELD separately are not (Dale & Henderson, 1987; McLoughlin & Gullo, 1984). Thus, the TELD fails to identify children with these specific problems.

Ironically, the PPVT-R and other seemingly similar vocabulary measures, such as the Picture Vocabulary subtest of the Test of Language Development-Primary (TOLD-P) (Hammill & Newcomer, 1982), the Expressive One Word Vocabulary Test (Gardner, 1979), and the Receptive One Word Vocabulary Test (Gardner, 1985) correlate only moderately for older preschool children (Channell & Peek, 1989).

Nor does positive correlation mean that tests are acceptable substitutions for each other. The TOLD-P does not provide a sufficient sample to allow it to substitute for the results of the PPVT-R (Friend & Channell, 1987).

Tests also can differ in their levels of difficulty. The Test of Adolescent Language (TOAL) (Hammill, Brown, Larsen, & Wiederholt, 1980), the Clinical Evaluation of Language Functions (CELF) (Semel & Wiig, 1980), and the Fullerton Language Test for Adolescents (Thorum, 1980) seem inordinately difficult, whereas the Screening Test of Adolescent Language (STAL) (Prather, Breecher, Stafford, & Wallace, 1980) identifies a more appropriate number of students (about one-fifth) as having difficulty (Lieberman, Heffron, West, Hutchinson, & Swem, 1987).

All tests are not created equal and should be carefully researched by speech-language pathologists before being used. The following section explores some of these differences, specifically test content, and some of the common misuses of tests. Finally, the variables that should be considered in test selection are discussed.

Content

The major criticism of existing instruments is the inadequacy of the content covered in both breadth and depth (Launer & Lahey, 1981). Two issues relative to content validity, *relevance* and *coverage,* must be addressed in test construction (Messick, 1980). Content relevance is the precision with which a certain aspect of language is delineated or defined. This is necessary to determine the dimensions of that aspect and its members. For example, tests of syntax may be organized based on transformational grammar, Brown's (1973) 14 morphemes, and semantic-syntactic categories, or on no recognizable rationale. Without a framework, content items may be selected on ''an unprincipled, arbitrary, and impressionistic basis'' (Lieberman & Michael, 1986, p. 77).

Content coverage is the representativeness with which an aspect of language is sampled. Theoretically, coverage of language features should reflect general use. Some features may be more significant than others, although this fact can be verified only through statistical analysis. Otherwise, subtle language impairments may go undetected. For example, the Test of Language Development (TOLD) (Newcomer & Hammill, 1977), the Carrow Elicited Language Inventory (CELI) (Carrow, 1974), and the Clinical Evaluation of Language Functions (CELF) (Semel & Wiig, 1980) emphasize early language development while missing more subtle later developing features. A single test's rather limited sample of a child's skills is an inadequate base on which to build a sound remedial program (Lieberman & Michael, 1986).

The psychometric testing model produces data on minimal portions of behavior, thus reducing language to simple, often irrelevant dimensions that may not reflect the qualities of that language overall (Muma, 1983: Oller, 1979). By fragmenting language into observable and measurable features, tests may highlight skills only tangentially related to language ability. Tests tend to emphasize structural components of language because they are easy to observe. Although structured testing may reveal the child's ability to use language in one context, it reveals very little about the child's language as it is needed and used in everyday communication (Cole, 1982).

By isolating language performance from the conversational context, tests may be measuring skills other than those they claim to measure. In fact, "language use in isolation often bears little resemblance to language use in context" (Newman, Lovett, & Dennis, 1986, p. 31). For example, the child may use interrogatives throughout the day to obtain information, desired objects, and needed assistance but may be unable to form interrogatives in isolation when given a group of words to include. In addition, the process of the test situation may be so foreign to the child or alien to the child's everyday communication environment that it influences the language the child produces. Performance may also be affected by factors as diverse as the child's state of health on the day the test is administered, attention level and comprehension of the instructions, and perception of the test administrator.

In short, norm-referenced approaches offer "canned" assessment with little consideration for the individual needs of the child with whom they are used. There is a tendency for assessment procedures to take priority over the child, with test selection based on commercial availability or clinical popularity (Duchan, 1982b; Kamhi, 1984). Tests are a priori and product oriented, offering little information on the appropriateness of the features being tested. The test results, in turn, offer little assistance in identifying individual problems and in planning intervention.

Misuse of Normative Testing

Norm-referenced tests should be used with caution. Lieberman and Michael warn "Let the clinician beware" (1986, p. 71). The best advice is to be an "informed clinician" (Siegel & Broen, 1976) and a wise consumer. Clinicians should be mindful of the frequent misuse of these instruments (McCauley & Swisher, 1983, 1984b; Lieberman & Michael, 1986; Stephens & Montgomery, 1985), among them: (a) misuse of scores as a summary of a child's performance, (b) use of inappropriate norms, (c) inappropriate assumptions based on test results, (d) use of specific test items to plan intervention goals, and (e) use of tests to assess therapy progress.

Misuse of Scores

The most frequent score used on standardized measures is the mean or average score. It is important to recall that a wide scoring area about the mean, called *standard deviation,* is considered to fall within the normal range. The mean is the average score. When plotted, the total number of individuals receiving each score will form the familiar *bell-shaped curve*, represented in Figure 2.1. Approximately two-thirds of the population will score within one standard deviation on either side of the mean score. The speech-language pathologist who uses this index for separating normal from non-normal will find that nearly one-third of the population, approximately 16% above and 16% below, fails to fall within this range. Two standard deviations is a better index of deviancy, leaving approximately 3% of the population above and 3% below those within the normal range. Test scores that are extreme or that represent the performance of children whose ages are at the extremes for the norming population should not be considered as reliable as more central measures.

Age-equivalent scores, or the average age of children getting a certain number of items right, seem to be less reliable than are other indices, such as standard scores and percentile ranks, and less sensitive to individual differences. Often, specific age-equivalent scores are determined by test makers through interpolation from the scores achieved by children at various ages.

The use of age-equivalent scores can lead to erroneous assumptions about children's behavior. The equality of scores does not translate to an equality of behavior and offers an inadequate description of that behavior (Longhurst, 1984). A child who achieves the same score as a younger child may not make the same kinds of errors. If these scores are used there should be some explanation of their value.

Speech-language pathologists should habitually check the standard error of measure (SEm) for information about the confidence of test scores (Brown, 1989). Because tests are less than perfectly reliable, a certain amount of error is reflected in each score. In short, the larger the SEm, the less confidence one can have in the test's results.

The SEm can be added to and subtracted from a test score to establish a band of confidence. For example, assume that a child received a score of 75 on two different tests with confidence intervals of 2 and 6 respectively. On the first

FIGURE 2.1
Parameters of the normal distribution

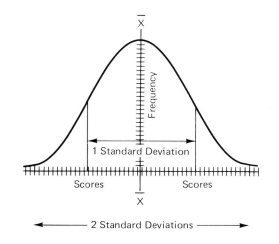

test, the child's error-free or true score is most probably 73–77, on the second, it is 69–81. The speech-language pathologist can have more confidence that the score of 75 on the first test is closer to the child's actual performance.

Larger SEm values may also mean that scores that seem very different actually overlap, as shown in Figure 2.2. Child A received a score of 81 and child B received a score of 90. A SEm of 6 applied to each score results in an overlap. Therefore, the children's actual abilities may be much more similar than the test results indicate.

The speech-language pathologist should check the test manual to obtain the SEm. Because this information is not always available, the speech-language pathologist may wish to determine this value from Table 2.1 (Brown, 1989). The entering values of standard deviation and reliability coefficient are usually provided in the test manual.

Speech-language pathologists should read, understand, and evaluate the manual accompanying the test and be knowledgeable of test construction and administration (Stephens & Montgomery, 1985). The literature about a certain test should be studied thoroughly before the test is used.

Inappropriate Norms

Often, the norming sample does not represent the population on which the clinician is using the assessment procedure. In this situation, the norms are inappropriate and should not be used. This situation occurs most frequently with minority or rural children or with children from lower socioeconomic groups. In these cases, local norms should be prepared following the norming procedure described in the test manual. Some tests, such as the Test of Language Development-Intermediate (TOLD-I) and the CELF, explain this process in detail.

Incorrect Assumptions

Test scores may represent only scores and not actual differences in linguistic ability. It is possible for two children to receive the same score and have very different linguistic abilities. Therefore, the speech-language pathologist must analyze each child's performance on different aspects or subtests in order to obtain descriptive information. Subtest scores should be interpreted independently from each other so as not to influence their interpretation. Because test items represent only a

FIGURE 2.2
A comparison of scores using standard error of measure

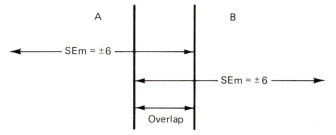

TABLE 2.1
Table of standard error of measure reliability and standard deviation values to estimate the standard error of measurement (SEm).

Standard Deviation	Reliability Coefficient								
	.95	.90	.85	.80	.75	.70	.65	.60	.55
30	6.7	9.5	11.6	13.4	15.0	16.4	17.7	19.0	20.1
28	6.3	8.9	10.8	12.5	14.0	15.3	16.6	17.7	18.8
26	5.8	8.2	10.1	11.6	13.0	14.2	15.4	16.4	17.4
24	5.4	7.6	9.3	10.7	12.0	13.1	14.2	15.2	16.1
22	4.9	7.0	8.5	9.8	11.0	12.0	13.0	13.9	14.8
20	4.5	6.3	7.7	8.9	10.0	11.0	11.8	12.7	13.4
18	4.0	5.7	7.0	8.0	9.0	9.9	10.6	11.4	12.1
16	3.6	5.1	6.2	7.2	8.0	8.8	9.5	10.1	10.7
14	3.1	4.4	5.4	6.3	7.0	7.7	8.3	8.9	9.4
12	2.7	3.8	4.6	5.4	6.0	6.6	7.1	7.6	8.0
10	2.2	3.2	3.9	4.5	5.0	5.5	5.9	6.3	6.7
8	1.8	2.5	3.1	3.6	4.0	4.4	4.7	5.1	5.4
6	1.3	1.9	2.3	2.7	3.0	3.3	3.6	3.8	4.0
4	.9	1.3	1.5	1.8	2.0	2.2	2.4	2.5	2.7
2	.4	.6	.8	.9	1.0	1.1	1.2	1.3	1.3

Note: This table of standard error of measurement is based on the formula $SEm = SD \sqrt{1 - r_{11}}$ where SD is the standard deviation of the test scores and r_{11} is the reliability coefficient for internal consistency of the tes t scores.
Source: Brown, J. (1989). The truth about scores children achieve on tests. *Language, Speech and Hearing Services in Schools, 20*, 366–371. Reprinted with permission.

small portion of language, they do not provide enough information on which to base therapy goals. The speech-language pathologist should be cautious in extrapolating global language development from scores on language tests, especially those that sample only one or two aspects of language (McLoughlin & Gullo, 1984). The PPVT is an excellent receptive vocabulary test, but it does not address other aspects of language or indicate overall language use.

Identifying Intervention Goals
As discussed in Chapters 4 and 5, a thorough description of the child's behavior is needed before the clinician can identify areas needing intervention. Individual test items or subtests do not provide an adequate sample of that behavior. At the very least, more than one psychometric assessment procedure should be used because of the variability of some children across tests (Rizzo & Stephens, 1981; Stephens & Montgomery, 1985). The more test scores available, the more reliable the assessment. Nor will test scores describe how children function within their everyday communication environment. Only through the use of a number of assessment protocols can the speech-language pathologist hope to determine intervention objectives. Psychometric tests are only a portion of the assessment process.

Measuring Therapy Progress

The continued use of norm-referenced tests to assess therapy progress may result in the child's learning the test, thus producing artificially high results. Assessment tools are designed for determining average and less-than-average performance. However, widely spaced testing or the use of different forms of the same test or of different but highly correlated tests can demonstrate changes in behavior over time (McCauley & Swisher, 1984b). Criterion-referenced tests are more appropriate for measuring individual progress.

Variables in Test Selection

The speech-language pathologist should be a wise consumer of intervention materials and should base test selection on several factors. Of particular interest are test reliability and validity, as discussed previously.

Other considerations in test selection include appropriateness of the test for a particular child, the manner of presentation and comprehensiveness, and the type and sensitivity of the test results. A test should be appropriate to the child's age or functioning level. In addition, the norming population should be sufficiently large and varied to include representatives of the child's racioethnic and socioecomonic background. If the child is from an identifiable minority, the clinician should check to see if the norming information gives data by such groups.

Appropriateness may also relate to manner of presentation. Some children perform better under certain conditions than they do under others. For example, children with a language learning disability can perform better if there is visual input accompanying the verbal. The manner of presentation may reflect the overall theoretical basis of the test. A sentence imitation test, for example, relies on auditory processing of verbal stimuli rather than on picture cues. Other practical issues related to presentation include the number of items and the content coverage discussed previously.

In turn, too few or poorly discriminatory items can lead to less sensitive scoring, in which one question can change the child's performance score several percentage points. The type of result, whether percentage, percentile, or age equivalent, is also a practical consideration in test selection. Depending on the test, the interpretive value of such scores may be very limited.

Summary

Perceptive individuals decry overdependence on and poor interpretation of the results of testing. Although standardized tests, especially those in language, have been frequently maligned (Darley, 1979; Dever, 1978; McCauley & Swisher, 1984a, 1984b), clinicians are often required to incorporate the results of these procedures in their overall assessments. It is important for clinicians to recognize that tests are informative but not the be-all and end-all of evaluation. Awareness of a test's shortcomings can greatly aid the interpretation of a child's performance (Stephens & Montgomery, 1985).

The issue of testing is central to the purpose of assessment. Data gathered in an assessment should be relevant to the initial clinical complaint, to the determination that a problem exists, to individual differences and individual processing, to the nature of the problem, to prognosis, to intervention implications, and to accountability (Muma, 1986). Otherwise, according to Muma, it's just a *numbers game*.

DESCRIPTIVE APPROACHES

The descriptive approach, usually based on a conversational sample of the child's language, is a widely taught method of defining children's communicative abilities. Unfortunately, because of time constraints, the method is not widely used, although it is gaining favor (McCauley & Swisher, 1984b; Muma, Lubinski, & Pierce, 1982; Muma, Pierce, & Muma, 1983; Newhoff & Leonard, 1983; Rees, 1978). Descriptive approaches have the potential of allowing clinicians to regard the language process while maintaining contextual integrity and individual differences (Muma, 1986).

Spontaneous sampling alone is best used as an indicator of the child's overall language functioning rather than as a device for noting specific language problems. More specific data can be obtained by probing the child's conversational behavior. In general, data from a language sample correlates significantly with results from elicited imitation and sentence completion tasks, although the syntactic structural patterns vary widely (Fujiki & Willbrand, 1982).

The advantages of the descriptive approach are that the speech-language pathologist can apply her own theoretical model to the assessment process and can probe and assess areas that seem most handicapping to the child (Kamhi, 1984; Duchan, 1982b). For example, the speech-language pathologist who follows a sociolinguistic model of language is free to explore the pragmatic and conversational aspects of the child's language. "By gathering clinical data and formulating and testing hypotheses based on these data, the clinician ensures that the clinical process remains flexible and attuned to the client's changing needs" (Kamhi, 1984, p. 227). To do this the speech-language pathologist must understand the complex interaction of constitutional—biological, cognitive, psychological, and social—and environmental forces.

The continuous speech sample has several advantages over more formal structured-response measures. Although testing reveals some information, "it reveals very little about the function, content, and form of the child's language in the various circumstances in which language is needed and employed in daily living" (Cole, 1982, p. 93). For example, single-word responses on a test may not be as adequate a data base for phonological analysis as a longer conversational response might be, although there is some disagreement on this point (Ingram, 1976; Klein, 1984; Shriberg & Kwiatkowski, 1980). Some phonological processes,

such as final consonant deletion, neutralization, stopping, and weak syllable deletion, may not be exhibited in single-word responses. Possibly these processes
are the most sensitive to linguistic and extralinguistic factors found in continuous
speech (Klein, 1984).

The disadvantages of the descriptive approach are (a) the level of language
expertise needed by the speech-language pathologist in order to elicit and analyze the child's language, (b) the length of time needed to collect and analyze the
child's language, and (c) the reliability and validity of the sample (Kelly & Rice,
1986). Although a number of descriptive protocols exist, the speech-language pathologist may not feel sufficiently well versed in all the aspects of language to
choose those appropriate for each child. For example, some protocols emphasize
form or content, although these alone will not ensure appropriate use (Roth &
Spekman, 1984a). For many theoreticians, the communicative value of each language event lies in the pragmatic functions of each utterance (Prutting & Kirchner, 1983). Yet, clinicians may not be comfortable with the pragmatic aspects of
language. In addition, a large caseload may preclude the use of lengthy descriptive procedures. Finally, as in psychometric testing, the clinician may not elicit a
valid sample of the child's usual language usage.

Reliability and Validity

Language samples are more susceptible than are standardized measures to clinician bias (Nye et al., 1987). This problem is especially critical when such measures
are used to assess intervention effectiveness. The speech-language pathologist
must attempt to analyze the language sample in the most objective manner possible. Descriptions of the physical behaviors observed are generally more reliable
than are subjective judgments of the causes or reasons for these behaviors. One
way to increase reliability is to separate the actual events from inferences based
on these events and to base decisions on the data from these events (Duncan &
Fiske, 1977).

According to Duncan & Fiske (1977), reliability across observations can be
increased by taking the following three precautions:

1. Define the behaviors to be observed as explicitly as possible and train
   observers to ensure good inter- and intra-observer reliability. The selection of the taxonomy of behavior categories to be observed will affect
   the validity of the observation. For example, a taxonomy of preschool
   speech acts would not be appropriate for rating the behavior of adolescents functioning above the preschool range. Accuracy can also be controlled by making point-to-point comparisons between the ratings of
   two observers. This type of analysis helps to sharpen definitions and
   to highlight possible areas of confusion.

2. Make judgments on only one type of behavior at a time. This procedure may require the use of videotaping so that a language sample can
   be replayed often for additional judgments on other behaviors.

3. Do not make summation judgments while observing ''on-line.'' It is too easy for preconceived notions of the child to influence our interpretation. Judgments about overall behavior are best made after assessing the accumulated data.

Some threats to validity are found within the sample itself. For example, preschool children vary in their attentiveness and disposition to talk moment by moment (Shriberg & Kwiatkowski, 1985). Given this condition, the possible threats to validity in a speech sample, even with older children, are *productivity*, or the amount produced; *intelligibility*, or the amount understood by the listener; *representativeness*, or the typicality of the sample; and *reactivity*, or the response of the child to differing stimuli (Shriberg & Kwiatkowski, 1985).

Productivity
The uncommunicative child or the child who produces only a few utterances will not give the clinician a productive sample from which to work, even though such a sample may accurately reflect the child's typical output. The child may have little language with which to talk. The key to greater production is for the speech-language pathologist to plan a variety of elicitation tasks that serve the purpose of gathering the sample (Wren, 1985).

Intelligibility
Intelligibility is the amount of agreement between what the speaker intended to say and what the listener interpreted from the sample. If much of the sample is untelligible, few utterances will be suitable for analysis. In general, intelligibility can be increased with increased clinician control over the content of the child's utterances. In short, the clinician who knows the topic can more easily determine what the child said.

Representativeness
A sample may not represent the child's typical behavior. Language samples are often collected in an atypical context, for example, a clinical room with the speech-language pathologist as the conversational partner. Much of the sample may be atypical when removed from the child's typical conversational context (Roth & Spekman, 1984b). Three issues are relative to the representativeness of the conversational sample: *spontaneity, variability of context,* and *stability of the structure/function sampled* (Muma, 1983).

Spontaneity is increased if the child is allowed to establish the topic. Interesting and varied stimulus materials can provide an excellent basis for spontaneous conversation and can elicit a variety of forms and functions.

Variability of the context and stimulus items will elicit a greater variety of child behaviors theoretically more representative of the child's everyday behavior. Data should be collected in a variety of settings, with a variety of partners, and on a variety of child-based conversational topics to ensure versatility (John-son, Johnston, & Weinrich, 1984). Because quantity and complexity vary with the task, no single task will yield a representative sample of the child's language (Wren, 1985).

Unrepresentative samples may reflect other-than-normal usage by the child. In this situation, the structures or functions sampled may vary widely from one situation to another. Everyday situations are most likely to elicit typical use and thus provide some stability across situations.

There is some debate as to whether clinicians should try to elicit typical or maximum production from the child. This debate is fueled by the often-reported gaps between what language-disordered children are capable of doing with their language and what they typically do (Wiig & Semel, 1976; Wren, 1981, 1982). The clinician must decide whether to use storytelling tasks that yield a larger average or mean length of utterance (MLU) or picture interpretation tasks that elicit greater language quantity (Atkins & Cartwright, 1982; Stallnaker & Creaghead, 1982).

Reactivity
The child's reaction to the techniques and the materials will also affect the overall validity of the sample produced. Sampling conditions and the nature of the content or stimuli available can greatly affect the sample. A directed condition, such as one in which the clinician uses a questioning technique, allows the examiner more control over the content being discussed and may in turn increase intelligibility (Weeks, 1971). Unfortunately, this improved intelligibility may sacrifice productivity and representativeness. In general, too much control restricts the child's output. For example, sentence-building tasks in which the child is asked to ''Make a sentence with the word *X*'' elicit the least typical language and very short sentences (Wren, 1985).

Words or structures divorced from dialogue, as in the previous example, require high-level metalinguistic skills to manipulate and thus are difficult for the child with language disorders. Other tasks, such as sentence repetition, sentence completion, and judgment of grammaticality, are unreliable and should not be used without a spontaneous conversational sample (Fujiki & Willbrand, 1982). Yet, even though the more open-ended conversation may be more representative, it is usually less intelligibile and may be difficult for some language-impaired children. For example, children with learning disabilities exhibit difficulty with conversations as with other assessment protocols (Bryan, Donahue, & Pearl, 1981; Bryan, Donahue, Pearl, & Herzog, 1981; Donahue, 1984; Noel, 1980; Roth, 1986; Spekman, 1981).

Similarly, specific stimulus items may increase intelligibility by controlling the topics discussed. In addition, the use of these items may enable the clinician to repeat stimulus conditions in subsequent evaluations. Again, increased intelligibility may result in decreased productivity of a variety of forms and functions and limited content. Further, the child may develop or already have a stereotypic pattern of responding to the item. For example, a doll may elicit a reduced style similar to "motherese."

The items chosen and the directions given may also affect the validity of the sample. For example, pictures can be used to elicit language, but the instructions given to the child often affect the quantity of language produced. The typical directive "Tell me about this picture" elicits less language than does a more directive style (Wren, 1985), such as the following:

> I'd like you to make up a story from this picture. I want you to tell me a whole story that has a beginning and an end. Start with "Once upon a time" and tell me the whole story.

The best advice for any speech-language pathologist is to remain flexible in order to shift between contexts and content and elicit the kinds of language behavior desired. "The examiner needs to have on hand a variety of stimulus materials and be skillful in identifying and discussing a range of topics of potential interest to the child whose speech is being sampled" (Shriberg & Kwiatkowski, 1985, p. 330).

Summary

Descriptive approaches are not without problems. Although they are potentially more representative of the child's everyday performance than is formal testing, this potential is not guaranteed. In addition, descriptive approaches require that the clinician have considerable knowledge of language and of the variables that affect children's language performance. Skillful manipulation of these variables by the speech-language pathologist can enhance the potential intervention value of descriptive methods.

AN INTEGRATED FUNCTIONAL ASSESSMENT STRATEGY

Adequate evaluation is one of the most difficult and demanding tasks faced by the speech-language pathologist. The goal—much more complex than providing a score or label—is to describe the very complex language system of the child. Each child has a unique pattern of language rules and behaviors to be revealed and described.

A number of speech-language professionals have suggested a combined assessment approach, although the exact components of each differ (Cole, 1982; Kelly & Rice, 1986; Klein, 1984; McCauley & Swisher, 1984b). Almost universally, speech-language professionals would agree that no single measure or session is adequate (Emerich & Haynes, 1986).

It is helpful to consider assessment procedures as existing along a continuum from formal, structured protocols to informal, less structured approaches. In general, the more structured the elicitation session, the less variety of structures and meanings expressed (Miller, 1978). Language elicited in more structured tasks is usually shorter and less complex, especially with younger children, than is language sampled in less controlled situations (Fey, Leonard, & Wilcox, 1981; Longhurst & Grubb, 1974).

Generally, the more specific the information desired, the more structured the approach. In this way formal assessments can help the clinician sharpen and focus what was observed. Even formal tests or portions of tests can be used in an informal way as a probe of specific behavior. Naturally, normative data cannot be used when the test procedure is altered in any way.

The clinician must consider the following seven variables in designing and implementing the assessment process (Kelly & Rice, 1986).

1. The child's chronological and functional age
2. The state of the child's sensory system (vision, hearing, etc.)
3. Caregiver concerns
4. Status of the child's psychological functioning
5. Child's interests and materials available
6. Child's activity level
7. Child's attention span

"Judicious manipulation of these subject and setting variables facilitates elicitation of a representative sample of the child's receptive and expressive communicative functioning" (Kelly & Rice, 1986, p. 89). In general, alternation of structured and less structured tasks keeps the child's attention and provides variety and relief from clinician demands. The clinician should readily adapt the methods to the child and be mindful that the child will respond differently to different adults.

The speech-language pathologist should keep in mind the why, what, and how of assessment (Miller, 1978). Considering why the child is being assessed helps the speech-language pathologist clarify the purpose. This, in turn, enables the clinician to decide what specific behaviors to assess and the best evaluative methods to use. The reasons for assessment can be grouped as (a) identification of children with potential problems, (b) establishment of baseline functioning, and (c) measurement of change. Baseline functioning enables the speech-language pathologist to determine the present level of performance, the extent of the language impairment, and the nature of the problem.

The combined or integrated assessment approach provides the most thorough evaluation. A combined approach should include a caregiver interview, a caregiver-child observation, a clinician-directed formal psychometric assessment, and a child-directed informal assessment consisting of a conversational sample from the child. The actual components will differ with each child. Each component is discussed in the remainder of this chapter.

The data-gathering process is scientific in nature in that it must be unbiased and objective. This collection process should be precise and measurable with very little intrusion by the clinician's conclusions. It is important, however, not to lose

FIGURE 2.3
A model of the assessment process

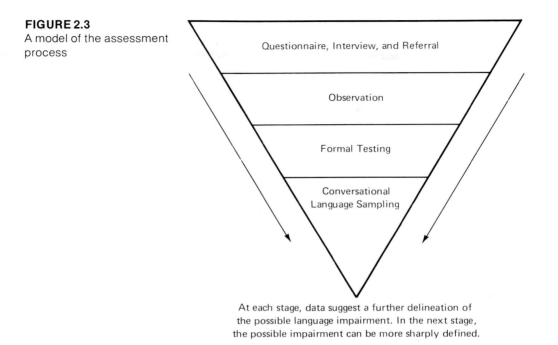

At each stage, data suggest a further delineation of
the possible language impairment. In the next stage,
the possible impairment can be more sharply defined.

the child in the mass of data, and clinical intuition is an important factor in summarizing data and in determining which aspects of language to evaluate.

At each diagnostic step, objectives should be derived from the information collected to this point. Thus, each step becomes more focused, and the possible language problems are highlighted. Figure 2.3 suggests a possible stage process of collecting data toward the goal of providing recommendations for intervention or modifications in ongoing programming. At each stage, the process becomes more focused. The following discussion deals with a number of assessment steps, both formal and informal, that are aspects of an overall integrated functional model.

Questionnaire, Interview, and Referral

Caregivers—parents, teachers, and others—are central to a functional assessment and intervention process (Kelly & Rice, 1986). Teachers can be a valuable referral source and should be encouraged to be alert for children with potential language problems (Siegel, 1979). Initial caregiver involvement helps to build rapport, increases the validity of the assessment results, and introduces the caregivers to the intervention process.

A caregiver interview or questionnaire can be a valuable source of initial information on client functioning and on the perceived problem from the

caregiver's perspective. Caregiver expectations for the child also provide an indication of the caregiver's willingness and perceived need to work with the child.

It is best to ask questions in a straightforward manner with no hesitation
that might signal embarassment or discomfort. The speech-language pathologist
avoids tag questions (e.g., ''You don't . . . , do you?'') that seek agreement rather
than confirmation or information. Responses should be treated matter-of-factly
with little comment that might discourage the caregiver from talking. A list of
possible questions is presented in Table 2.2 (Brinton & Fujiki, 1989; Cole, 1982;
Lund & Duchan, 1988; Spinelli & Terrell, 1984).

Caregiver responses should be analyzed and hypotheses formed before deciding on the strategy for the remainder of the assessment. Potential language
problems should be researched thoroughly throughout the remainder of the assessment process.

Observation

For the most natural interaction, the speech-language pathologist will want to
observe the caregiver(s) and child in such everyday settings as the home and
classroom. In the classroom, the speech-language pathologist might observe the
child participating in a number of different activities. This situation is not always
possible. Time may not permit observation alone. In this case, the speech-language pathologist may wish to observe closely while collecting a language sample
and may form tentative hypotheses for later confirmation from the analyzed sample.

If observation occurs in a more clinical setting, appropriate toys and both
structured and nonstructured activities should be provided for the child and caregiver. The caregiver should be encouraged to bring familiar objects and the child's
favorite toys from home or the classroom. The clinician may also wish to observe
the child's behavior with various communication partners. Caregivers should be
encouraged to ask questions.

The speech-language pathologist should instruct caregivers to interact as
typically as possible with the child. It is essential that caregivers not quiz or direct
the child to perform during the observation (Cole, 1982). Optimum performance
is attained if the clinician unobtrusively remains in the room or leaves and observes from outside via observation windows or video monitors.

The style of interaction is more than just the frequency of various forms of
behavior. More important are the ways in which the child uses the various features of the interactional style. The key question is, How does the child interact
with others?

Routinized situations may provide the child with a scaffold within which
processing becomes automatized before the child is capable of more elaborate formulation (Lieven, 1984). The clinician needs to assess the child's familiarity with
the situation and the degree to which that situation provides a prop for the child's
language.

TABLE 2.2
Interview or questionnaire format

Questions relative to language uses:
How does the child let you know items desired? What does the child request most
    frequently?
What does the child do when requesting that you do something?
    When wants you to pay attention?
    When wants something?
    When wants to direct your attention?
Does the child ask for information?
How does the child express emotion or tell about feelings?
    What emotions does the child express?
Does the child make noises when playing alone? Does the child engage in monologues
    while playing? Does the child prefer to play alone or with others?
Does the child describe things in the environment? How?
Does the child discuss events in the past, future, or outside of the immediate context?

Questions relative to conversational skill:
When does the child communicate best?
How does the child respond when you say something? How does the child respond to
    others? Does the child interact more readily with certain people and in certain
    situations, and if so, with whom and when?
With whom and when does the child communicate most frequently?
Does the child initiate conversations or activities with you and with others? What is the
    child's most frequent topic?
Does the child join in when others initiate conversations or activities?
Does the child get your attention before saying something to you?
    How does the child do this? Does the child maintain eye contact while talking to you?
Does the child take turns when talking? Does the child interrupt? Are there long gaps
    between your utterances and the child's responses? Will the child take a turn without
    being instructed to do so or without being asked a question?
When the child speaks to you, is there an expectation of a response? What does the child
    do if you do not respond?
When the child responds to you, does the response usually match or is it relevant to what
    you said?
How does the child ask for clarification? How frequently does this occur?
If you ask the child for more information or for clarification, what happens? Does the child
    demonstrate frustration when not understood?
When the child asks for or tells you something, is there usually enough information for
    you to understand?
When the child tells you more complex information or relates an event or story, is it
    organized enough for you to follow the train of thought?
Does the child have different ways of talking to different people, such as adults and small
    children? Does the child phrase things in different ways with different listeners? Is the
    child more polite in some situations?
Does the child seem confused at times? What does the child do if confused?

(continued)

...inued)

...tive to form and content:

... to understand simple directions?

...now the names of common events, objects, and people in the

...? What types of information does the child provide about these (actions,

...le, descriptions, locations, causation, functions, etc.)?

...seem to rely on gestures, sounds, or the immediate environment to be

...understood?

Does the child speak in single words, phrases, or sentences? How long is a typical utterance? Does the child leave out words? Are the child's sentences complex or simple? How does the child ask questions?

Does the child use pronouns and articles to distinguish old and new information?

Does the child use words for time, such as *tomorrow, yesterday,* or *last night?* Does the child use verb tenses?

Can the child put several sentences together to form complex descriptions and explanations?

Source: Compiled from Brinton & Fujiki (1989), Cole (1982), Lund & Duchan (1988), and Spinelli & Terrell (1984).

The INREAL/Outreach Program of the University of Colorado recommends an observation strategy called SOUL. The acronym stands for silence, observation, understanding, and listening. The adult remains silent for periods of time, assessing the situation before talking. Observation of the child's play and interactions with other people occurs prior to forming hypotheses. Understanding is insight into the child that comes from the distillation of data collected during observation. Finally, listening requires total involvement by the adult and the use of responses appropriate to the functioning level of the child.

The reliability of observation is increased if the clinician's descriptions detail as closely as possible the actual observed behavior (Duncan & Fiske, 1977). Inferences and hypotheses come later. The speech-language pathologist obtains from the caregiver interview some notion of what to observe. It is best if the observation is videotaped or audiotaped for later referral.

Table 2.3 lists some features that the speech-language pathologist might observe. This list is not exhaustive. Each category is discussed in some detail in Chapters 4 and 5, where we consider the analysis of a conversational sample. The purpose of observation is to note within the larger scope of interaction the language characteristics to be tested, collected, and analyzed later in the assessment.

Reliability of observation is not fortuitous. Speech-language pathologists should train together thoroughly so that their observations are as accurate and as objective as possible. This accuracy and objectivity can be accomplished by repeated observation and scoring of videotaped samples by more than one clinician. Scoring can then be compared, discussed, and modified in light of re-observation of taped samples.

TABLE 2.3
Features to note while observing the child

Form of language. Does the child use single words, phrases, or sentences primarily? Are the sentences of the subject-verb-object form exclusively? Are there mature negatives, interrogatives, and passive sentences? Does the child elaborate the noun or verb phrase? Is there evidence of embedding and conjoining?

Understanding of semantic intent. Does the child respond appropriately to the various question forms (what, where, who, when, why, how)? Does the child confuse words from different semantic classes?

Language use. Does the child display a range of illocutionary functions, such as asking for information, help, and objects, replying, making statements, providing information, etc.? Does the child take conversational turns? Does the child introduce topics and maintain them through several turns? Does the child signal the status of the communication and make repairs?

Rate of speaking. Is the rate inordinately slow or fast? Are there noticeable or lengthy pauses between the caregiver and child's turn? Are there noticeable or lengthy pauses between the child's adjacent utterances? Does the child use fillers frequently or pause before producing certain words? Are there frequent word substitutions?

Sequencing. Does the child relate events in a sequential fashion based on the order of occurrence? Can the child discuss the recent past or recount stories?

Formal Testing

In general, the role of testing is twofold: (a) to identify the child with potential language problems based on normative testing and (b) to begin a description of the child's language performance. Although screening tests may crudely address the first issue, they certainly do not address the second. Except as a tool for eliminating consideration of impairments in certain aspects of language, screening tests are of little diagnostic value.

Within the evaluation, a change to more formal tasks might be accomplished through the use of a nonthreatening receptive task, such as the Peabody Picture Vocabulary Test-Revised (PPVT-R) (Dunn & Dunn, 1981). Such a task allows the child to become accustomed to the clinician's direction. It is important, however, that the clinician make a thorough assessment of all aspects of language. This task may necessitate more than one session with the child and caregivers. Table 2.4 presents some of the more widely used language tests organized by areas assessed by each. Issues relative to each aspect of language are discussed following the table.

Syntax

Syntactic testing can be extremely complicated because of the complexity and diversity of the syntactic system. Speech-language pathologists may wish to use

TABLE 2.4

Aspects of language covered by commonly used tests

Test Name	Test Type		Aspect of Language					Mode	
	Screening	Diagnostic	Syntax	Morphology	Phonology	Semantics	Pragmatics	Receptive	Expressive
Adolescent Language Screening Test	X		X	X	X	X	X	X	X
Analysis of the Language of Learning		X	X	X	X	X			X
Assessment of Phonological Processes	X	X			X				X
Bankson Language Screening Test	X		X	X				X	X
Berko Test of English Morphology		X	X	X					X
Carrow Elicited Language Inventory		X	X	X			X		
Clark-Madison Oral Language Test		X	X	X			X		
Clinical Evaluation of Language Functions	X	X	X	X		X		X	X
Compton Phonological Assessment of Children	X	X			X			X	X
Evaluating Communicative Competence		X	X			X	X	X	X

Fullerton Language Test
for Adolescents

Full-Range Picture Vocabulary
Test

Interpersonal Language Skills
Assessment

Language Processing Test

Let's Talk Inventory for Children

Miller-Yoder Language
Comprehension Test

Multilevel Informal Language
Inventory

Northwest Syntax Screening Test

Oral Language Sentence
Imitation Diagnostic Inventory

Patterned Elicitation Syntax
Screening Test

Peabody Picture Vocabulary Test

Phonological Process Analysis

Test of Adolescent Language

Test of Auditory Comprehension
of Language—Revised

Test of Language Development—
Intermediary

Test of Language Development—
Primary

The Word Test

entire test batteries or portions of several tests. The latter strategy is recommended for in-depth probing of potential problem areas. Appendix A offers an item analysis of several of the more widely used syntactic tests to aid clinicians in item selection. Naturally, when tests are used in a nonstandard manner or combined with other subtests, the norms can no longer be used. Results must be described accurately and interpreted in light of the tasks involved.

In general, comprehension of syntactic forms precedes production. Thus, a thorough language assessment should include evaluation of both aspects. Although the receptive procedures used and the structures assessed vary widely across tests, the common element is that the child demonstrates understanding—usually by pointing or following directions—while producing only minimal language, if any.

Syntactic production is typically tested using either a structured elicitation or a sentence imitation format. In structured elicitation, the child may be asked to describe a picture following a model by the test administrator. The model sentence establishes the sentence form to be used but differs from the desired sentence by the structure being tested. In sentence imitation, the child gives an immediate repetition of the administrator's sentence.

The underlying assumption of elicited imitation procedures is that sentences that exceed the child's immediate memory span will be reproduced according to the child's own linguistic rule system, which the child must use as a processing aid. Theoretically, the child's sentence should be very similar to the one the child would produce spontaneously. Conversely, the imitated sentence will not contain any structures absent in the child's spontaneous language production.

Although elicited imitation serves as the basis of a number of diagnostic instruments (Carrow, 1974; Gray & Ryan, 1973; Zackman, Huisingh, Jorgensen, & Barrett, 1978a & b) and as a portion of several other tools (Bankson, 1977; Foster, Giddan, & Stark, 1973; Hendrick, Prather, & Tobin, 1975; Mecham, Jex, & Jones, 1967; Newcomer & Hammill, 1977; Semel & Wiig, 1980), the validity of the procedure has been frequently questioned. In part, the issue in elicited imitation is one of scoring. Whereas most tests are interested merely in the accuracy of repetition, the Carrow Elicited Language Inventory (CELI) (Carrow, 1974) attempts to analyze the changes language-impaired children make when they repeat.

The imitative procedure may underestimate, overestimate, or correctly estimate the child's actual language abilities (Prutting & Connolly, 1976). For example, although the performance of language-disordered children on elicited imitation tests can be enhanced by the addition of contextual cues, such as pictures or object manipulation (Hale-Haniff & Siegel, 1981; Nelson & Weber-Olsen, 1980; Weber-Olsen, Putnam-Sims & Gannon, 1983), their imitations are still simpler than their spontaneous language production (Connell & Myles-Zitler, 1982). In part, this disparity may result from the fact that assumptions about the performance of nonimpaired children may not apply to language-impaired children (Miller, 1978).

Because the relationship between elicited imitation and spontaneously produced language is a very complex one, speech-language pathologists are advised

to use elicited imitation results with caution and to rely on the data from spontaneous samples when the two differ (Fujiki & Brinton, 1987). Elicited imitation responses should be analyzed for the specific ways that they differ from the model.
Table 2.5 provides a method of scoring sentence imitation tasks that maximizes
the available information for clinical use (Mattes, 1982). Each response is scored
for grammatical acceptability, type of syntactic error, semantic equivalence, and
quality of response.

Morphology

Morphological testing usually focuses on bound morphemes or inflections in the
form of prefixes and suffixes. Most tests emphasize suffixes, such as tense markers, plurals, possessives, and comparators, because of their high usage and relatively early development. The two most common test formats for morphology are
cloze or sentence completion and sentence imitation. Tests use either actual words
or nonsense words. The rationale for nonsense words is that their use will not
bias performance by previous exposure. In general, children who have mental
retardation or learning disabilities have greater difficulty than do nonhandicapped children with nonsense words.

Phonology

Commonly used sampling techniques for phonological analysis include spontaneous labeling of pictures and objects (Fisher & Logemann, 1987; Fudala, 1970;
Goldman & Fristoe, 1986; Hodson, 1980; Klein, 1984; Templin & Darley, 1969),
conversation and narration (Shriber & Kwiatkowski, 1980), and imitation (Weiner, 1979). Different methods of collection yield different results in the amount
and type of errors produced (Andrews & Fey, 1986; Johnson, Winney, & Pederson, 1980). Labeling tasks produce the greatest variety and allow for the greatest
clinician control of phonological contexts. In addition, the known targets increase
the clinician's ability to analyze unintelligible utterances (Hodson, 1980; Paden &
Moss, 1985). On the other hand, speech sounds in conversation may also be important.

Speech in conversation contains more speech sound errors (Dubois &
Bernthal, 1978; Klein, 1984) and more clinically significant results (Andrews &
Fey, 1986) than does speech sampled in isolated words. Single-word production
tasks do not correlate well with the results of connected speech analysis (Dubois
& Bernthal, 1978; Simmons-Miles, 1983; Shriberg & Kwiatkowski, 1980). Thus,
clinicians may miss some significant clinical information by concentrating only on
production in isolated contexts. Most professionals agree on the need for more
than single-word test performance because of coarticulation and the need to assess in the use context of ongoing conversation (Daniloff & Moll, 1968; Haynes,
Haynes, & Jackson, 1982; Panagos, Quine, & Klich, 1979; Schmauch, Panagos, &
Klich, 1978).

Ease of identification and caseload constraints would suggest that clinicians
apply an initial strategy in which articulation test results are analyzed for phonological processes when a phonological disorder is suspected (Haynes & Steed,

TABLE 2.5
Elicited language analysis procedures

Format

Student's Name: _____

Birthdate: _____ Examiner: _____ Test Date: _____

Test item #	Instructions: Record the child's responses in the spaces below. Score responses in terms of grammatical acceptability, syntactic usage, vocabulary usage and response quality by placing a check mark in the boxes which most accurately describe the response.	Grammatical Acceptability	Syntactic Usage on Structure Tested								Vocabulary			Response Quality		Comments
			Correct: Identical	Correct: Nonidentical	Substitution Error	Deletion Error	Insertion Error	Modification Error	Word Sequence Error	Non-Attempt Error	Equivalent in Meaning	Related in Meaning	Unrelated in Meaning	Delayed Response	Self-Corrected Response	Perseverative Response	

The child's elicited imitation is written in the appropriate column at the left. Omissions, substitutions, changes in meaning and the like are noted by marking the appropriate column. The errors and target structures can be recorded under the comments column, such as "Omit past tense -ed" or "Change passive voice to active." Such analysis may help delineate unlearned structures and the cognitive-linguistic knowledge base.

Response Categories

Grammatical acceptability. Child's response is a complete and grammatically correct sentence.

Syntactic usage on structure tested. The manner in which the grammatical structure tested is produced.

A. *Correct production: identical sentence frame.* Child's response is an identical word-for-word reproduction of the model.

B. *Correct production; nonidentical sentence frame.* The grammatical structure being tested is produced correctly, although the sentence frame differs from the model.

C. *Substitution error.* The child substitutes an inappropriate grammatical form for the structure being tested.

D. *Deletion error.* The child inappropriately omits the grammatical structure being tested.

E. *Insertion error.* The child inserts the gramatical structure being tested within a sentence frame where it is inappropriate.

(continued)

TABLE 2.5 (*continued*)

F. *Modification error.* The child produces a modification of the grammatical structure being tested that is not acceptable in any context (ex. *him's, ain't, it's is*).

G. *Word sequence error.* The child produces the grammatical structure being tested in an inappropriate position within the response.

H. *Non-attempt error.* Performance can not be evaluated (ex. *I don't know*).

Vocabulary usage. Manner in which the child's response relates semantically to the stimulus sentence.

A. *Equivalent in meaning.* Although the specific vocabulary used by the child is not identical to the model, the response is identical in meaning.

B. *Related in meaning.* The child produces a response which is partially related to the meaning of the model. The child may omit essential elements or modify vocabulary.

C. *Unrelated in meaning.* The child produces a nonmeaningful response or one that is unrelated to the model.

Response quality.

A. *Delayed correct response.* The child produces a correct response which is nonimmediate, requires a repetition of the model, or is produced after hesitation during response.

B. *Self-corrected response.* The child self-corrects an incorrect response without prompting by the examiner.

C. *Perseverative response.* The child produces a response that resembles that used on a previous test item but inappropriate for this item.

Source: Mattes, L. (1982). The elicited language analysis procedure: A method for scoring sentence imitation tasks. *Language, Speech, and Hearing Services in the Schools, 13*, 37–41. Reprinted with permission.

1987; Klein, 1984). For example, the Khan-Lewis (1987) might be used to reanalyze the results of the Goldman-Fristoe Test of Articulation (Goldman & Fristoe, 1986).

Most articulation tests sample each sound once in each of the positions in which it appears in words. Other appearances are not scored. By carefully transcribing each word spoken in the test, however, the clinician can increase the data base and have additional productions to analyze for possible phonological processes. Table 2.6 is a form to use with the Goldman-Fristoe Test of Articulation. Blank spaces on this table are used to note those phonological processes demonstrated by the child. The processes are explained in the table. Developmental and normative information is included in Chapter 4.

Imitation tasks may also offer a compromise between efficiency and thoroughness. Several studies have found a positive correlation across single-word free speech and imitation samples and across connected speech and sentence imitation samples (Haynes & Steed, 1987; Paynter & Bumpas, 1977; Siegel, Winitz, & Conkey, 1963). Subsequently, clinicians can collect and analyze conversational

TABLE 2.6 (pages 52–54)
Phonological analysis of articulation test results

Name _____

Age _____

Date _____

Goldman-Fristoe Items

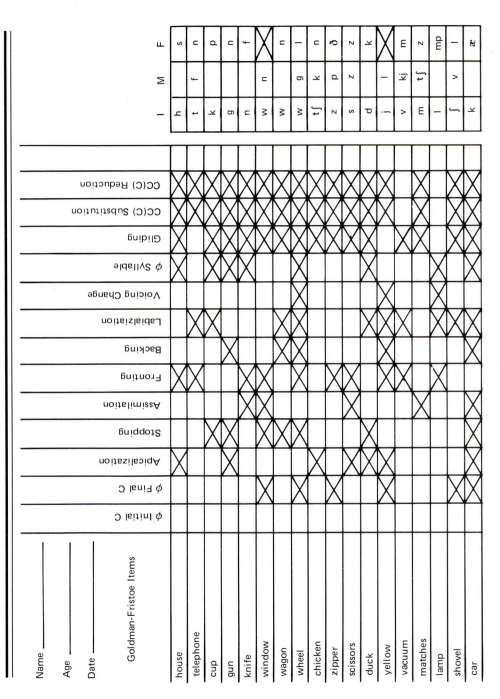

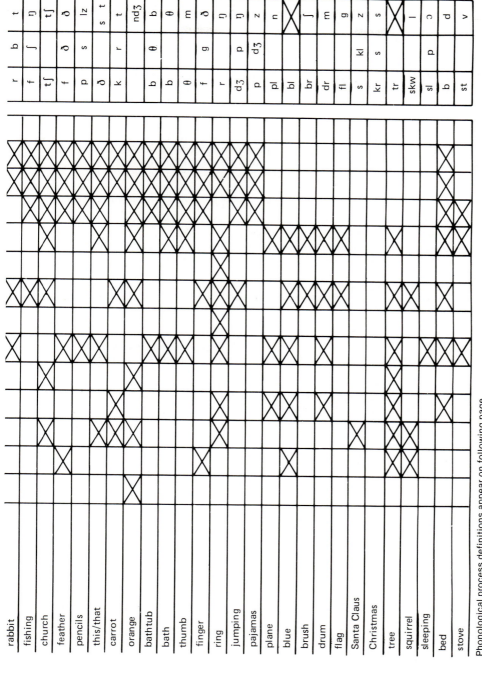

Phonological process definitions appear on following page.

TABLE 2.6 *(continued)*

Phonological process definitions

φ**Initial C** Initial consonant deletion occurs when the initial consonant of a target word is omitted in the child's production. Example: /bot/ goes to [ot]

φ**Final C** Deletion of final consonant occurs when a target word ending with a consonant is produced with that final consonant omitted. Example: /bot/ goes to [bo]

Apicalization In apicalization a labial consonant is replaced by a tongue-tip consonant. Example: /fud/ goes to [sud]

Stopping The process of stopping involves the replacement of a fricative, affricate or semi-vowel with a stop consonant. Example: /sop/ goes to [top]

Assimilation Assimilation refers to the influence that speech sounds can have on the production of other speech sounds. Thus if a speech sound changes to be more like another speech sound in its near environment, assimilation has occurred. The assimilation can be to other speech sounds that precede or follow the changed phone. Example: /fit/ goes to [pit] because of the influence of the stop /t/.

Fronting Fronting occurs when a velar stop or palatal affricate or fricative is replaced by an alveolar speech sound. Example: /kap/ goes to [tap]

Backing The process of backing occurs when an anterior consonant is replaced by a velar or glottal consonant. Example: /to/ goes [ko]

Labialization Labialization involves the replacement of a tongue-made articulation with a speech sound made with one or both of the lips. A common instance is the replacement of /θ/ with /f/. When the sound change only occurs in the presence of a labial consonant it is a form of assimilation.

Voicing Change Voicing change occurs whenever a speech sound changes in its voicing feature. The addition of voicing is marked by a plus sign (+). Devoicing is marked by a minus sign (−).

φ**Syllable** Syllable deletion can occur only in polysyllabic words. Typically, the unstressed syllable is deleted. Example: /patedo/ goes to [tedo]

Gliding Gliding entails the replacement of a liquid with a glide. Example: /lo/ goes to [wo]

CC(C) Substitution/Reduction In this process a two-or three-member cluster has a member substituted or deleted. Typically, the marked member is the one substituted for or deleted. Example: /stov/ goes to [tov] or /blu/ goes [bwu]

Source: Lowe, R. (1986). Phonological Process Analysis Using Three Position Tests. *Language, Speech, and Hearing Services in Schools, 17,* 72–79. Reprinted with permission.

samples in order to revise their hypotheses and to plan intervention (Andrews & Fey, 1986).

Semantics

Testing of semantic abilities is usually confined to word definitions and word categories. Of interest are the child's comprehension and theoretically smaller production vocabularies. Comprehension vocabulary is usually measured by having the child point to a picture(s) that best represents the word produced by the test administrator. Such tests tell the speech-language pathologist very little about the depth or breadth of the child's understanding of the concept named. Comprehension of longer utterances is usually assessed by having the child follow simple commands or directives.

Expressive or productive vocabulary is usually tested by having the child name pictures or supply a definition. Categorical understanding is assessed by asking the child to supply an antonym or synonym or to name related words in a category. Between ages 5 and 9, the child undergoes a change in the organization of language from a syntactic to a more categorical system. Thus, category membership and related words should be tested with all children in late elementary and high school.

Many individuals, especially children with learning disabilities or closed head trauma, exhibit word-finding and substitution difficulties. Usually, the words substituted share some visual attributes with the target word referent, such as saying *sheet* for *cape* and *net* for *screen*. Late elementary school children with learning disabilities exhibit more visually related word substitution errors than do non-LD children (German, 1982). Additional word-finding substitutions found in children with learning disabilities include functional descriptions, such as *bookholder* for *shelf* (Denckla & Rudel, 1976; Johnson & Myklebust, 1967).

Diagnostically, use of these word-finding strategies indicates that the child comprehends the word but has difficulty retrieving it (German, 1982). Although testing may reveal a deficit in visual confrontation naming skills, such tests rarely indicate the nature of the deficit. Identification of the word retrieval strategies of these children may aid in the design of remediation techniques directly related to these strategies.

One method for attaining more information from tests is a double naming technique (Fried-Oken, 1987). In this procedure, a standard naming test is administered twice. The results are examined to identify error response groups that occur once and twice. The double error group or errors that occur on both administrations require further analysis.

The clinician administers a number of cues with the double error words to determine if the errors are related to word-finding difficulties and to identify naming strategies. In this procedure, cues are administrated in the following order (Fried-Oken, 1987):

1. *General question.* The child is asked a general, open-ended question, such as ''Can you think of another word for this?'' or ''What is this again?'' that provides no additional linguistic information.

2. *Semantic/phonemic facilitator.* Two cues, based on additional semantic and phonemic information, are administered. The order of presentation varies, but the clinician should carefully record the order and the response. The semantic cue describes the object's function, provides a superordinate label (categorical), or states the location. For example, if the picture shows a sofa, the clinician might say ''It's something you sit on,'' ''It's a piece of furniture,'' or ''You find it in the living room.'' The child's response and the type of semantic facilitator should be noted.

   The phonemic cue includes the initial phoneme of the desired label (''The word starts with a /__/.'') This type of cue requires certain metalinguistic skills in order for the child to use the information.

TABLE 2.7
Naming error categorization

Naming Strategy	Example
Phonological	foon/SPOON
Perceptual	lampshade/SKIRT
Semantic	tortoise/OCTOPUS
Semantic + perceptual	broom/MOP
	shirt/JACKET
Part/Whole	shoelace/SHOE
Functional circumlocution	you can play songs/PIANO
Descriptive circumlocution	it has numbers and hands/CLOCK
Contextual circumlocution	in a band/TAMBOURINE
Superordinate	food/CRACKERS
Subordinate	shetland pony/HORSE
Unrelated perseveration	canoe/HARMONICA
	canoe/MUSHROOM
Comment	I don't know/GLOVE
No answer	10 + seconds of silence/MITTEN
Gesture	"strumming"/GUITAR

Source: Fried-Oken, M. (1987). Qualitative examination of children's naming skills through test adaptations. *Language, Speech, and Hearing Services in Schools, 18,* 206–216. Reprinted with permission.

3. *Verification.* If the child is still incorrect, the clinician provides the correct label and asks whether the child has ever seen this object before in order to verify whether the word is in the child's repertoire.

The child's responses and the cues are analyzed to determine the qualitative nature of the errors and the child's naming strategy. Possible naming strategies of 4- to 9-year-old children are listed in Table 2.7 (Fried-Oken, 1984).

Pragmatics

Very few tests are available that assess the child's conversational skills. In general, there are two varieties, a storytelling format and topic discussion. In the latter, as exemplified by Let's Talk (Bray & Wiig, 1987; Wiig, 1982), various topics and situations are presented to the children, and they are expected to respond appropriately. In all of these test situations, the essential feature of conversational relevance is strained, and it is doubtful that a true description of the child's abilities is attained. For example, this format makes it difficult to assess question comprehension with commercially available tests (Moeller, Osberger, & Eccarius, 1986). In general, questioning is inadequately sampled, restricted in type, and lacking in variation of communicative contexts (Parnell & Amerman, 1983).

The nature of pragmatics makes formal testing difficult. At present, it seems more appropriate to use a conversational sample to assess children's language use.

Testing with Minority and Handicapped Children

In two judicial decisions regarding placement of Mexican-American and African-American children in classes for the educably mentally retarded (*Diana v. State Board of Education*, 1970; *Larry P. v. Riles*, 1972), the courts ruled that judgments made on the basis of responses to tests whose norming populations are inappropriate for these children are discriminatory. Many of the tests widely used in speech-language pathology (i.e., Carrow, 1973; Carrow, 1974; Kirk, McCarthy, & Winifield, 1968; Lee, 1971; Dunn, 1959; Mecham, Jex, & Jones, 1967) are normed on population samples with a disproportionately high number of white and middle-class children. Thus, older versions of the Peabody Picture Vocabulary Test (PPVT) (Dunn, 1959), for example, have been shown to yield lower scores for lower socioeconomic groups and for middle-class African-American children (Cazden, 1972; Kresheck & Nicolosi, 1973). Error analysis suggests that some test items may be culturally biased against African-American children. There are few, if any, standardized language tests that are nonbiased for evaluating bidialectal and bilingual children (Bernstein, 1989).

Typically, speech-language pathologists make two common errors with nonstandard children. Either the children are incorrectly identified as having a language disorder or those with a disorder are missed. For example, African-American children from rural Alabama who speak the Black English dialect common to that area continue to delete final consonants beyond the age for predominantly white children (Haynes & Moran, 1989). The speech-language pathologist who is unaware of this difference might incorrectly conclude that these children exhibit a phonological disorder. Common phonologic, syntactic, and pragmatic differences found in Black English and Hispanic English and in the English of some Asian speakers are listed in Appendix B.

The following five guidelines should be considered prior to using standardized tests with nonstandard children (Musselwhite, 1983):

1. What is the relationship of the norming population and the client? For example, with retarded children and other children functioning below their chronological age, it is more realistic to use cognitive development rather than chronological age for interpreting language and communication performance (Miller, 1978). Children in the United States who are bilingual Spanish-English or who use Spanish only may perform very differently even from each other (Wilcox & McGuinn-Aasby, 1988). These differences may reflect U.S. regional differences, country of origin, or socioeconomic differences (Norris, Juarez, & Perkins, 1989).

2. What is the relationship of the child's experience and the content areas of the test? Items using farm content, for example, may have little relevance for inner-city children.

3. What is the relationship of the language and/or dialect being tested

and the child's language and/or dialect dominance? This issue is critical in determining language impairment. The determining factor should be the child's ability to function within her or his own linguistic or dialectal community (Iglesias, 1986).

4. Is there detailed specification of idiomatic or metaphoric language used in the test? In other words, will the language of the test penalize a nonstandard child?

5. Is the child penalized for a particular pattern of learning or style of problem solving? Data indicate that a child with mental retardation or a language learning disability has a different information processing style.

Dual sets of norms can be used to compare minority and handicapped children's performance to the standard group and to their peer group (Musselwhite, 1983). Some tests have been normed on different population samples, such as English- and Spanish-speaking children. In general, these tests must be used very cautiously, because they assess structures important for English speakers and ignore those of the other language. The standardized norms could be used to identify children with language differences. Children who exhibit language disorders relative to their peer group could be identified by use of the peer group norms. Even this procedure may bias some results, given the diversity of some populations, such as Hispanics. Locally prepared norms may be more appropriate. Norris et al. (1989) present a procedure for adapting standard instruments for bilingual or bidialectal populations.

The speech-language pathologist is encouraged to use language tests normed on a population that reflects the child's background. Appendix C contains a partial list of commercially available tests for bidialectal and bilingual children.

The accuracy of testing with bilingual children for whom English is a second language may also be increased by using interpreters who speak the child's primary language (Watson, Omark, Gronell, & Heller, 1986). When an interpreter is not available or when the child speaks a nonstandard American English dialect, family members can aid the clinician. Accuracy may also be increased by sampling the child's language in a variety of situations (Bernstein, 1989).

Conversational Language Sampling

Conversational samples have the potential for providing the most accurate description of the child's language as it is actually used in conversational exchange. The next several chapters discuss the best ways to maximize the information from this source through design of collection situations and analysis methods.

CONCLUSION

Too often, a battery of readily available tests, given to every child regardless of possible language impairment, passes for thorough assessment. As with intervention, assessment procedures must be designed for the individual client. Standardized tests are only a portion of this process. Language tests are aids to the clinician. They cannot, as Siegel (1975) cautions, ''substitute for informed clinical judgment'' (p. 212).

A thorough assessment includes a variety of procedures designed to heighten awareness of the problem and enable the speech-language clinician to delineate more clearly the language abilities and impairments of the child. For training to be truly functional, there must be a thorough description of the child and the child's language.

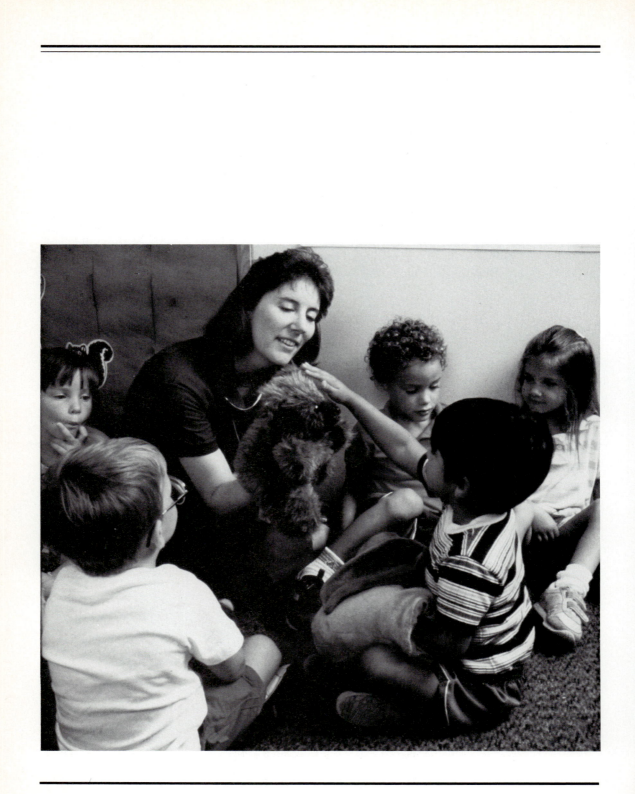

3
Language Sampling

Language sampling provides specific information for planning intervention because it includes both the content and context of language use (Blau, Lahey, & Oleksiuk-Velez, 1984). If the goal of language intervention is generalization to the language used by the child in everyday situations, it is essential that the speech-language pathologist collect a language sample that is a good reflection of that language in actual use.

Good language samples do not just occur. They are the result of careful planning and execution. The speech-language pathologist can design the assessment session so that the context fits the purpose of collecting the desired sample. The result is usually a combination of free conversation sampling and some evocative techniques.

The speech-language pathologist must make several decisions before collecting the sample. After studying the interview, observational, and testing results, decisions must be made relative to the context, participants, materials, and conversational techniques to be used. It should be remembered that ''there is no way to 'make' children talk . . . [the clinician] can only make them want to talk by creating a situation in which there is a reason to talk and an atmosphere that conveys the message that . . . [the clinician is] interested in what they have to say'' (Lund & Duchan, 1988, p. 23), This chapter covers the planning, collection, recording, and transcription of conversational samples.

PLANNING AND COLLECTING A REPRESENTATIVE SAMPLE

Several issues are of importance when planning and collecting a language sample. Among the most prominent are the representativeness of the sample and the effect of conversational settings, tasks, partners, and topics. In addition, collection of several language forms and functions may require the use of evocative techniques.

Representativeness

Representativeness can be addressed by ensuring spontaneity and by collecting samples under a variety of conditions. Spontaneity can be achieved if the child and conversational partner engage in real conversations on topics of interest to the child. To ensure spontaneity, the clinician can follow the (LCC)[3] formula for (a) *less clinician control,* (b) *less clinician contrivance,* and (c) *a less conscious child* (Cochrane, 1983).

The speech-language pathologist's control of the context should be weak so as not to restrict the child's linguistic output in quantity or quality. Although there is some indication that clinician style has little effect on gross measures, such as MLU and Developmental Sentence scores (Johnston, Trainor, Casey, & Hagler, 1981), more subtle measures may be affected to a greater degree. Control devices, such as the use of questions and decisions of topic, may cause the child to adopt a passive conversational role.

Not all children will participate freely in such exchanges, and other approaches may be required. In general, the speech-language pathologist can elicit longer and more complex language with picture interpretation tasks than with imperatives or story recapitulation (Atkins & Cartwright, 1982). In storytelling, the use of pictures can enhance the length and complexity of the sample, especially if the speech-language pathologist gives cues, such as ''Tell me a story about this picture. Begin with 'Once upon a time.' '' The least spontaneous condition involves the specific linguistic tasks of answering questions or completing sentences. The clinician can relinquish some control by placing these tasks within a less formal or play format.

The sample will be less contrived if the clinician follows the child's lead and adopts the child's topics for conversation. More contrived situations, such as ''Tell me about this picture'' or ''Explain the rules of Monopoly,'' do not elicit spontaneous everyday speech. The most contrived situation occurs when the clinician relies on a tried-and-true, never-fail list of standard questions for all clients, reqardless of age, sex, or interests.

Finally, if the child is less conscious of the process of producing language, the sample will be more spontaneous. Asking the child to produce sentences containing certain elements, for example, makes the linguistic process very conscious and may be very difficult, especially out of context. Whereas a child may not be able to produce a sentence with *has been* on demand, the same child may be able to relate the story of the three bears with ''Someone *has been* sleeping in my bed.'' The former task requires metalinguistic or abstract linguistic skills that may be beyond the child's abilities.

The child's caregivers can offer suggestions to the speech-language pathologist on contexts, partners, and materials or topics to help obtain a representative sample. It may be desirable for caregivers to serve as partners, especially with young children. After the sample has been collected, caregivers can review the data and comment on the typicality of the child's behavior.

A Variety of Settings, Tasks, Partners, and Topics

The sampling environment can contribute to representativeness if there are a variety of settings, tasks, partners, and topics. Variety ensures that the sample will not be gathered in one atypical situation. Instead, variety can reflect a sampling of the many interactional situations in which the child functions. Although variety is desirable, it is not always practical, especially in the public school setting. Tapes collected by the parent or teacher can provide an acceptable substitute.

Settings and Tasks

The best context is a meaningful activity containing a variety of elicitation tasks. In general, the child who is more familiar with the situation will give the most representative sample. Familiar routines provide a linguistic and/or nonlinguistic script that guides the child's behavior. For young children, play is one of these routine situations.

Language is a natural part of many routine events. Consider the linguistic sequence of behaviors that occur when one person calls another on the telephone.

The speech-language pathologist needs to decide whether the child's typical or optimal production is desired. For example, storytelling without picture cues yields a large MLU from preschoolers but does not elicit the quantity of language associated with picture interpretation or explanation tasks. This decision on type of production is critical, because language-impaired children often perform well below their linguistic knowledge level.

Settings should not be contrived. Familiar, meaningful situations with a variety of age-appropriate and motivating activities will provide greater variety and thus will be more representative (Kunze, Lockhart, Didow, & Caterson, 1983; Roth & Spekman, 1984b). Good settings for preschoolers include the free play mentioned earlier, snack time, and show-and-tell. School-aged children can be sampled during group activities, class presentations, or field trips. Generally, the child involved in some activity produces more language than the child who is watching others or conversing about pictures. It is better if the sample consists of two different settings in which different activities are occurring.

The materials used should be interesting, age-appropriate, and capable of eliciting the type of language desired. Interest can be piqued if the child is allowed to choose from a preselected group of toys or objects. Parents can also bring the child's toys from home in order to increase the validity of the sample (MacDonald, 1978).

In general, children around age 2 respond well to blocks, dishes, pull and wind-up toys, and dolls. Three-year-olds prefer books, clothes, puppets, and such toys as a barn with animals or a street with houses and stores. These toys encourage role playing and language production. Kindergarten and early elementary school children respond best to toys with many pieces and to puppets and action figures. Finally, older children will usually converse without the use of objects and can be encouraged to talk about themselves and their interests or to provide narratives. Narratives, a special type of language production, are discussed in Chapter 6.

The selection of clinical materials can affect the pragmatic performance of young children by modifying the physical context in which the sample is collected (Gallagher, 1983; Wanska, Bedrosian, & Pohlman, 1986). This selection is especially important given the current emphasis on the use of play in pragmatic assessment and intervention (Craig, 1983; McCune-Nicolich & Carroll, 1981). When no toys are present, children are more likely to initiate memory-related topics (Bedrosian & Willis, 1987).

The speech-language pathologist should consider the nature of the toys to be used in a play assessment (Wanska et al., 1986). For example, toys with construction properties, such as Legos, Play Doh, or clay, might be used to determine whether the child can remove the conversation from the present. Such toys are more likely to elicit more displaced topics, especially as objects are being constructed (Chapman, 1981).

On the other hand, toys that encourage role play might be used to elicit more verbalizations or vocalizations for objects, events, and actions. Compared to construction-type toys, a toy hospital elicits more discussion of the here and now and more fantasy topics and is more conducive to sociodramatic play and verbal representations of events and actions (Wanska et al., 1986).

Toys may also assist in eliciting specific linguistic structures. For example, children are more likely to produce spatial terms in play with objects than in conversation (Washington & Naremore, 1978). Object movement and manipulation can serve as nonlinguistic cues for the child. Since children's cognitive knowledge and linguistic performance of spatial relationships may differ markedly, manipulation of toys can aid the speech-language pathologist in assessing the child's comprehension (Cox & Richardson, 1985; Harris, Morris, & Terwog, 1986). The toys and positions should be varied so as not to suggest answers to children (Messick, 1988).

Conversational Partners

Because the speech-language pathologist is interested in the child's use of language, the unit of analysis becomes the conversational dyad of the facilitator and the child and their interactive behaviors in a given context (Prutting & Kirchner, 1983). The dyadic context enables the clinician to view the child's communication within the applied situation of the natural environment (Tiegerman & Siperstein, 1984).

Conversational partners are also carefully selected and instructed in their role. It is especially important to use familiar conversational partners with children under age 3 because these children often respond poorly to strangers. Parents of young children or children with acknowledged handicaps may need special instruction to avoid having their children ''perform.'' Uninstructed parents may feel compelled to quiz their child or to have their child recite stereotypic verbal routines, such as nursery rhymes, to enhance the child's linguistic output. The problem with such recitations is that they may have little to do with the conversational abilities of the child.

In general, it is best to involve the parent or caregiver and child in some activity. Caregivers can be instructed to talk about what they and the child are doing. Toys, such as doll houses, action figure playsets, farms and towns, and puppets, encourage interactional and role play.

Familiar conversational situations are chosen as well in order to attain the most typical spontaneous sample with the child conversing as naturally as possible. Interaction may involve one adult or child, or a small group of children, engaged in sharing, playing, or working in the home or classroom.

The child should be assessed across several familiar persons with different interactive styles because of the effect conversational partners—either individually or in small groups—have on the child's verbal output (Mirenda & Donnellan, 1986; Prizant & Rentschler, 1983). For example, peer interaction usually involves more equal status between participants than do adult-child interactions (Mishler, 1975; Youniss, 1980). Adults tend to guide and control the topic when conversing with children, whereas child-child conversations are presumably more equal (Bloom, Rocissano, & Hood, 1976; Chapman, Miller, MacKenzie, & Bedrosian, 1981). As one might expect, these two conditions result in very different interactive styles for the child. If two children are talking, the adult should leave the room because children who are unsure of the situation will defer to the adult and thus skew the data.

The language performance of children below age 3, of minority children, and of children with language learning disabilities may deteriorate in the presence of an authority figure, such as an unfamiliar adult. This does not mean that the speech-language pathologist cannot act as a conversational partner. In many ways, the speech-language pathologist is the best conversational partner because of her knowledge of language and of interactions.

The speech-language pathologist and all other participating adults need to be mindful of the inherent problems in adult-child conversations and act to reduce the authority figure persona. The adult can accomplish this by accepting the child's activity, agenda, and topics and by participating with the child. With young children, participation may necessitate using the floor for play.

The speech-language pathologist as the conversational partner can set the tone of the interaction by being nondirective, interesting, interested, and responsive. She should respond to the content of the child's language, not to the way in which it is said. At this point, the purpose is to collect data, not change behavior. Our goal is collecting, not correcting.

The speech-language pathologist can manipulate the situation skillfully in order to probe for a greater range of information (Spinelli & Terrell, 1984). Initially, interaction may be dampened because the speech-language pathologist is not the child's usual communication partner. Therefore, it is important for the speech-language pathologist to get acquainted slowly and in a nonthreatening manner. This is best accomplished by meeting the child on his or her terms through play and by following the child's lead.

The speech-language pathologist possesses the clinical skill to elicit a variety of functions, introduce various topics, and ask questions about experiences. Role play, dolls, and puppet play provide information about the child's event knowledge in a range of situations. There is the potential to elicit a greater variety of language than might be possible when the child and parent communicate.

The best way to attain a semblance of equal authority is for the speech-language pathologist and child to engage in a play interaction. Instead of being directive, the speech-language pathologist comments on their ongoing activity.

Children who are reluctant to talk to adults may be more willing to interact with a puppet or doll. I have found that small animals, such as guinea pigs, make excellent communication partners for children. After explaining to the child that she must leave to run a short errand, the speech-language pathologist introduces the guinea pig and asks the child to talk to it so that it will not get lonely. The child should be observed while the clinician is absent.

Despite conventional wisdom, neither the race of the conversational partner nor the race depicted in stimulus materials seems to affect language performance as measured by response length and response latency (Seymour, Ashton, & Wheeler, 1986). This is not to say that all children, particularly minority children, will be unaffected. Speech-language pathologists should be aware of potential difficulties and should approach each child with an open mind. Racial incompatibilities should not be expected, but the speech-language pathologist should be conscious of this potential.

The speech-language pathologist attempts to get the greatest variety of partners possible. Parents, teachers, and peers can fill this role, either alone or in small groups.

Topics
Children have a wide variety of interests, and the conversational partners must be careful to enable the child to talk about them. Children are more spontaneous and produce more language when they are allowed to initiate the topics of discussion.

The speech-language pathologist should be prepared to shift topics as readily as activities. Therefore, the speech-language pathologist must be conversant in topics of interest to children, such as school activities, holidays, television programs, fads and fashions, and rock music.

Summary
Child variables, such as recent past experience and mood, can greatly affect language sampling because the child is often the initiator in this protocol and because there are few performance constraints (Hess, Sefton, & Landry, 1986; Klee & Fitzgerald, 1985). To get the most representative sample possible, therefore, the clinician should use familiar situations, persons, and tasks or topics. Repre-

sentativeness is enhanced if the conversational sample is collected in more than one setting, with different conversational partners and tasks or topics in each.

It may be helpful to think of interactional situations along a continuum from relatively nondirected or free to more controlled or scripted (Shriberg & Kwiatkowski, 1985). Such toys as a dollhouse, a farm, action figures, bubbles, or dress-up clothes are rather open-ended, especially when the partner has suggested, ''Let's talk and play with these things.'' Books or colorforms offer more control and can be used to elicit particular words, forms, or narratives. Familiar routines, such as doing the dishes, can also be used along with such cues as ''What are you going to do now?'' to elicit more specific behavior. Interviews, picture labeling, and responding to questions offer the most control but at the sacrifice of spontaneity and representativeness. These latter techniques are more appropriately considered evocative techniques used to elicit specific behaviors.

Evocative Conversational Techniques

Although the sample should represent the everyday language used by the child, free samples may have limitations, such as low frequency or nonappearance of certain linguistic features and conversational behaviors (Roth & Spekman, 1984b). Absence or low incidence does not mean that the child does not possess these features or behaviors. Therefore, it may be necessary to supplement the sample with evocative procedures specifically designed to elicit them. Test protocols might also be modified to obtain more structured samples (Thomas, 1989).

The speech-language pathologist may need to plan both the linguistic and nonlinguistic contexts for elicitation of various functions and forms. At first, some procedures may seem stiff and formal, even forced. Initially, the clinician may need to role play the sampling situation and memorize conversational openers and replies. Once familiar with the many ways of eliciting a variety of functions and forms, she can relax and use the techniques more naturally as opportunities arise within the interaction.

Specific tasks that are within the child's experience can be used to elicit specific language forms (Roth & Spekman, 1984b). This approach allows a broad range of pragmatic functions to occur (Kunze et al., 1983). For example, a mock birthday party can be used to elicit plurals, past tense, and questions (Wren, 1985). The clinician might elicit plurals by saying the following:

> Today is X's birthday. Let's have a party. What are some things that we'll need? (Or, Here are some things we need. What are these?)

The pathologist can use plates, spoons, glasses, candles, presents, and so on. Thus, the child's utterances are placed within some context. Within the same situation, past tense might be elicited by dropping dishes and asking what happened or by reviewing whether you did everything to get ready (''Okay, now tell me what you did to get ready for the party. I washed the dishes''). Finally, questions can be elicited by a party game variation of Ask the Old Lady (Brown, 1973).

Let's play a question game. This is X (puppet, doll, action figure). I want you to ask X some questions about his birthday party. I wonder how old he is. You ask him.

The child may need a demonstration before being able to complete the question task.

Our interest in generalization of intervention to everyday use necessitates an interest in the pragmatic organizational framework of the sample. Some areas of interest include the intentions of individual utterances, the presuppositions or the inferential behavior of the speaker in forming the message to the assumed needs of the listener, and the social organization of the discourse that maintains the dialogue (Roth & Spekman, 1984a). Specific procedures and activities can be used to elicit a variety of communication intentions, examples of presupposition, and the underlying social organization of discourse within a variety of situations. Table 3.1 gives examples of situations that each elicit a variety of language functions.

Intentions or Illocutionary Functions

Illocutionary functions are the intentions of each utterance. Most utterances clearly demonstrate the speaker's intent. For example, ''I would like a cookie, please'' clearly demonstrates a desire or request for some entity. Likewise, ''What time is it?'' demonstrates a desire for information. However, the relationship is not always so obvious. ''What time is it?'' might be used as an excuse. For example, the speaker who does not wish to do something and knows that time is limited might use this utterance to establish the time factor for other people.

Well, I don't know . . ., it's getting late. What time is it? (Reply) Oh, well, I really better be going.

Utterances may also express more than one intention. For example, the speaker might respond to a piece of art with ''What do you call that *thing*?'' Here, the speaker requests information and also makes an evaluation.

TABLE 3.1
Situations with the potential to elicit a variety of language functions

---

Dress-up
Playing house or farm
Dolls, puppets, adventure or action figures
Farm set or street scene
Simulated grocery store, gas station, fast-food restaurant, beauty parlor
Role playing
Playing school
Acting out stories, television shows, movies
Imaginary play
Simulated TV talk show

A number of existing taxonomies of communication intentions can be applied to the language sample. Table 3.2 lists some taxonomies that have been used clinically with child language samples. It is best to determine the range of functions expected for the child's developmental level before organizing activities to try to elicit these intentions. Guidance regarding the intentions expected at certain ages is presented in Table 3.3.

Similar to asking the child to produce a sentence with *has been,* asking the child to form a question about a certain topic or to make a statement out of context may require metalinguistic skills beyond the child's abilities. The following are a broad range of intentions and accompanying activities that may elicit language functions or intentions within a conversational or situational context (Creaghead, 1984; Kunze et al., 1983; Roth & Spekman, 1984b):

Answering/responding.   The speech-language pathologist asks the child a variety of questions while engaged in play (''Where shall we put the houses?'' ''Who is that?'' ''What's in his hand?''). Note the type of question and the response.

Calling/Greeting.   The speech-language pathologist leaves and reenters the situation, role plays people entering and leaving a business, calls on the telephone, or uses dolls, puppets, or action figures to elicit greetings. If she turns away from the child with a favorite toy, the child may also call.

Continuance.   Continuance is turn filling that lets the speaker know that the listener is attending to the conversation. Typical continuants include ''uh-huh,'' ''yeah,'' ''okay,'' and ''right.'' These can be observed throughout the session. The speech-language pathologist notes when the child seems to rely on this function rather than contribute anything new or relevant to the conversation.

Expressing feelings.   The speech-language pathologist models feeling-type responses throughout the play interaction. Dolls, puppets, or action figures are described as having certain feelings and the child is asked to help. For example, she could say, ''Oh, Big Bird is sad. Can you talk to him and make him feel better?''

Hypothesizing.   The speech-language pathologist poses a physical problem for the child, such as ''How can we get everyone to the party on time?'' or ''How can we get Batman out of the cage?'' The child proposes solutions to the problem.

Making choices.   The speech-language pathologist presents the child with alternatives, such as ''I don't know whether you'd rather have a peanut butter sandwich with jelly or fluff.''

Predicting.   In sequential activities, the speech-language pathologist can ponder, ''I wonder what will happen now'' or ''I wonder what we'll do next.''

Protesting.   The speech-language pathologist can elicit protesting by putting away toys or taking away snacks before the child is finished. She can also hand the child something other than what the child requested.

TABLE 3.2
Taxonomies of the illocutionary functions of children

Early Symbolic (Below age 2)	Symbolic (Age 2–7 years)
Dore (1974), Halliday (1975), Owens (1978)	Chapman (1981), Dore (1986), Folger & Chapman (1978)
Requesting action	Requests (for)
	Action
Form: Command, demand	Form: Question, command, embedded command, indirect request, suggestion
	Permission
Regulation	Regulation
Protesting	Protesting
	Rule setting
Requesting information	Requesting information
	Form: Choice (yes/no), product (what, which, who . . .), Process (how, why . . .)
Replying	Replying
Continuants	Acknowledgments
	Qualifications
	Agreements
Comments	Comments
	Assertives
Naming	Identifications
	Descriptions
Personal feelings	Personal feelings
Declarations	Statements
	Reports
	Evaluations
	Attributions
	Explanations
	Hypotheses
	Reasons
	Predictions
	Declarations
	Procedurals
	Choice makings
	Claims
Answers	Answers
	Providing information
	Form: Choice, product process
	Clarification
	Compliance
	Conversational organization
Calling/Greeting	Attention getters
	Speaker selection
	Rhetorical questions
	Clarification questions
	Boundary markers
	Politeness
	Exclamations
Repeating	Repetitions
Practicing	Elicited imitations

As children become older, they add new functions and continue to diversify those they already possess.

TABLE 3.3
Intentions and age of mastery

Within Brown's Stage I (MLU 1.0–1.99) (Usually prior to 24 months)	Answering/Responding Continuance Declaring/Citing Denying Making choices Naming/Labeling Protesting Repeating
Emerging within Brown's Stages II and III (MLU 2.0–3.0) (Usually between 24–36 months)	Calling/Greeting Detailing Predicting Replying Requesting assistance/Directing Requesting clarification Requesting information Requesting objects
After Brown's Stage III (MLU 3.0+) (Usually after 36 months)	Expressing feelings Giving reasons Hypothesizing

Sources: Carpenter & Strong (1988), Owens (1978)

Reasoning.   The speech-language pathologist attempts to solve a problem, such as "I wonder why the boy ran away" or "I wonder what we did wrong."

Repeating.   The speech-language pathologist should note the amount of repetition of self and of the partner. This can take the form of empty comments in a conversation in which the child adds no new information, for example:

> ADULT: Did your class go to the zoo yesterday?
> CHILD: Yeah, zoo.
> ADULT: What did you like best? The monkeys?
> CHILD: Monkeys.
> ADULT: Monkeys are my favorite too. They're so funny.
> CHILD: Monkeys funny.

Replying.   The speech-language pathologist should note occasions when the child responds to the content of what she has said without being required to do so. This behavior is one of the mainstays of conversation as each speaker builds on the comment of the previous speaker.

Reporting.   Reporting can include several functions.

Declaring/citing.   While engaged in an activity, the child spontaneously comments on the present action. The speech-language pathologist models this behavior (''Car goes up the ramp'') but does not attempt to cue a response because declaring/citing is a spontaneous function. She can also engage in unexpected or unusual behavior and await the child's comment.

Detailing.   The speech-language pathologist presents the child with two objects that are of different size or color. If the child takes one and says nothing, the clinician models (''I'll take the little one'' or ''Here's a green truck'') and presents other objects later. The clinician does not attempt to cue a response because detailing is a spontaneous function.

Naming/Labeling.   The speech-language pathologist presents a novel object or points to pictures in a book and remarks, ''Oh, look.'' If the child does not label the object or picture, the speech-language pathologist models the response (''Look. A clown'') and goes on. The child may do so on subsequent exposure to other novel objects. The speech-language pathologist does not cue a response because labeling is a spontaneous function.

Requesting assistance/directing.   The speech-language pathologist presents interesting toys that require adult help to open or use. For example, she can place objects in clear plastic containers or drawstring bags that require help to open, give the child one portion of a toy while keeping the other on a shelf, or let wind-up toys run down. The pathologist makes such comments as ''I wish we could play with this; it would be fun,'' ''Oh, we could use more parts,'' or ''Gee, we need to fix that.'' In another situation, the child helps two puppets or dolls solve a problem in which one will not share a special toy with the other. The speech-language pathologist can also present the child with situations that require a solution, such as taped scissors, pencils with broken points, toys with missing pieces, or paints without brushes. During interactions the speech-language pathologist should note self-directing or self-talk accompanying play. This behavior can be modeled.

Requesting clarification.   This intention can be elicited when the speech-language pathologist mumbles or makes an inaccurate statement.

Requesting information.   Place novel but unknown objects in front of the child. Naming the object correctly is labeling and the speech-language pathologist should confirm. If the child labels incorrectly, the speech-language pathologist says ''No, it's not an X'' or ''No, can you guess what it is?'' The responses ''What's that?'' or ''What?'' and those with rising intonation (''Frog?'') should be considered requests for information.

The speech-language pathologist might also direct the child to use an object not in the situation or not in the expected location. If modeling is required, the speech-language pathologist can ask a question, such as ''Do you have the scissors?'' When the child answers negatively, she can direct the child by saying, ''Ask Sally if she does.''

Requesting objects.   The speech-language pathologist exposes the child to enticing objects or edibles that are just out of reach.

Creaghead (1984) has developed an elicitation protocol that targets several communication intentions and conversational devices within two different structured activities. Table 3.4 outlines the two protocols. The speech-language pathologist uses each protocol as a script to elicit the intentions and devices.

Some intentions are responsive in nature, for example, answering a question or following a directive or request for action. In addition to the child's production level of such requests, it is helpful to know the child's level of response (Roth & Spekman, 1984b).

With responsive functions, the speech-language pathologist must not interpret noncompliance as noncomprehension. The child simply may not want to comply or may choose to ignore the request. The speech-language pathologist first should be certain that the child can perform the behavior requested. The ages at which children comprehend different levels of request are listed in Table 3.5.

It might be helpful for the speech-language pathologist to use two children in an ask-and-tell situation so that each child can act as a model for the other. In a similar manner, the clinician and child can switch roles as questioner (or director) and respondent.

These are just a few suggestions for eliciting a variety of communication intentions. In summary, the speech-language pathologist must consider the type of intentions displayed, their forms, the means of transmission, and the social conventions that affect these means. For example, some situations may call for the use of nonverbal means; others may not.

Presuppositional and Deictic Skills

Whereas intentions are noted at the individual level, other linguistic aspects, such as presupposition and deixis, underlie the entire conversational interaction. *Presupposition* is the speaker's assumption about the knowledge level of the listener and the tailoring of language to that supposed level. *Deixis* is the interpretation of information from the perspective of the speaker. When a speaker says ''Come here,'' this must be interpreted as a point close to the speaker, not as a point with reference to the listener. Deictic terms include, but are not limited to, *here/there, this/that,* and *come/go.*

Presuppositional and deictic skills can be assessed in *referential communication tasks* (Roth & Spekman, 1984b). In referential tasks, one partner describes something or gives directions to the other partner, who is usually on the other side of an opaque barrier or unable to see the speaker (see Figure 3.1). Variations include blindfold games or telephone conversations. As a rule, preschoolers perform better if describing real objects rather than abstract shapes.

TABLE 3.4
Elicitation protocol for communication intentions and conversational devices

Test Procedures—Format 1	Test Procedures—Format 2
As child enters the room—check GREETING	As child leaves the room—check CLOSING
Have cookies and crackers in jar within child's view but out of reach—check REQUEST FOR OBJECT	Give the child and yourself a piece of paper and tell him to draw "mumble"—check REQUEST FOR CLARIFICATION
Hand child the tightly closed jar containing the cookies—check REQUEST FOR ACTION (help opening the jar)	After clarifying, do not give him a crayon—check REQUESTING AN OBJECT
Ask child, "How do you think we can get the jar open?"—check HYPOTHESIZING	Ask the child if he wants a red or blue crayon—check MAKING CHOICES
Say "Do you want "mumble?"—check REQUEST FOR CLARIFICATION	Put on big glasses and then show the child a picture of a person and call it a dog—check COMMENTING ON OBJECT and DENIAL
Ask the child if he wants peanut butter or jelly on his cracker—check MAKING CHOICES	Ask the child "Do you want to play with "mumble"— check REQUEST FOR CLARIFICATION
Hand the child the opposite of what he chose—check DENIAL	Tell the child to get the telephones, which are not in sight—check REQUEST FOR INFORMATION
Put the peanut butter and jelly on the table. Ask the child "What are we going to do now?"—check PREDICTING	Ask the child "What are we going to do?"—check PREDICTING
Tell the child to put peanut butter or jelly on the cracker—check REQUEST FOR OBJECT (knife)	The tester calls the child, then the child calls the tester on the telephone—check GREETING and CLOSING
Tell the child to get the knife, which is not in sight— check REQUEST FOR INFORMATION	Hold a conversation with the child. During this, make a remote-controlled toy move. The toy should be out of the sight of the tester and covered with a cloth—check COMMENT ON ACTION
Put the peanut butter and/or jelly on the cracker and eat it. Get out extra big toothbrush and pretend to brush teeth—check COMMENT ON OBJECT	Ask the child "What happened"—check DESCRIBING EVENT
Hold a conversation with the child. During this, pull invisible string so that rag doll falls off the table—check COMMENT ON ACTION	Ask the child "What do you think is under the cloth?"—check HYPOTHESIZING
Ask the child "What happened?"—check DESCRIBING EVENT	Ask the child "Why did it move?"—check GIVING REASON
Ask the child "Why did it fall?"—check GIVING REASON	Make the toy move briefly—check REQUEST FOR ACTION
During conversation—check ANSWERING, VOLUNTEERING TO COMMUNICATE, ATTENDING TO THE SPEAKER, TAKING TURNS, ACKNOWLEDGING, SPECIFYING A TOPIC, CHANGING A TOPIC, MAINTAINING A TOPIC, GIVING EXPANDED ANSWERS	During conversation—check ANSWERING, VOLUNTEERING TO COMMUNICATE, ATTENDING TO THE SPEAKER, TAKING TURNS, ACKNOWLEDGING, SPECIFYING A TOPIC, CHANGING TOPIC, MAINTAINING A TOPIC, GIVING EXPANDED ANSWERS
Stop leading the conversation and be silent—check ASKING CONVERSATIONAL QUESTIONS	Stop leading conversation and remain silent—check ASKING CONVERSATIONAL QUESTIONS
Request clarification—check CLARIFYING	

Note: These protocols may be used as suggested scripts for efficient elicitation of several communication intentions and conversational devices.
Source: Creaghead, N. (1984). Strategies for evaluating and targeting pragmatic behaviors in young children. *Seminars in Speech and Language, 5,* 241–251. Reprinted with permission.

TABLE 3.5
Age and comprehension of requests

Age in years	Comprehension
2	I need a ____ .
	Give me a ____ .
3	Could you give me a ____?
	May I have a ____?
	Have you got a ____?
4	He hurt me. (Hint)
	The ____ is all gone. (Hint)
4 1/2	Begin to comprehend indirect requests: Why don't you ____ or
	Don't forget to ____ . Mastery takes several years.
5	Inferred requests in which the goal is totally masked are now
	comprehended. In this example, the speaker desires some juice:
	Now you make breakfast like you're the mommy.

Source: Adapted from Ervin-Tripp, S. (1977). Wait for me roller skate. In S. Ervin-Tripp & C. Mitchell-Kernan (Eds.), *Child Discourse.* New York: Academic Press.

In these tasks, the speech-language pathologist must be alert to the use of direct/indirect reference. In direct reference, the speaker considers the audience and clearly identifies the entity being mentioned. Indirect reference typically follows direct reference and refers to entities through the use of pronouns or such terms as *that one*. The child with poor presuppositional skills may use indirect reference without prior direct reference.

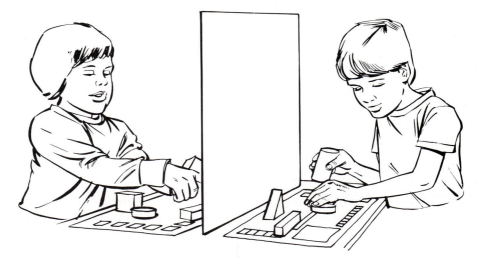

FIGURE 3.1
Barrier tasks

Additional presuppositional information can be gathered by varying the roles, topics, partners, and communication channels available in the sampling situation. Roles can be varied so the child has an opportunity to act as listener and speaker. Assessment of both roles is essential. For example, the LLD child will generally ask few questions for clarification, even when there is little understanding of what has been said. As speakers, these children make limited use of descriptors, provide very little specific information, and are less effective than non-LLD children.

The choice of topics can also influence presuppositional behavior and provide for a variety of role taking. Children can be asked to describe events about which the speech-language pathologist or partner is ignorant (e.g., a family outing). In this situation, the child must determine the amount of information necessary for the listener to understand the topic. The partner who asks the child to explain something that the partner already understands violates the principle that communication should make sense. There is no sense in explaining something that someone already understands.

As the number of communication channels decreases, the speaker is forced to rely more heavily on the remaining ones. For example, the use of a telephone requires the speaker to rely almost exclusively on the verbal communication channel. This situation is a challenge even for the nonimpaired language user. Imagine how difficult it would be to teach someone over the phone to tie a shoelace.

The use and nonuse of barriers will permit such verbal-only and verbal-plus communication. If the listener provides no feedback in verbal-only communication, the speaker must take an extremely active role in the conversation. In addition, barrier activities require listeners to adapt the speaker's perspective.

Several other activities can be used to elicit presuppositional skills. Of interest is whether the child can encode the most informative or uncertain elements in a situation. In general, human beings tend to comment on entities and events that are new, changing, or unexpected. In the sampling situation, novel items can be introduced into repetitive activities. The clinician must attend to the child's behavior to see if the child refers to the novel stimulus.

I know of one clinic where a kitten is abruptly introduced into the sampling situation. The clinician says nothing but waits to see if the child will comment and in what manner.

In general, young language-impaired children encode novel information less frequently than do nonimpaired children. Older school-aged, language-impaired children tend to use more pronouns with less identification of the referent than do nonimpaired children.

Pictures or objects, identical except for one element, can also be used. The child can be asked to explain how the two differ. Hide-and-seek with objects can be used to assess comprehension and expression of deictic terms as the clinician and child direct each other to find the objects.

Games and stories can be used to elicit indirect/direct reference. For example, a story can be told and then questions asked to elicit indefinite and definite articles and/or nouns and pronouns. The child can also retell a story to a second child who has not heard it. Any portion of extended discourse, such as describing a movie, explaining how to accomplish a task, or telling a story, will be valuable clinical data (Roth & Spekman, 1984b).

The clinician is interested in the lexical items used and also in the ambiguity of the referent. Of interest is the number of times the child mentions the referent by name or by the use of pronouns. Some children overuse the referent name, whereas others rely on the pronoun without sufficient return to the referent name to avoid confusion.

Finally, role-playing activities with very specific situations can also be helpful. The child in the following situation faces very definite behavioral constraints.

> Imagine that you and a friend are trying to find a drinking fountain. You see a man coming down the street. While your friend remains seated on a park bench, you try to find out about the fountain. I'll be the man. What would you say? (Child responds.) Now, I'm your friend. What would you tell me?

Discourse Organization

Discourse has internal organization. For example, a telephone conversation has a recognizable pattern, as does the telling of a personal event. The social organization of discourse can be assessed within familiar activities that provide a scaffolding for dialogue (Roth & Spekman, 1984b). The clinician may be interested in the amount of social and nonsocial speech. For example, preschool children frequently engage in nonsocial monologues in play, in contrast to older children, who participate more in dialogues or in social monologues. This change signals a growing awareness of the social nature of speech and language use. With the retarded, acquisition of conversational rules is more closely related to social-experiential factors, such as chronological age, than to expressive language ability as measured by average utterance length (Leifer & Lewis, 1984).

The speech-language pathologist can provide opportunities for the child to initiate conversation, to take turns, and to repair in response to self-feedback or the feedback of others in different situations. By failing to respond to the child or by responding inappropriately, mumbling, failing to establish a referent, or providing insufficient information, the speech-language pathologist may elicit contingent queries or requests for clarification from the child.

RECORDING THE SAMPLE

There is no ideal length for a conversational sample. Length varies with the purpose of collection (Bloom & Lahey, 1978; Crystal, Fletcher, & Garman, 1978; Lee, 1974). For example, a 50-utterance sample may be adequate for lexical evaluation because it will contain 73% to 83% of the lexical information found in a 100-utterance sample (Cole, Mills, & Dale, 1989).

Given the constraints of the clinical sample, 50 or 100 child utterances are considered adequate, providing there is some variety of setting, partners, tasks, or topics and that other data collection methods are used. At least two different samples should be included (Cole et al., 1989).

Occasionally, children fall into repetitive patterns of responding, such as naming pictures in a book. This kind of activity provides very little variation in the child's behavior. It is best either to limit this type of interaction or not use it for analysis. If, on the other hand, the child frequently exhibits perseverative or stereotypic patterns, they should be recorded for analysis, saved for supporting data, or commented on in the assessment report.

The sample is permanently recorded using videotape, audiotape, event transcription, or a combination of these (Roth & Spekman, 1984b). Taping is essential because the interaction must be repeatedly reviewed for information.

Although videotaping can be intrusive and expensive, especially the initial equipment purchase, it yields the best data for describing the verbal and nonverbal behaviors observed. The alternatives to videotaping are not as reliable, thus increasing the variability in the behavior recorded. Even if videotape is used, the speech-language pathologist may find a simultaneous audiotape helpful for transcribing the speech and language portion. The following recording methods are listed in order of decreasing desirability:

1. Simultaneous videotaping and audiotaping
2. Simultaneous audiotaping with pathologist descriptions of non-linguistic behaviors recorded in one and the linguistic interaction in the other.
3. Simultaneous audiotaping and written data recording on time sheets (see Table 3.6). Having more than one observer may help ensure that no behaviors are overlooked and may increase the reliability of description of those that are observed. Writing data as the interaction progresses is extremely tedious but necessary.

It is important that data collection methods begin at the same time for later transcription. This should be accomplished as unobtrusively as possible. A cough or some similar signal can alert observers that recording has begun.

TRANSCRIBING THE SAMPLE

The conversational sample is transcribed as soon after recording as possible. This ensures that the speech-language pathologist brings to the task as much memory of the situation as possible.

The format of the transcript varies with the purpose of the assessment. For example, there is little need to transcribe the partner's utterances if the speech-language pathologist is interested only in phonological analysis. For most other purposes, however, the type of format shown in Table 3.7 is suggested.

TABLE 3.6
Time form for recording the nonlinguistic context

			Minute _____
Time (sec.)	Child's Behavior	Partner's Behavior	Other
0			
.			
.			
.			
10			
.	Looks at partner		
.	Points to truck		
20			
.	Reaches for truck		
.		Hands truck	
30			
.			
.	Pushes car		
40	Looks at partner		
.	Points to gas station		
.			
.		Moves car to gas station	
50		Moves car to gas station	
.			
.			
.			
60			

The speech-language pathologist transcribes the linguistic behavior of both the child and the conversational partner along with the nonlinguistic behaviors of each. Phonetic transcription can be used if there is concern about use of phonological rules. The timesheet format enables the speech-language pathologist to evaluate delays or latencies on the part of the child.

All of the child's utterances, including false starts, nonfluencies, and fillers, are transcribed. Although these linguistic elements may not be used for calcula-

TABLE 3.7
Transcription format

			Minute _____
Time (sec)	Child's Utterances	Partner's Utterances	Nonlinguistic
0			
.		What do you need now?	
.			
10			
.	Can I have the truck?		C. looks at partner
.			C. points to truck
.			
20		Which one?	
.	That one.		
.		Oh, the red one.	C. reaches for truck
.		Okay.	P. hands truck
30		Now can we go on vacation?	
.	Bro-o-om		C. pushes car
40	We need gas first.		C. looks at partner
.			C. points to gas station
.		Well, then...	P. moves car to gas station
50		I'll drive my car over, too.	C. moves car to gas station.
.		What else do we need?	
60	Gotta get soda and chips.		

tion of average or mean utterance length, they are extremely important in determining language and communication difficulties.

All utterances of the conversational partner(s) are also transcribed. These are important in assessing the manner and style of the conversational partners. The speech-language pathologist is interested in the amount of control and the amount of talking exhibited by the partner.

Determining utterance boundaries is often difficult. This is not an exact science, and the artistry of the speech-language pathologist is needed at this point.

An utterance is a complete thought that is divided from other utterances by sentence boundaries, pauses, and/or a drop in the voice. Table 3.8 contains examples of utterance boundaries.

Declaring sentences to be utterances is easy. Most of what is said, however, is not in complete sentence form. For example, the response to a question often omits shared information and might consist of such responses as ''No,'' ''Cookie,'' and ''Okay.'' Each of these is a complete utterance. Longer responses, such as ''No, later'' or ''No, let's go later,'' are also single utterances. This might change if the child were to respond with a pause and drop in the voice

TABLE 3.8
Utterance boundaries

A sentence is an utterance.
  Mommy went to the doctor's tomor . . . yesterday.

Run-on sentences with *and* should contain no more than one *and* joining clauses.
  We went in a bus and we saw monkeys and we had a picnic and we petted the sheeps and one sheep sneezed on me and we had sodas and we came home.

  Utterances:
  1. We went in a bus and we saw monkeys.
  2. (And) we had a picnic and we petted the sheeps.
  3. (And) one sheep sneezed on me and we had sodas.
  4. (And) we came home.

  Other complex or compound sentences should be treated as one utterance.
  He was mad because his mommy spanked him because he broke the lamp and spilled the doggie's water.

Imperative sentences are utterances.
  Go home.

Pauses, voice drops, and/or inhalations mark boundaries.
  Eat (pause and voice drop) . . . chocolate candy.
    Two utterances: Eat. Chocolate candy.
  Eat (momentary delay) . . . chocolate candy.
    One utterance: Eat chocolate candy.

Situational and nonlinguistic cues help to determine boundaries.
  Eat (hands plate to partner insistently) . . . chocolate candy (points to candy dish).
    Two utterances: Eat. Chocolate candy.
  Want (reaches unsuccessfully) . . . mommy (turns to look).
    Two utterances: Want. Mommy.
  Want mommy (reaches unsuccessfully).
    One utterance: Want, mommy.

The linguistic context also helps.
  Partner: Well, what do you want?
  Child: Candy (pause) . . . you get it.
    Two utterances: Candy. You get it.

after ''No.'' ''No (pause and drop voice). Let's go later.'' Now there are two utterances.

Partial sentences or phrases, nonfluent units, and run-on sentences are
even more difficult. A partial sentence might consist of the child pointing to an
object and saying ''Doggie.'' This would count as an utterance. In the following
exchange, the child makes an internal repair:

> PARTNER: I like to play mommy.
> CHILD: No, you not . . . me the . . . you baby.

The entire unit is an utterance and will be analyzed in different ways using all or
part of what the child said.

For run-on sentences, the speech-language pathologist can follow the general rule that allows two clauses to be joined together in a sentence. In the following example, sentence/utterance boundaries have been marked as they might be
on a transcript:

> [I went to the party, and we ate pizza] [(and) We played games, and I won a prize]
> [(and) We had cake and ice cream.]

Division can be aided by the child's pauses and breath patterns. Children in the
late preschool years often make long strings of clauses with *and* meaning *and then*.
Counting these as a single utterance inflates the mean utterance length. Once the
sample is transcribed, it can be analyzed.

CONCLUSION

Collecting a representative language sample that demonstrates the child's diverse abilities is a difficult task. Careful planning and execution are required, as
are exacting methods of recording and transcription. Although these procedures
may seem difficult and time-consuming initially, they can be accomplished easily
and relatively quickly with practice. A properly planned and executed sampling
and a thorough transcription will yield an abundance of linguistic and nonlinguistic information.

Guides for collecting a language sample include the following:

☐ Establish a positive relationship with the child before recording the language sample.

☐ Reduce your authority figure persona to ensure more participation by
the child. A child is more likely to respond naturally with someone who
is an equal.

☐ Be unobtrusive while collecting the sample so that the child is less conscious of the process.

☐ The conversational partner should keep talking to a minimum. Although clinicians abhor a vacuum, when possible they should wait out
the child.

☐ Avoid yes/no questions and constituent questions that require only a one-word response from the child. Ask process rather than product questions.

☐ Follow the child's lead in play and in the selection of topic. Determine the child's interests before beginning the collection process. Select those materials at the child's interest level that are likely to stimulate interest.

☐ If the child does not talk or responds in a very repetitive or stereotypic manner, model reponses for the child or have another person model.

Only through sampling the child's linguistic abilities in a conversational context can the speech-language pathologist gain insight into how the child's language works for the child. This is the first step in designing intervention that is relevant to the child and thus more likely to generalize.

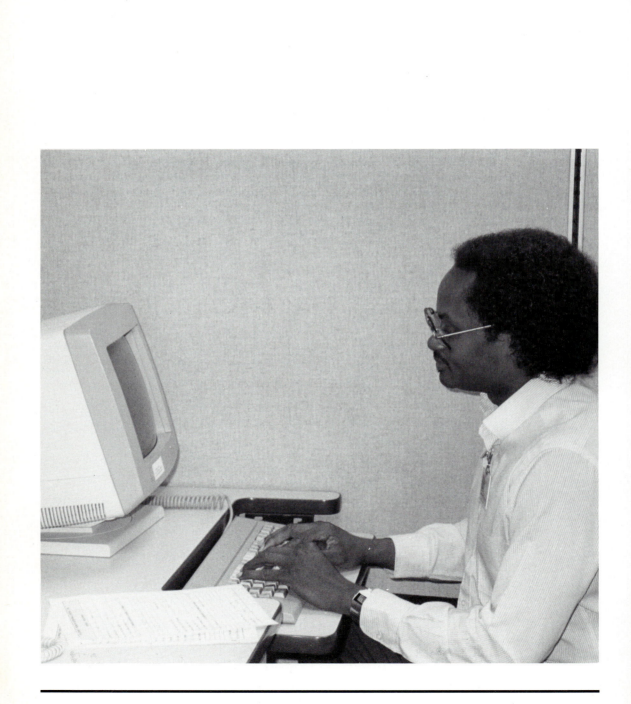

TABLE 4.1
Analysis at th

4

Analyzing a Language Sample at the Utterance Level

Language is a complex symbol system, and the analysis methods used with a conversational sample reflect this complexity. For this reason, analysis of a language sample should not be a fishing expedition for possible problems. Language analysis is best used to explore certain aspects of the child's behavior brought into question through other data collection methods. If a language disorder exists, it can be confirmed by descriptive analysis of a sample of the unique language pattern of the language-impaired child.

Typical or traditional language sample analysis has concentrated almost exclusively on language form. This limited analysis may miss many very important aspects of language and language use in conversation. Language must be appropriate for the listener and for the context; it must be polite enough but not too polite; and it must provide sufficient information, be relevant, and be sufficiently truthful (Grice, 1975). In addition, language must incorporate the rules for discourse, such as initiating, maintaining, and closing a conversation; establishing, maintaining, and changing a topic; using appropriate register; and signaling pragmatic information with syntactic forms.

Traditional analysis has focused exclusively on the utterance or sentence as the unit of analysis. Although this type of analysis is appropriate for many language features, it may not be the best way to assess behaviors that transcend these units. For example, an analysis of a child's use of pronouns necessitates crossing utterance boundaries in order to describe the child's introduction of new information and reference to old or established information, which may have been introduced by the child or the conversational partner.

utterance level   Illocutionary functions or intentions
                      Frequency, range, and appropriateness
                  Form
                      Quantitative measures: MLU (mean length of utterance), T-units
                      Morphological analysis of selected morphemes
                      Syntactic analysis
                          Noun phrase
                          Verb phrase
                          Sentence types
                          Embedding and conjoining
                      Phonological analysis
                          Word and phoneme level
                  Content
                      Lexical
                          Type-token ratio
                          Over- and underextensions
                          Word relationships
                          Semantic categories
                      Intrasentential relations
                      Figurative language

This chapter considers the analysis of language that can be easily accomplished within utterances, noting significant aspects of use, form, and content. These aspects are outlined in Table 4.1. Chapter 5 discusses analysis across utterances and partners and by conversational event. This three-tiered analysis method seems appropriate for describing the interactive qualities of language use within the context of conversation.

Each utterance can be analyzed within use, form, and content categories following a variety of analysis formats (Johnson et al., 1984; Lund & Duchan, 1988). Individual utterances can yield the frequency and range of various features. Some data will be descriptive, whereas other data will be more normative. This situation reflects the research information available and the type of analysis desired.

ILLOCUTIONARY FUNCTIONS OR INTENTIONS

At the individual utterance level, pragmatic analysis is limited to a description of the illocutionary functions or intentions expressed and understood. The frequency and range of these intentions can be described and compared to those of other children at the same age. The appropriateness and form of these intentions are also of interest. Although there is little normative data on the sophistication of intention form, each intention can be analyzed for its form and means of transmission.

Very little normative data are available on the frequency and range of intentions (Roth & Spekman, 1984a). This reflects the contextual variability of intentions and the lack of agreement by professionals on the intentions expressed at various ages. Intentions are heavily influenced by and heavily influence the conversational context.

Frequency and Range

A number of taxonomies of illocutionary functions are available, reflecting different ages and contextual situations (Chapman, 1981; Dore, 1974, 1976; Owens, 1978; Prutting, Bagshaw, Goldstein, Juskowitz, & Umen, 1978; Rodgon, Jankowski, & Alenskas, 1977). Tables 3.2 and 3.3 attempt to equate these functions and to demonstrate possible changes over time. The speech-language pathologist may wish to develop a taxonomy based on one or a combination of the taxonomies presented.

The range of intentions changes with age, becoming wider and more complex with increasing age. In addition, with maturity, the child may express multiple intentions within a single utterance. Thus, the more mature speaker's ability to express different functions is more flexible. With maturity, the speaker discusses more emotions and feelings, includes such phrases as ''I think . . .'', and provides justifications.

After selecting the most comfortable taxonomy or combination of taxonomies, the speech-language pathologist rates each utterance of the child and conversational partner for the intentions expressed. The normative data available, although only limited, do demonstrate that within a conversation partners use a wide range of intentions; no intention predominates unless warranted by the situation. The nonimpaired child will initiate conversation and reply to the initiations of the partner, seek information and provide it, ask for assistance, and volunteer information. In contrast, some children, such as those with autism, may initiate communication only rarely and respond with minimal replies (Loveland, Landry, Hughes, Hall, & McEvoy, 1988).

Occasionally, adults or children fall into perseverative patterns of communicating, for example, the parent who constantly quizzes her child to name the pictures in a book or the child who keeps repeating a pleasing or tantrum phrase. Perseverative behavior can skew the data and allow one type of intention, such as answers, to predominate. These patterns should be noted during conversational sample collection, and the situations gently changed. The use of different situations and different partners may ensure a better distribution of intentions.

Some children, such as the incessant questioner, use only a limited range of illocutionary functions. If this behavior persists across a number of situations and partners, the speech-language pathologist can be reasonably certain that this narrow range of functions represents the child's typical behavior. As suggested in Chapter 3, a number of situations can be used in an attempt to elicit a variety of illocutionary functions.

Appropriateness

A very narrow intentional range may indicate inappropriate use of language. Although some contexts may require the almost exclusive use of one type of function, most conversational exchanges include a wide variety of intentions. The question of appropriateness must be judged against other factors, such as age, race or ethnicity, region of the country, socioeconomic status, gender, and most important, the communication context.

The language sample can confirm the caregiver's observation that "John seems to ask questions all of the time, even when he knows the answers." Although the observation may not be unfounded, only data from the language sample can offer concrete proof.

The child who responds inappropriately may not know the linguistic context and may need more contextual cues. For example, language-impaired children have more difficulty responding to *wh-* questions than do nonimpaired children (Parnell, Amerman, & Harting, 1986). These children have more difficulty with both the accuracy of their answers and the functional appropriateness. Analysis of both of these types of errors is discussed in the section on contingency in Chapter 5. In general, language-impaired children fail to recognize the request for information inherent in questions. Even relatively simple *What + be* questions are difficult when they concern nonimmediate or noncontextual referential sources. Thus, analysis of the context within which *wh-* questions are asked is as important diagnostically as is the analysis of the variety of *wh-* questions produced and comprehended.

Encoding

Intentions can also be analyzed using a means of transmission format, such as verbal/vocal/nonverbal (Roth & Spekman, 1984a). The transition from linguistic through paralinguistic to nonlinguistic can be used to describe a hierarchy of competency or effectiveness based on the child's developmental level. The nonlinguistic context and behaviors of the conversational partners must be transcribed to make this information available.

In general, the child with poor linguistic skills will rely on other means of communicating intentions. Although some very sophisticated information can be communicated nonlinguistically, as in the popularly named *pregnant pause,* less mature language users tend to depend on nonlinguistic and paralinguistic means more than do mature users. As with the various intentions expressed, there should be a range of transmission means exhibited by the child and partner.

If the child uses an augmentative form of communication, that form should be specified even more and might include physical manipulation of object, physical manipulation of partner, gestures, and sign or other augmentative device. Two children described as nonverbal may have very different means of communicating their intentions.

FORM

Language form includes syntax, morphology, and phonology or the means used to encode the intentions of the speaker. Even though most language analysis methods concentrate on this aspect of language, very little normative data are available. The task is partially normative and partially descriptive, involving both quantitative and qualitative analysis.

Quantitative Measures

Quantitative measures include mean length of utterance (MLU), T-units, type-token ratios, and the density of sentence forms. The last measure is discussed under syntactic analysis.

Mean Length of Utterance

Mean length of utterance is the average length in morphemes of the speaker's utterances. Up to an average of 4.0, some linguists believe MLU to be a good measure of language complexity available. Not all linguists agree (Crystal, Fletcher, & Garman, 1976; Johnston & Kamhi, 1984; Klee & Fitzgerald, 1985). In general, there is less variability in MLU below 4.0 (Rondal, Ghiotto, Bredart, & Bachelet, 1987). This mean is reached by the nonimpaired child at around age 4½. At lower MLUs, new structures added to the child's utterances increase the complexity of those sentences. After this level of development, much of the growth in complexity is the result of internal reorganization of utterance form rather than addition of new structures. This explanation of the relationship between length and complexity is extremely simplified, and there are many related factors.

In order to calculate MLU, the speech-language pathologist divides the language sample into utterances. It is best not to include in analysis the portions of conversation that occurred while the child was adjusting to the partner or to the situation. Determination of utterance boundaries is discussed in Chapter 3. The number of morphemes in each utterance is counted and totalled for the entire sample. Rules for counting morphemes, based on the order of development with nonimpaired children, are included in Table 4.2. Brief rationales for these rules are included where appropriate.

The total number of morphemes is divided by the number of utterances from which it was derived to determine the MLU. This value can then be compared to the age data in Table 4.3. It is obvious from this table that a wide variability and a wide range of ages are considered within the normal range. Even so, the need to collect a typical sample is very important. If data have been collected in two or more settings, the MLUs from each can be compared to assess the stability of the overall data.

Although age and MLU are correlated as shown in Table 4.3, some interesting data suggest cautious acceptance of this correlation. First, the relationship of

TABLE 4.2

Rules for counting morphemes relative to preschool and school-age children

Structure	Example	Count		Rationale
		Psch.	Sch.	
Each recurrence of a word for emphasis	No, no, no.	1 each	1 each	
Compound words (2 or more free morphemes)	Railroad, birthday	1	2+	Compound words learned as a unit by preschoolers
Proper names	Bugs Bunny, Uncle Fred	1	2+	Proper names, even those with titles, learned as a unit by preschoolers
Ritualized reduplications	Choo-choo, Night-night	1	1	
Irregular past tense verbs	Went, ate, got, came	1	2	Verb tense learned as new word by preschoolers, not as *verb* + *ed*.
Diminutives	Doggie, horsie	1	2	Phonological form CVCV easier than CVC for preschoolers and does not denote smallness
Auxiliary verbs and catenatives	Is, have, do; gonna, wanna, gotta	1	1+	Preschoolers do not know that such words as *gonna* are *going to*
Contracted negatives	Don't, can't, won't	1–2	2	Because negatives *don't, can't, and won't* develop before *do, can,* and *will,* count as one until the positive form appears. Then count the negative forms as two morphemes.
Possessive marker (-'_s_)	Tom's, mom's	1	1	
Plural marker (-_s_)	Cats, dogs	1	1	
Third-person singular present tense marker (-_s_)	Walks, eats	1	1	
Regular past tense marker (-_ed_)	Walked, jumped	1	1	
Present progressive marker (-_ing_)	Walking, eating	1	1	
Dysfluencies	C-c-candy, b-b-baby	1+	1+	*Count only the final complete form.
Fillers	Um-m, ah-h	0	0	

*In the example "I want can . . . I want can . . . I want candy," only the last full production is counted, being 3 morphemes.

TABLE 4.3
Age and mean length of utterance relationship

Age in months	MLU	x̄ Range
18	1.1	1.0–1.2
21	1.6	1.1–1.8
24	1.9	1.6–2.2
27	2.1	1.9–2.3
30	2.5	2.4–2.6
33	2.8	2.7–2.9
36	3.1	3.0–3.3
39	3.3	3.2–3.5
42	3.6	3.3–3.9
45	3.8	3.4–4.3
48	3.9	3.6–4.7
51	4.1	3.7–5.1
54	4.2	3.8–5.4
57	4.3	3.9–5.8
60	4.4	4.0–6.0

Sources: Klee, Schaffer, May, Membrino, & Mougey (1989), Miller (1981), Scarborough, Wyckoff, & Davidson (1986), Wells (1985).

rate of MLU and age change is not a constant, as seen in Table 4.3. Second, language impairments are not necessarily evidenced by delays in MLU as might be expected (Klee, Schaffer, May, Membrino, & Mougey, 1989).

T-units
Expressive language syntax of older children can be measured in T-units (minimal terminal units) (Hunt, 1970) consisting of one main clause plus any attached or embedded subordinate clause or nonclausal structure. Thus, the unit has shifted from the utterance to the sentence. For example, the sentences ''I want ice cream'' and ''I want the one that is hidden in the blue box'' constitute T-units with varying numbers of words and clauses. The T-unit is more sensitive than MLU to the types of language differences seen after age 5, such as phrasal embedding and various types of subordinate clauses (O'Donnell, Griffin, & Norris, 1967).

Children's language can then be described in words per T-unit, clauses per T-unit, and words per clause. There is a gradual and progressive increase in words and clauses per T-unit and in words per clause in spontaneous speech with increased age through childhood and adolescence, although the values change only gradually during early school years (Klecan-Aker, 1985):

Units	Age 6	Age 9
Words/T-unit	9.03	10.15
Clauses/T-unit	1.26	1.31
Words/clause	7.14	7.75

To calculate these values, the speech-language pathologist divides the sample into sentences, each equaling one T-unit. The number of words and clauses can then be determined for each and divided by the number of T-units to calculate an average. The words per clause can be similarly determined.

Syntactic and Morphologic Analysis

Many disordered populations experience difficulty with syntax and morphology. For example, children who are mildly-to-moderately behaviorally disordered seem to have word-order difficulties (Camarata, Hughes, & Ruhl, 1988).

A number of computer-assisted and unassisted analysis methods are available for syntax and morphology (Miller & Chapman, 1985; Crystal, Fletcher, & Garman, 1978; Lee, 1974; Lund & Duchan, 1988; Miller, 1981; Tyack & Gottsleben, 1977). Although each method yields different data, none presents a total picture of a child's language. In general, the more normative the results, the less descriptive and prescriptive, and vice versa. Each analysis method is described in Appendix D. A generic analysis method might borrow useful portions from several of these.

It should be noted that some utterances defy analysis, such as those containing contrasting stress used to negate. For example, one speaker might say, "Penny went," only to be corrected by the other speaker with "*Mary* went." At a syntactic level, these two sentences would appear to be similar.

Morphological Analysis

The speech-language pathologist is interested in intraword development as well as in sentence development. With preschool children, she will want to analyze Brown's 14 morphemes as suggested by Miller (1981). These are listed in Table 4.4. Other morphemes, such as pronouns, may also be of interest. Older children may use a variety of morphological prefixes and suffixes. A list of the more common prefixes and suffixes is included in Appendix E.

Correct usage of Brown's 14 grammatical morphemes can be a clinical aid for establishing the developmental stage of preschool children (Miller, 1981). Table 4.4 lists the morphemes by stage of mastery, the stage in which each morpheme is produced correctly by children in 90% of the obligatory contexts.

The percent correct value is determined by dividing the number of correct appearances by the total number of obligatory contexts. In obligatory contexts, the child might use the morpheme correctly, make an error substitution, or omit the morpheme. Table 4.5 presents selected portions of a language sample and the calculation of percent correct for the regular plural marker.

The percent correct yields only limited data. More descriptive information can be gained. For example, the clinician who calculated only the percent correct for past tense *-ed* still would not know if errors were related to nonuse of *-ed* where required or to use of *-ed* on irregular past tense verbs. The pronoun error analysis format in Table 4.6 offers guidance for analysis with other forms.

After calculating percent correct, the speech-language pathologist can at-

TABLE 4.4
Brown's fourteen morphemes by stage of mastery

Stage of Mastery	Morpheme	Example	Age Range of Mastery* (in months)
II	Present progressive -ing, (no auxiliary verb)	Mommy driving.	19–28
	In	Ball in cup.	27–30
	On	Doggie on sofa.	27–30
	Regular plural -s	Kitties eat my ice cream.	24–33
		Forms: /s/, /z/, and /Iz/	
		Cats (/kæts/)	
		Dogs (/dↄgz/)	
		Classes (/klæsIz/), wishes (/wIʃIz/)	
III	Irregular past	Came, fell, broke, sat, went	25–46
	Possessive 's	Mommy's balloon broke.	26–40
		Forms: /s/, /z/, and /Iz/ as in regular plural	
IV	Uncontractible copula (verb to be as main verb)	He is. (response to "Who's sick?")	27–39
	Articles	I see a kitty.	28–46
		I throw the ball to daddy.	
	Regular past -ed	Mommy pulled the wagon.	26–48
		Forms: /d/, /t/, and /Id/	
		Pulled (/pʊld/)	
		Walked (/wↄkt/)	
		Glided (/glaIdId/)	
	Regular third person -s	Kathy hits.	
		Forms: /s/, /z/, and /Iz/ as in regular plural	
V+	Irregular third person	Does, has	28–50
	Uncontractible auxiliary	He is. (response to "Who's wearing your hat?")	29–48
	Contractible copula	Man's big.	29–49
		Man is big.	
	Contractible auxiliary	Daddy's drinking juice.	30–50
		Daddy is drinking juice.	

*Used correctly 90% of the time in obligatory contexts. Adapted from Bellugi (1964), R. Brown (1973), and Miller (1981).

tempt to describe the child's stage of language development. This is not an exact science. Rarely is the determination clear-cut or is one and only one stage identified.

Morphological markers are applied to word classes. For example, the past tense -ed marker is confined to verbs. Therefore, the speech-language pathologist should also note word classes in which errors occur. Occasionally, errors are con-

TABLE 4.5
Calculating percent correct for plural

Utterance	Correct	Incorrect	Type of Error
2. Want more cookies.	x		
3. Three cookie.		x	Not marked
4. No, one big cookies.		x	Marked singular
22. Dogs.	x		
27. Give the pencils to me.	x		
28. I want two pencils.	x		
31. You color the foots.		x	Marked irregular
40. What blue crayons?	x		
TOTAL	5	3	

$$\text{Percent correct} = \frac{\text{Total of correct}}{\text{Total of correct} + \text{incorrect}} = \frac{5}{8} = 62.5\%$$

fined to only one word class, such as verbs. Nouns would be affected by such markers as plural regular and irregular, possessive, and articles. Verb markers include third person singular, past tense regular and irregular, present progressive, modals, *do* + verb, copula (*am, are, is, was, were*), and perfective (*have* + *be* + verb). Finally, adjective and adverb markers include, but are not limited to, comparative and superlative and adverbial *-ly*.

The speech-language pathologist should be mindful of phonological rules regarding these morphemes and their location in words and of dialectal and bilingual variations. Even though a child omits a morphological ending, it cannot be assumed that the child does not understand or is not able to produce the morpheme. For example, children who speak Black English may omit some word endings for phonological reasons. Others may be omitted because they are redundant, such as the plural *-s* when the noun is preceded by a number as in *ten cent*. The bidialectal or bilingual child's abilities must be established by testing of both the marker and the concept associated with it.

The only standard for comparison of children's performance is the communication community of each child. A child's language is disordered to the extent that he or she is unable to communicate effectively in that community. Two errors that occur in language assessment are (a) mistaking dialectal variations for disorders, and (b) overlooking disorders mistakenly assumed to be dialectal variations. In general, dialectal variations develop by age 5 with few noticeable at age 3 (Battles, 1990).

Pronouns offer a special case of morphological analysis because of the complex nature of the underlying semantic and pragmatic functions. If the child's strategy is "when in doubt, use the noun," then it will be difficult to find errors in pronoun substitution (Haas & Owens, 1985). More in-depth analysis is required, possibly similar to that presented in Table 4.6. The types of errors made reveal the underlying rules that the child is using. Pronouns are discussed in more detail in Chapter 5 in the section concerning analysis across utterances and partners.

Syntactic Analysis

Analysis is also accomplished at the intraclausal and clausal levels. For this type of analysis it is best to exclude imitations, short answers to questions, and stereotypic or rote responses because these types of utterances are not usually clinically significant.

For analysis purposes, it is helpful to separate sentences and nonsentences. Sentences are grouped as declarative, negative declarative, imperative, negative imperative, interrogative, and negative interrogative. Sentences can then be grouped for further analysis by length or structure. For example, declarative sentences can be categorized as subject-verb, subject-verb-object, subject-verb-complement, and multiple clauses, either embedded or conjoined. The form of the child's sentences can be compared to some normative data, such as that in Table 4.7, to best determine the child's stage of development, although descriptive data are also valuable. The speech-language pathologist should note intrasentential noun and verb phrase development, sentence types, and embedding and conjoining.

The speech-language pathologist can use Table 4.7 in a comparative fashion. For example, let's assume that the child said, ''I want a big doggie.'' The noun phrase *a big doggie* has been expanded by the addition of an article and an adjective. This noun phrase occurs in the object position of the sentence. Expansion of the noun phrase in the object position is an example of structure occuring at Stage II and above, according to the intrasentential column of Table 4.7. The verb phrase is unelaborated as is the subject noun phrase. These represent structures at the Stage I level or above. No analysis is required for negative, interrogative, embedding, or conjoining with this example.

Noun phrase.   Noun phrase elaboration is assessed by describing the number and variety of noun phrase elements. The order of the elements within the noun phrase is relatively fixed, although the order of development is not so definite. The noun function is obligatory, and the other modifiers are nonobligatory. In order of mention within the noun phrase, the elements are initiator(s), determiner(s), adjectival(s), noun, and post-noun modifier(s) (Crystal et al., 1978; Dever, 1978). Some or all of these elements may be present in the noun phrase, as shown in Table 4.8. Some elements may be used in combination, whereas the use of others is more exclusive.

Initiators consist of a small core of words that limit or quantify the following phrase. Examples include *only, a few of,* and *merely.* Most of these words can also serve as adverbs. The speech-language pathologist must be careful to identify the accompanying noun phrase.

Determiners come in many varieties and include, in order of mention, quan-

TABLE 4.6
Possible pronoun analysis method

Stage	Pronoun	Correct	Incorrect	Total	Percent Correct	Substitution				Omission	Ambiguous Referent	Overuse of Nominal
						Case	Gender	Person	Number			
I (MLU: 1.0–2.0)	I											
	me											
II (MLU: 2.0–2.5)	my											
	it (subj.)											
	t (obj.)											
III (MLU: 2.5–3.0)	you (subj.)i											
	your											
	she											
	them											
	he											
	we											
	her (poss.)											

Sub-analysis of Incorrect Responses

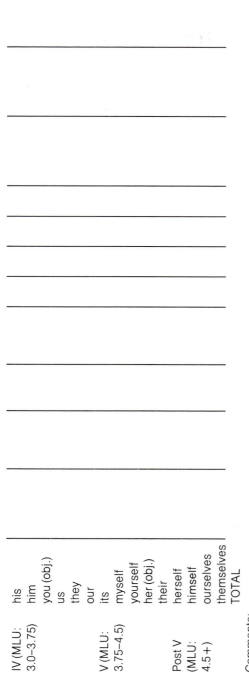

IV (MLU: 3.0–3.75)	his							
	him							
	you (obj.)							
	us							
	they							
	our							
V (MLU: 3.75–4.5)	its							
	myself							
	yourself							
	her (obj.)							
	their							
Post V (MLU: 4.5+)	herself							
	himself							
	ourselves							
	themselves							
	TOTAL							

Comments:

Note: Pronouns, arranged by stage of acquisition, are scored as correct or incorrect, although the total and percent columns are initially left blank. Incorrect pronoun use is then analyzed as a substitution or omission error. Substitution may be multiple, as when *she* is used for *his*, demonstrating substitutions of case and gender. When this step is completed, the sample is checked to ensure that the referent has been clearly identified for each pronoun and that the child has not overused the referent name in place of a pronoun. These are also errors, and once noted, they should be added to the incorrect total on the left. When this step is completed, the total and percent correct columns can be completed.

TABLE 4.7
Language analysis based on Brown's stages of development

Stage	Approx. Age	Negative	Interrogative
Early I (MLU:1–1.5)	12–22 mos.	Single word - *no, all gone, gone* Negative + X. ("No eat")	Yes/no asked with rising intonation on single word. *What* and *where.*
Late I (MLU:1.5–2.0)	22–26 mos.	*No* and *not* interchangeably.	That + X. *What* + noun phrase + (doing)?
Early II (MLU:2.0–2.25)	27–28 mos.		*Where* + noun phrase + (going)?
Late II (MLU:2.25–2.5)	29–30 mos.	*No, not, don't,* and *can't* inter- changeably. Negative element placed between subject and predicate.	*What* or *where* + subject + predicate.
Early III (MLU:2.5–2.75)	31–32 mos.		
Late III (MLU:2.75–3.0)	33–34 mos.	*Won't* appears. Develops auxiliary forms *can, do, does, did, will,* and *be.*	Begins to use auxiliary verbs in questions (*be, can, will, do*). ("You are going?")
Early IV (MLU 3.0–3.5)	35–37 mos.		
Late IV (MLU:3.5–3.75)	38–40 mos.	Adds *isn't, aren't, doesn't* and *didn't.*	Begins to invert auxiliary verb and subject ("Are you going?"). Adds *when, how,* and *why.*
Stage V (MLU:3.75–4.5)	41–46 mos.	Adds *wasn't, wouldn't, couldn't,* and *shouldn't.*	Adds modal auxiliary verbs (*would, could, should,* etc.) Stabilizes inverted auxiliary.
Post-V (MLU:4.5+)	47 + mos.	Adds *nobody, no one, none,* and *nothing.* Difficulty with double negatives. ("Nobody don't . . .")	

TABLE 4.7 *(continued)*

Embedding	Conjoining	Intrasentential
	Serial naming without *and.* ("Coat, hat.")	Pronouns *I* and *mine.* Only Isolated nouns elaborated. (Art./Adj. + Noun)
Prepositions *in* and *on.* *Gonna, wanna, gotta,* etc. appear. Infinitive phrases (*to* + verb) appear in the object position.	And ("Coat *and* hat")	Pronouns *me, my,* and *it, this,* and *that.* Progressive *-ing* and plural *-s* markers acquired. Noun elaboration in object position only. (Art./Adj./Dem./Poss. + Noun)
	But, so, or, and *if* appear. Begin clauses with *and.*	Pronouns *she, he, her, we, you, your, yours,* and *them.* Possessive *-s* marker acquired. Noun elaboration in subject and object positions. [Art. + (Mod) + Noun.] Other modifiers *alot, some,* and *two.*
Subordinate clauses after such verbs as *like, think, guess, show, remember, pretend,* etc. ("Pretend you do it.")	*Because* appears. Clauses joined with *and* appear (not until late V that most children can produce this form.)	Pronouns *his, him, hers, us,* and *they.* Noun phrase may include demonstrative or article plus adjective, possessive, or modifiers such as *something, other,* or *another.*
Subordinate clauses appear in object position. Multiple embeddings by late V.	Clauses joined with *if* appear.	Pronouns *our, ours, its, their, theirs, myself,* and *yourself.* Articles *a* and *the,* past *-ed* and third person *-s* markers, uncontractable copula acquired.
Subordinate clauses attached to the subject. Embedding and conjoining within same sentence beyond MLU of 5.0.	*When, because, but,* and *so* in clause joining beyond MLU of 5.0.	Remaining reflexive pronouns. Irregular third *has* and *does,* contractable copula and auxiliary (be), uncontractable auxiliary (be) acquired.

TABLE 4.8
Elements of the noun phrase

Initiator	+	Determiner	+	Adjective	+	Noun	+	Post-noun Modifier
Only, a few of, just, at least, less than, nearly, especially, partially, even, merely, almost		**Quantifier:** All, both, half, no, one-tenth, some, any, either, each, every, twice, triple		**Possessive Nouns:** Mommy's, children's		**Pronoun:** I, you, he, she, it, we, you, they,		**Prepositional Phrase:** On the car, in the box,
				Ordinal: First, next, next to last, last, final, second		mine, yours, his, hers, its, ours, theirs		in the gray flannel, suit,
		Article: The, a, an				**Noun:** Boys, dog, feet, sheep, men and women, city of New York, Port of Chicago, leap of faith, matter of conscience		**Adjectival:** Next door, pictured by, Renoir, eaten by, Martians, loved by, her friends,
		Possessive: My, your, his, her, its, our, your, their		**Adjective:** Blue, big, little, fat, old, fast, circular, challenging				
		Demonstratives: This, that, these, those		**Descriptor:** *Shopping,* (center), *Baseball,* (game), *hot dog,* (stand)				**Adverb:** Here, there, Embedded
		Numerical Term: One, two, thirty, one thousand						**Clause:** Who went with you, that you saw

Examples:

Nearly . . . . all the one
                    hundred . . . . old college . . . . alumni . . . . attending the
                                                                                                event

Almost
all of . . . . .her thirty . . . . former . . . . clients

Nearly . . . . half of your . . . . brother's
                    old baseball . . . . uniforms . . . . .in the closet

tifiers; articles, possessive pronouns, or demonstratives; and numerical terms, such as *two, twenty,* or *one hundred*. Quantifiers include such words as *all, both, half, twice,* and *triple*. In combination with initiators, determiners can yield *nearly all, at least half,* and *less than one-third*. Articles include common forms, such as *the, a,* and *an*. Possessive pronouns include *my, your,* and *their*. Demonstratives serve as articles but are interpreted from the perspective of the speaker as in *this, that these,* and *those*.

In order of appearance, adjectivals consist of nouns marking possession, as in *mommy's* sock, ordinals, such as *first, next,* and *final*; adjectives, such as *little, big,* and *blond*; and nouns used as descriptors, as in *hot dog* stand and *cowboy* hat. Thus, a speaker might say "brother's first little cowboy hat." The exact order of adjectivals is more complex, requiring more explanation than space allows. (See Crystal, Fletcher, & Garman, 1978 or Dever, 1978.)

The noun function can be filled by subjective pronouns, such as *I, you,* and *they*; objective pronouns, such as *me, you,* and *them*; genitive pronouns, such as *mine, yours,* and *theirs*; simple singular and plural nouns, such as *boy, girls,* and *women*; and mass nouns that have no distinction between singular and plural, as in *sand, water,* and *police.* When a pronoun is used, the noun to which it refers usually has already been identified. Therefore, few noun modifiers are used, and the noun phrase is relatively simple. The noun function may also be complex or may consist of a phrase, as in *Statue of Liberty, need to succeed,* and *City of Los Angeles,* or a compound, as in *Tom and Bob* and *duty and responsibility.* Finally, if the noun is understood by both the speaker and listener, it may be omitted, as in the following exchange:

> "What did you and Barb do last night?"
> "(We) Went to that movie at the mall."

Finally, post-noun modifiers may take many forms including prepositional phrases (*in the gray flannel suit*), embedded clauses (*who lives next door*), adjectivals (*next door* and *driven by my mother*), and adverbs (*here* and *there*). Post-noun modifiers may be used singly or in combination, for example, "The man *who lives in the green house on the next block* bought all of the candy that I was selling." The development of elements of the noun phrase takes most nonimpaired children many years. As noted in Table 4.7, elaboration begins in isolation and then moves to the object position in the sentence before appearing in the subject position. This pattern is only the beginning of the development process; with increasing age the child should use more and more noun elaborations. Adjectives and determiners appear at the two-word stage for both language-impaired and nonimpaired children (Morehead & Ingram, 1976). Initiators and post-noun modifiers appear later, with language-impaired children exhibiting a marked delay (Morehead & Ingram, 1976). For nonimpaired children, clausal post-noun modifiers appear in late stage IV and V (Table 4.7). The speech-language pathologist is interested in the distribution of these elaborations in these positions and the average number of morphemes within noun phrases. It may be helpful for the speech-language pathologist to use a format of analysis similar to that in Table 4.8.

Verb phrase. Verb phrase elaboration consists of the verb and associated words, including noun phrases used as complements or as direct or indirect objects. The speech-language pathologist is concerned with the verbs used and those that are missing or incomplete. Other elements of the verb phrase that are present or absent are also important and reflect the maturity of the speaker's language system.

Predicates or verb statements show the relationship of the various sentence elements to each other. This relationship takes three forms: intransitive, in which the verb cannot take an object; transitive, in which the verb can take an object, and equative, which consists of the copula (*to be*) plus a complement of a noun, adjective, or adverb. Although these forms are relatively simple initially, increasing maturity results in increasing verb complexity with the use of auxiliaries, modals, and complex progressive forms, such as *have been going*. There is also increasing use of adverbs and adverbial forms. Verb phrases can be described by the length and range of types, as demonstrated in Table 4.9.

Simple transitive (*Mommy throw*) and equative verb phrases (*Doggie big*) appear at an MLU of about 1.5 (Kamhi & Nelson, 1988). At this stage, the verbs are

TABLE 4.9
Elements of the verb phrase

Modal Auxiliary	+	Perfective Auxiliary	+	Verb to be	+	Negative*	+	Passive	+	Verb	+	Prepositional Phrase, Noun Phrase, Noun Complement, Adverbial Phrase
May, can, shall, will, must, might should, would, could		Have, has, had		Am, is, are, was, were, be, been		Not,		Been, being		Run, walk, eat, throw, see, write		On the floor, the ball, our old friend, a doctor, on time, late

Examples:
Transitive (May have direct object)

May.....................have..wanted.....a cookie
Should..not..throw........the ball in the house

Intransitive (Does not take direct object)

Might.................have.................been...walking.....to the inn
Could...not...talk..........with you

Equative (Verb *to be* as main verb)

....is....................not...a doctor
....was...late
....were..on the sofa
May..be..ill

* When modal auxiliaries are used, the negative is placed between the modal and other auxiliary forms, for example, "Might not have been going."

unmarked for tense or person, and the copula is omitted. As language becomes more complex, verbs become marked, the copula appears, and intransitive verb phrases appear. By Stage II, the progressive -*ing* marker and catenatives (*gonna, wanna, gotta, hafta*) appear. The perfective form (*have + verb-en*) and the passive voice begin to be used by Stage IV. Adverbial phrases also appear in Stage IV. In general, language-impaired children who exhibit these more complex structures tend to use them less frequently than nonimpaired children (Johnston & Kamhi, 1984).

Tense markers are used to describe the temporal relationships between events. For example, if the event being described is taking place while the speaker mentions it, the speaker uses the present progressive verb form (auxiliary + verb-*ing*) to indicate an ongoing activity (*walking, eating*). In contrast, the perfect form of the verb (have + verb-*en*) indicates that the action is being described in relation to the present. Thus, ''I have been working here for two years'' implies that this action is still occurring, whereas ''I *have eaten* my dinner'' implies that the action is now complete. Verb tense analysis can be accomplished in a form similar to that presented in Table 4.9. Table 4.7 identifies the ages at which most children acquire auxiliary and modal auxiliary verbs.

Adverbs also mark temporal relations, in addition to manner and result. Temporal relations can be expressed between two events (*before, next, during, meanwhile*), with the continuation of an event (*for the past year, all week*), in the recent past (*recently, just a minute ago*), and with repetition (*many times, again*).

Verb aspect indicates temporal notions, such as momentary actions, duration, and repetition. Momentary actions are of short duration (*fall, break, hit*). In contrast, duration is marked by verbs of longer action with definite beginnings and ends (*sleep, build, make*). Phrases may also be used to convey a definite act (*sing a song*), and an act without a well-defined terminal point (*sing for your own enjoyment*). Still other verbs describe repetitive actions (*tap, knock, hammer*).

The development of tense markers seems to be related to the temporal aspect of the verb. The speech-language pathologist should investigate the relationship between tenses the child uses and the verbs to which these tenses are applied. No doubt, this analysis will require a sample larger than a 50 to 100 utterance sample.

Modal auxiliary verbs, such as *can, could, will, should, shall, may, might,* and *must,* are used to express the speaker's attitude (Bliss, 1987). Syntactically, modals function in the formation of questions and negatives. They are also used in such statements as ''I *will* do it tomorrow.''

As with the pronoun system, modals represent a complex interaction of form, content, and use that is reflected in the slow rate of acquisition, which usually lasts from age 2 to age 8 (Fletcher, 1975; Kuczaj, 1982; Major, 1974; Miller, 1981). Semantic categories of modals include wish or intention (*will, would*), necessity or obligation (*must, should*), ability or permission (*can*), certainty (*will*), and probability or possibility (*may, might*) (Bliss, 1987).

Those modals associated with action, such as *can* and *will* (ability, intention, and permission request), are acquired first. During the third year, the number of modals and the categories increases. Beyond age 4, the child clarifies the different forms and their uses (Hirst & Weil, 1982).

Language-impaired children rarely use modal auxiliaries (Menyuk & Looney, 1972; Trantham & Pedersen, 1976), possibly because of the linguistic subtleties expressed. In general, language-impaired children have more difficulty with catenatives, modals, and auxiliary verbs than their language level would suggest (Johnston & Kamhi, 1984). The speech-language pathologist is interested in the range and frequency of modals the child exhibits. When analyzing a sample, the pathologist pays particular attention to the level of development, the range of semantic concepts, the variety of usage, and the types of errors (Bliss, 1987). Variety of usage is noted with different pronouns, verb tenses, negative and positive statements, and sentence types.

Sentence types.   A single event may be described by the agent that originates the action, the action or state changes, and/or the recipient or object of that action (Duchan, 1986b). The agent as a noun or noun phrase is usually first, followed by the action word or verb, which in turn is followed by the recipient or object of that action in the form of a noun or noun phrase (e.g., ''John threw the ball'' or ''Mother ate the cookie'').

If the agent performs the action for the benefit of some other person, that beneficiary either precedes or follows the noun phrase describing the object of the action. For example, in ''He painted the picture for mother,'' *for mother* follows the object of the sentence. Instruments used to complete the action are usually placed after the action and follow the preposition *with*, as in ''He painted *with a brush.''*

Sentences that differ from the predominant subject-verb-object format may be difficult for the language-impaired child to decipher and form. Often, overreliance on the S-V-O strategy is not noted until the child begins school. The language-impaired child may resist rearrangement or interruption of this form and may attach other structures only at the beginning or end. Yes/no questions may be asked with rising intonation rather than through transformation of the subject and verb elements. Passive sentences, which use an object-verb-subject form, may be misinterpreted.

The speech-language pathologist is interested in the range of internal sentence forms and in the different sentence types. Sentence types include positive and negative forms of the declarative, interrogative, and imperative. Declarative sentences are statements (''He likes ice cream'' or ''She does not want to go'').

Interrogatives include three types of questions, including yes/no, *wh-* or constituent, and tag. Yes/no questions ask for confirmation or denial in the form of a yes or no response, as in ''Did you fix the light?'' The form of yes/no questions may vary from a statement with rising intonation (''You went to the store?'') to a transformation using the copula or an auxiliary verb (''Is he happy?'' or ''Did she eat her pie?'').

Wh- questions require more information and begin with such words as *what, where, who, why, when,* and *how.* Either the copula or auxiliary verb and the subject are transformed from their order in a statement (e.g., ''What is her age?'' or ''Why did he go?''). A less mature form that can be used with some *wh-* questions places the *wh-* word at the end of the sentence (e.g., ''She likes *what*?''). These types are typically used for clarification, however, and are discussed later.

Tag questions are statements with question tags attached (''She's lovely, isn't she?''). These questions seek only agreement.

The development of questions is given in Table 4.7. Mature tag questions, because of their complex nature and infrequent use, are acquired much later than are yes/no and *wh-* interrogatives. Some nonimpaired children do not master the mature tag form until midelementary school (Dennis, Sugar, & Whitaker, 1982; Reich, 1986). A less mature form using *okay* or *alright* (or the Canadian *eh*) may appear in preschool (''I do this, okay'').

The range of sentence types and the maturity of form are of interest to the speech-language pathologist. These are listed in Table 4.7.

With more mature speakers, the speech-language pathologist must consider the use of emphasis, pauses, and intonation to mark different meanings for the same form. Pauses mark the end of conceptual units and direct the listener in the type of response required. For example, ''Do you like football (pause) or baseball?'' requires a very different response from ''Do you like football or baseball?'' Rising intonation is used on an entire word for unexpected or surprise events, and falling intonation for the expected. As mentioned previously, rising intonation at the end of a word or sentence signifies a question, and falling intonation a statement.

Imperatives are commands (e.g., ''Eat your dinner'' or ''Stop that''). The subject, *you*, is understood. Speech-language pathologists must be careful not to confuse these sentence types with utterances in which the child omits the subject. The child who repeatedly omits the subject in other sentences probably should not be credited with imperative forms.

The behavior of other people may also be influenced by requests. These are discussed in separate sections in Chapter 3 and in the illocutionary functions of this chapter because of the pragmatic aspects of this form.

Negative sentences, whether declarative, interrogative, or imperative, also possess characteristic developmental forms (Table 4.7). The nonimpaired child's first negatives are marked by *no* and slightly later by *not*. Initially, these two forms are used interchangeably. To these are added *don't* and *can't*, also used interchangeably, followed by *won't*. Positive forms of *do, can, will,* and *would* develop later, followed by negative forms for the verb *to be* and for other auxiliaries. By school age the child develops indefinite forms (e.g., *no one* and *nothing*) and indirect negative imperatives (''Watch out for the hole''). These do not require syntactic negative transformations. During the school-age years, the child masters such negative prefixes as *un-, non-,* and *ir-*.

Embedding and conjoining.   Both embedding and conjoining involve relationships between clauses. In addition, embedding also involves the relationships between phrases.

A clause consists of a noun phrase and a verb phrase. A clause that can stand alone is an independent clause or sentence, even though it contains only the noun and the verb ("John ran"). Some clauses contain both elements but are not independent. These clauses, such as "that you want," must be attached to an independent clause or sentence in a process called embedding. In this manner, "that you want" can be embedded in "The toy is on sale" to form "The toy *that you want* is on sale." Two or more independent clauses can be joined together in a process called conjoining.

Clausal embedding initially develops in the object position at the end of the sentence (Table 4.7). Called *object noun complements*, these dependent clauses take the place of the object following such words as *know, think,* and *feel* ("I know *that you can do it*"). Object noun complements using *that* (I think *that I like it*) appear at an MLU of 4.0, most frequently following the verb think (Tyack & Gottsleben, 1986). By an MLU of 5.0-5.9, this type of embedding accounts for only 6% of children's two-clause sentences. Object noun complements using what (I know *what you did*) account for 8% of these sentences. Relative clauses attached to nouns develop next, beginning in the object position, as in "I want the dog *that I saw last night.*" Finally, the relative clause moves to the center of the sentence, describing the subject, as in "The one *that you ate* was my favorite."

Relative clauses appear less frequently than other forms of clausal embedding among preschoolers, although by school age, 20 to 30% of two-clause sentences may be of this type (Scott, 1984). Relative clauses appear at about 48 months initially as post-noun modifiers for empty nouns, such as *one* or *thing* (Wells, 1985). The most common relative pronouns for preschoolers are *that* and *what.* During the school years, pronouns expand with the addition of *whose, whom,* and *in which.*

Phrases may also be embedded in clauses. A phrase is a group of related words that does not contain a subject and a verb. There are several different types, including prepositional, participial, infinitive, and gerund phrases. Such phrases take the place of nouns or modify nouns. Prepositional phrases may also be adverbial in nature, as in "She will arrive *in a minute.*" As in clausal embedding, phrasal embedding usually develops initially at the end of the sentence.

Infinitive phrases first appear in the object position, most frequently following *want* (I want *drink pop*). This form with the *to* omitted emerges at a median age of 30 months (Wells, 1985). Infinitives with a different subject than the main verb (Mommy I want you *to eat it*) appear somewhat later.

The speech-language pathologist is interested in the number and type of embeddings. Some developmental data are included in Table 4.7. The position of these embeddings within the sentence is also important, given the developmental significance of position.

Clausal conjoining appears relatively late in preschool development, although some conjunctions appear much earlier. Conjunctions express the relationships between two entities, such as words or clauses.

Usually, *and* is the first conjunction learned; it is used to join objects in a group. Throughout the preschool period *and* continues to be the most frequently used conjunction, being 5 to 20 times more common than *but* (Scott, 1988). Around 30 months of age children begin to sequence clauses using *and* as the initial word in each sentence (Bloom, Lahey, Hood, Lefter, & Fiess, 1980; Lust & Mervis, 1980). As noted in Table 4.7, *and* is also the first conjunction used to join clauses. At this point *and* is used for sequential events and is interpreted as *and then*. Even among school-age children, 50 to 80 percent of all narrative sentences begin with *and* (Scott, 1984, 1987). With age and an increase in written communication, use of *and* decreases. Between ages 11 and 14, only 20 percent of spoken narrative sentences begin with *and*. In written narratives, the rate is only about 5 percent (Scott, 1987). Other conjunctions may express a causal relationship (*because*), simultaneity (*while*), a contrasting relationship (*but*), and exclusion (*except*). Conjunctions develop in the following order: *and, because, when, if, so, until, before, after, since, although,* and *as* (Lee, 1974; Loban, 1976; Scott, 1987; Tyack & Gottsleben, 1986; Wells, 1985). The most frequently used conjunctions through age 12 are *and, because,* and *when.*

Early strategies that rely on the order of mention for interpretation may persist with the language-impaired child. Thus, the child ignores the conjunctions and their intended meanings. The sentences, ''Go to the market before you go to the movie'' and ''Go to the market after you go to the movie,'' are interpreted as having the same meaning.

The speech-language pathologist is interested in the range and frequency of the conjunctions used and in the amount of conjoining present in the sample. This information is especially important with more mature speakers and is discussed in the following chapter on narratives.

The speech-language pathologist should also note multiple embeddings and embedding and conjoining that occur within the same sentence. Again, this is much more characteristic of school-age language than of preschool language. The narratives of children 10 to 12 years old are easily distinguishable from those of preschoolers by the presence of multiple embedding and conjoining within the same sentence.

Phonologic Analysis

A phonological analysis should describe the child's phonetic inventory; the syllable structures or word shapes produced by the child; strategies, such as avoidance of certain sounds or use of favorite sounds; and the child's phonological processes (Edwards, 1984). Children with specific language impairment demonstrate difficulty with the regularities of the phonological system (Leonard, Schwartz, Allen, Swanson, & Loeb, 1989). All of these data may not be available from one or two conversational samples, although every sound in a word provides some data.

After applying the Assessment of Phonological Processes (Hodson, 1980), the Natural Process Analysis (Shriberg & Kwiatkowski, 1980), and a modified form of the Procedures for the Phonological Analysis of Children's Language (Ingram, 1981), Dyson and Robinson (1987) concluded that no one phonological analysis procedure provides the optimum amount of information for the selection of intervention targets. There seems to be little difference in the phonological processes identified by the three analysis procedures (Paden & Moss, 1985). Thus, a variety of processes should be sampled and a combination of procedures used.

It is important for the speech-language pathologist to recognize that phonological processes are not necessarily errors. For children at certain ages these rules or processes function as ways for them to produce sounds and sound combinations with which they have difficulty. These rules reflect ''natural processes'' (Oller, 1974) that act to simplify adult forms of verbal language for young children.

Just as young children simplify sentence structure, they may follow similar rules to simplify words. For example, the two-year-old who has difficulty with long words may adopt the strategies of dropping weak or unstressed syllables, simplifying consonant blends, and omitting final consonants. The resultant word may resemble the target only vaguely, if at all.

These processes are found in all developing children at some stage in their acquisition of verbal language. It is only when these processes do not evolve into more mature strategies that parents, teachers, and speech-language pathologists become concerned. The following section discusses the major phonological processes found in young children and the methods for analyzing data from a conversational sample.

Phonological Processes

With first words, children shift to greater control of articulation. Babbling requires less constrained production, but when children add meaning to sound they need some phonological consistency to transmit their messages. After the onset of meaningful speech, there is much individual variation in the pattern and rate of vocabulary growth, the use of invented words, and the syllable structure of words acquired.

Most first words are monosyllabic CV or VC units or CVCV constructions (Ferguson, 1978; Ingram, 1976). Within a given word, the consonants are usually the same or noncontrasting, such as baby or goggie (doggie). It is the vowels that initially vary. Consonant contrasts usually occur in less frequent CVC constructions, such as *cup* (Waterson, 1978).

Children produce great phonological variation in their early words. The same word may be produced consistently or may vary greatly. The most noticeable phonological patterns among toddlers relate to syllable structure and include open syllables and diminutives, reduplication, and cluster reduction (Table 4.10).

As with other aspects of language, children's phonological development progresses through a long period of language decoding and hypothesis building. During the preschool years, children not only acquire a phonetic inventory and a phonological system, but also develop ''the ability to determine which speech sounds are used to signal differences in meaning'' (Ingram, 1976, p. 22). Some sound contrasts are very difficult for children to perceive and to produce, whereas others are relatively simple. Much of the morphological production of

TABLE 4.10
Phonological processes of young children

Processes	Examples
Syllable structure	
Deletion of final consonants	*cu* (/kʌ/) for *cup*
Deletion of unstressed syllables	*nana* for *banana*
Reduplication	*mama, dada, wawa* (water)
Reduction of clusters	/s/ + consonant (*stop*) = delete /s/ (*top*)
Assimilation	
Contiguous	
Between consonants	be*ds* (/bɛdz/), be*ts* (/bɛts/)
Regressive VC (vowel alters toward	
some feature of C)	nasalization of vowels: *can*
Noncontiguous	
Back assimilation	*dog* becomes *gog*
	dark becomes *gawk*
Substitution	
Obstruants (plosives, fricatives, and affricatives)	
Stopping: replace sound with a plosive	*this* becomes *dis*
Fronting: replace palatals and velars	*Kenny* becomes *Tenny*
(/k/ and /g/) with alveolars (/t/ and /d/)	*go* becomes *do*
Nasals	
Fronting (/ŋ/ becomes /n/)	*something* becomes *somethin*
Liquids: replaced by	
Plosive	*yellow* becomes *yedow*
Glide	*rabbit* becomes *wabbit*
Another liquid	*girl* becomes *gaul* (/gɔl/)
Vowels	
Neutralization: vowels reduced to /ə/ or /a/	*want to* becomes *wanna*
Deletion of sounds	*balloon* becomes *ba-oon*

Source: Drawn from D. Ingram, *Phonological Disability in Children.* New York: Elsevier, 1976.

preschool children will depend on their ability to perceive and produce phonological units.

For this discussion, the phonological processes of children (Table 4.10) have been divided into processes relative to syllable structure, assimilation, and phoneme substitution. The greatest reduction in the use of phonological processes occurs between ages 3 and 4 (Haelsig & Madison, 1986), and most processes disappear by age 4.

Syllable structure processes. From the moment children begin babbling, the basic unit used is the open or CV syllable, one ending in a vowel. When they begin using words, children frequently attempt to simplify production by reducing words to this form or to a CV multisyllable structure.

This basic syllable structure form affects the final consonant (Ingram, 1976; Oller, 1974). Open syllables predominate. Words with final consonants or multisyllabic words are frequently produced in a CV or CV multisyllable form (Waterson, 1976). The final consonant may be deleted, producing a CV structure for a CVC (*cup* may become /k/), or followed by a vowel to produce a CVCV structure from a CVC (*cake* may become *cake-ah*). The diminutive, in which the child adds an /i/ to the end of a CVC word (producing *doggie* from *dog*), is another form of this process. Open syllable processes usually disappear in half of the children between ages 3 and 4.

The child may also delete unstressed syllables to simplify word production. Generally, initial unstressed syllables are deleted most frequently. This process usually disappears after age 4.

Reduplication appears to be a step in the acquisition of final consonants. Reduplication occurs when children attempt polysyllabic words (*water*) but are unable to produce the one syllable correctly (Ferguson, Peizer, & Weeks, 1973; Menn, 1971). They compensate by repeating another syllable (*wawa*). Usually, either the first or the stressed syllable is reproduced. This process usually disappears by age 3, but may occur occasionally with words that are difficult to produce.

Finally, consonant clusters may be reduced or simplified to one consonant, producing *top* for *stop*. These deletions are predictable and usually adhere to the following patterns:

Cluster	Deletion	Example
/s/ + plosive (/t, p, k/)	s	*stop* becomes *top*
plosive or fricative	liquid or glide	*bring* becomes *bing*
+ liquid or glide		*swim* becomes *sim*

Cluster reduction, which usually disappears after age 4, is often followed by a stage in which another sound is substituted for the omitted sound. Some children have continuing difficulty with consonant clusters, and we do not expect mastery until about age 7.

Assimilation processes.   Assimilation processes simplify production by enabling the child to produce different sounds in the same way. In short, one sound becomes similar to another in the same word. The process may occur on contiguous or noncontiguous sounds and may affect following or preceding sounds. For example, young children often produce doggie as doddie or goggie, demonstrating assimilation in either direction.

Substitution processes.   There are several types of substitution processes, including stopping, fronting, and backing. Most of these processes are reduced by half between ages 3 and 4 and disappear by age 4½. In stopping, plosives are substituted for other sounds. Stopping is most common in the initial position in words (Oller, 1974), as in *dat* for *that*.

In fronting, labial or alveolar sounds are substituted for palatals or velar sounds. For example, /t/ and /d/ might be substituted for /k/ and /g/ producing *tid* for *kid* and *dun* for *gun*. Within nasals, fronting might also result in /n/ being substituted for /ŋ/, producing *rinin* for *ringing*. The speech-language pathologist must be careful not to confuse dialectal variation, in which only the final sound is substituted (e.g., *walkin*), for fronting. In dialectal variation, the /ŋ/ would only be modified on the present progressive marker, producing *ringin* rather than *rinin*. Backing is the reverse of fronting, and back sounds are substituted.

Multiple processes. To make this puzzle even more difficult for those who must unscramble these phonological patterns, children often use more than one phonological process at a time. For example, *blanket* may become /bæki/ as a result of cluster reduction and open syllabification.

Analysis Steps

Unscrambling is a good term for describing the process of phonological process analysis. Because this analysis is difficult and time-consuming, it should be attempted only when a phonological disorder is suspected based on prior data. When analysis is undertaken, however, previously unrecognized patterns may reveal themselves.

The entire sample is transcribed phonetically with the addition of the applicable diacritical markers shown in Table 4.11. Target words and transcribed productions can then be transferred to an analysis sheet similar to that found in Table 4.12. Unintelligible patterns can be determined by having a familiar listener, such as a parent or teacher, interpret the child's speech from the audiotape.

Because phonological processes are found at the syllable and/or word levels, words are analyzed individually for the presence or absence of these processes. Casual, stylistic, or everyday patterns, such as *runnin'*, *wudja get?*, *get 'um*, and *j'eat yet?*, should not be analyzed for phonological processes because they represent a very different sort of behavior.

Words, syllables, and sounds are rated for evidence of various phonological processes. The speech-language pathologist must identify processes and describe the consistency of each. An individual word may be affected by one or more processes. Where substitutions are suspected, further analysis is attempted at the sound level.

Most individual sound errors will be inconsistent. The data from every consonant in question is evaluated. The following procedure of analysis is suggested (Edwards, 1984; Klein, 1984; Lund & Duchan, 1988):

1. Rate all productions using a form similar to Table 4.13.
2. Compute the percentage of correct production for each sound in question by dividing the number correct by the total number attempted. Note consonants that are never produced correctly.

TABLE 4.11
Diacritical markers

Marker	Meaning	Example
/:/	Full lengthening. Place to right of phoneme to indicate increased duration of production.	Adjacent identical sounds: last time /lst:alm/ Omission of final sound results in vowel lengthening: *car* /kↄ:/
/~/	Nasalization. Place above non-nasal phoneme to indicate nasalization.	*can* /kãn/ *nine* /naIn/
/÷/	Nasal emission. Place above phoneme to indicate audible emission through nares.	*Pete* /pit/
/n/	Dentalization. Place above phoneme to indicate consonant produced with tongue tip against upper teeth, as done correctly with the /d/ in *width.* Found in fronting processes and in frontal distortion or lisp.	*this* /ðIs/ *big* /bIg/
/ʌ/	Lateralization. Place above phoneme to indicate a release of air around the sides of the tongue, as in a lateral distortion or lisp.	*miss* /mIŝ/

3. Identify patterns by position in words, manner, place, and voicing of production. An arrangement such as that in Table 4.13 aids in summarizing these data.

4. Sounds that experience variability of substitution patterns should be analyzed for assimilation. This may necessitate a change in the initial portion of the analysis.

5. Note sounds that may be produced incorrectly when they occur but may also be substituted for other sounds.

Not all children with phonological disorders demonstrate the common processes noted in this section (Leonard, 1985). Occasionally, children form idiosyncratic rule systems. In this case, the speech-language pathologist should form hypotheses about the child's rule or rules and test these hypotheses through intervention (Fey & Stalker, 1986).

Selection of intervention targets can be based on different criteria suggested by a number of specialists (Dunn & Barron, 1982; Dyson & Robinson, 1987; Edwards, 1983; Grunwell, 1982; Hodson & Paden, 1983; Ingram, 1976, 1983; Shriberg, 1983; Shriberg & Kwiatkowski, 1980; Weiner, 1981). These criteria can be summarized as follows:

1. Select processes that occur frequently (at least 40% of the time) but are optional (less than 100% of the time).

TABLE 4.12
Sample phonological process analysis format

Target Word	Word Produced	No Process Evident	*Deletion of Consonants Not in Clusters			Deletion of Unstressed Syllable	Reduplica-tion	Reduction of Consonant Clusters			*Assimilation			*Substitution		
			Init.	Med.	Fin.			Init.	Med.	Final	Init.	Med.	Final	Init.	Med.	Final

Syllable Processes

*Individual phoneme analysis (See Table 4.13) is needed.

113

TABLE 4.13

Analysis of phonological processes affecting individual sounds

2. Select processes that affect stimulable sounds or sounds within the child's phonetic inventory.
3. Select processes that will have the greatest effect on intelligibility.
4. Select processes that affect early developing sounds.

Obviously, it is impossible to meet all of the criteria at once. The knowledgable speech-language pathologist will have to determine the most effective criteria for the clinical model.

CONTENT

The understanding of word meanings and word relationships is affected by many factors, such as age, sex, and regional and racial/ethnic differences. To know a word is to know more than just a definition. It means that the child understands that word's relationship to similar words of meaning and sound and to words of an opposite meaning and understands the semantic class into which the word can be placed.

Meaning extends beyond the word, however, and larger units of analysis, such as the phrase or sentence, must also be considered. The performative is the deep structure meaning and intent of the utterance from which the form flows. What is said, for example, "Don't hit me," may be very different from the intended message, which might be "Go away, I don't understand what you want."

Obviously, all of this information cannot be ascertained from a brief language sample. Word understanding can be assessed by playing games like Simon Says or by directing the child through a series of tasks. The clinician can make statements in which words are obviously used incorrectly in order to judge the child's reactions. Word games that solicit definitions or antonyms can also provide valuable information. Sorting and categorization tasks can be a part of a play situation and can provide information on the child's ability to categorize and classify. The child can be asked to name the members of a category or to deduce the category name from a list of members. The clinician can play the "fool" and make ridiculous comparisons ("A mouse is bigger than an elephant") or silly pairings ("The comb goes between his toes") to gauge the child's reactions.

Children with language impairments and with language learning disabilities usually do not have difficulty with referent-symbol tasks, such as those represented by the Peabody Picture Vocabulary Test. These children may have difficulties, however, with double meanings, abstract terms, synonyms, and nonliteral interpretation. In addition, the physical setting can be especially important for language impaired children because they depend much more on the context for support than do nonimpaired children. The child may understand a word only given certain physical situations.

Initially, word meanings are learned by a process called *fast mapping,* in which a hypothesized meaning is assigned to a word on first meeting. In general, children learn new words after only one exposure by forming an initial, albeit partial, understanding based on the linguistic and nonlinguistic contexts. This meaning is gradually refined or replaced with use over time. Children with language impairments and those who are nonimpaired seem to learn word meanings in this fashion, although some language-impaired children, such as those with a brain injury, may require more subsequent exposures than do nonimpaired children (Keefe, Feldman, & Holland, 1989; Rice, Buhr, & Nemeth, 1990). Another difficulty for language-impaired children is related to recall of the phonological shape or pattern of new words (Dollaghan, 1987b). This problem may also reflect the generally slower recall rate reported for language-impaired children (Sininger, Klatzky, & Kirchner, 1989).

Lexical Items

Obviously, there are several levels of semantic analysis relative to individual words and relations between words and larger units. At the word level, the child demonstrates individual word meanings and word classes. Several questions arise relative to word use and range of meanings and relationships.

Type-Token Ratio

The type-token ratio or the ratio of the number of different words to the total number of words is a quantitative measure with a checkered past of professional acceptance. This reflects recognition that the value may vary widely with the language sample size. In general, there is less variability across larger samples of 350 words or more (Hess, Sefton, & Landry, 1986). Multiple settings and more representative samples would yield theoretically more stable values, although there may be great situational variability for an individual child (Hess, Haug, & Landry, 1989).

Although the normative data are old, they still may be useful. Children between the ages of 3 and 8 years demonstrate ratios of 0.45 to 0.50 (Templin, 1957). Children who receive values greater than 0.5 have greater variability and flexibility in their language, whereas those below 0.45 tend to use the same words over and over again. Very low values might indicate perseverative or stereotypic behavior.

A low value may indicate overreliance on words with broad application but unspecified meaning (empty words) such as *thing* and *one*. Children with poor vocabularies or word-finding difficulties may use empty words rather than more specific words that are not at their disposal.

Two spontaneous language profiles emerge from the samples of children with word-finding problems (German, 1987). Some children exhibit word-finding difficulties both on structured naming tasks and in spontaneous samples. They exhibit reformulations, time fillers, empty words, repetitions, starters, and grammatical errors. Other language-impaired children exhibit these behaviors only on structured naming tasks, although they produce relatively less language in spontaneous samples than do nonimpaired children.

Mature speakers should possess a variety of words for describing sensory experiences, such as sight (*clearly*), sound (*loud*), smell (*stunk*), and feelings (*happy, tired*). They should be able to describe the environment in terms of time (*at five o'clock*) and location (*in front of*). Entities should possess physical qualities, such as shape (*sort of round*), size (*big*), number (*two, many, few*), substance (*metal, wood*), and condition (*new, ragged*). There should be terms for relationships, such as comparisons (*bigger than, as big as*) and qualifications (*nearly, not quite, only, enough*); and verbs for describing actions (*run, jump, eat*), states (*am, is, are*), and sensory processes (*feel, hear, see*). Finally, the speakers should be able to describe causation (*because …*) and motivation. As noted previously, these terms develop slowly. The full range is characteristic of the mature speaker.

Deictic terms or terms that must be interpreted from the perspective of the speaker (e.g., *here, there, this, that, come,* and *go*) offer a special problem for the language-impaired child. The shifting reference that occurs with each speaker change contributes to the child's difficulty. Children with language learning disabilities, autism, or emotional disturbances may lack either the listener or speaker perspective. These children may also refer to themselves by name and may echo the utterances of others.

Over-/Underextensions and Incorrect Usage

The speech-language pathologist should note all inaccurate uses of words that indicate some variation between the child's meaning and the conventional one. In general, meanings mature from the personal experiential ones found in preschool children to the shared conventional ones of adults.

Some children use words incorrectly because they do not know the shared conventional definition. Others use word substitutions that are incorrect. For example, a recent letter from a young adult with language learning disability included the following:

> I wish I could write as good as you. You know where to put paragraphs and how to use *punctuality* right.

Because I am usually late, I assume he meant *punctuation*. Further testing by the speech-language pathologist can reveal the basis of the child's substitutions. The child may miss the target word slightly, as in the above example, or may have word-finding difficulties, resulting in word substitutions.

Word Relationships

Each word in a language is related to other words in ways that account for the richness of that language. These relationships consist of word associations (e.g., *salt and pepper* or *king and queen*), synonyms, antonyms, and homonyms. Some of these associations are expressed in the conversational sample, whereas others need to be probed by the speech-language pathologist. These associations reflect underlying cognitive organizational strategies.

Semantic Categories

Semantic categories, such as agent, action, and location, are the earliest word classes children use. Indeed, most of the early language development of toddlers is concerned with semantic units.

Several categorization schema attempt to describe the semantic classes of young children and adults (Brown, 1973; Chafe, 1970; Clancy, Jacobsen, & Silva, 1976; Fillmore, 1968; Leonard, Bolders, & Miller, 1976). Table 4.14 is a composite of these semantic category schema. The speech-language pathologist is interested in the range of semantic categories expressed by the child.

Semantic knowledge or the underlying concepts about properties of entities may be a better framework than linguistic form for the assessment of children with nonstandard dialects (Wolfram & Christian, 1976). The adequacy of the semantic knowledge of these children is often questioned, based on the form of their language, despite evidence of the universal nature of semantic representation in such categories as action, state, location, and possession (Blake, 1984; Miller, 1982; Stockman & Vaughn-Cooke, 1982). It is incorrectly assumed that nonstandard speakers acquire concepts later than do speakers of dialects closer to Standard American English (SAE).

The developmental trends are very similar and suggest guidelines for assessment of the semantic features of nonstandard speakers (Stockman & Vaughn-Cooke, 1986). By age 30 months, working-class, nonstandard speakers use mostly two-word combinations and encode several semantic categories, such as existence, action, location, state, negation, attribution, notice, intention, and recurrence. These guidelines can be used to help identify nonstandard children who may need clinical intervention.

Intrasentence Relationships

In addition to an interest in the child's word meanings and relationships, the speech-language pathologist investigates other relationships expressed in the sentence through the use of conjunctions, negatives, and prepositions (Lund & Duchan, 1988), and various sentence forms, such as passive voice.

Four types of conjunctive relations are expressed in conjoined sentences (Bloom, Lahey, Hood, Lifter, & Fiess, 1980): additive, temporal, causal, and adversitive.

In the additive form, two clauses with no dependent relationship are simply joined to one another. In the sentence "John ate pie, and Mary drank coffee," neither event depends on the other for its existence.

In the temporal form, one clause depends on the other to precede or follow or occur at the same time, as in "I'm going out and I'm taking a very long walk" or "I'll rake the leaves while you finish painting the trim." Practically, a person

TABLE 4.14
Semantic categories

Semantic Function	Description	Example
Action	The predicate expresses action with a transitive or intransitive clause.	We *grew* pumpkins and squash. (Transitive) She *gave* us a dollar. (Transitive) He *swims* daily. (Intransitive)
State	The predicate makes a statement about the way things are with a transitive, intransitive, or equative clause.	I *want* a hot fudge sundae. (Transitive) Tigers *look* fierce. (Intransitive) She *is* tall. (Equative) My sister is now at Harvard. (Equative)
Agent or Actor	Animate instigator of action. Sometimes inanimate, especially if natural force. Usually the subject but may also be passive complement.	Mike threw the *ball*. *Termites* destroyed our cabin. *Wind* blew down the trees. The *cat* chased the dog. The dog was chased by the *cat*.
Instrument	Usually refers to the inanimate object used by the actor to effect the action stated in the verb. The actor is usually not stated but may be. The instrument function may also be adverbial, as in *on his drum*.	The *axe* split the wood. The building was erected by a *crane*. She used the *baseball bat* with great skill. The shaman kept rhythm on his *drum*.
Patient	The entity on which an action is performed. The patient may be a direct object in transitive clauses or the subject in intransiive clauses.	Mike threw the *ball*. *The lighthouse* withstood the hurricane.
Dative	The animate recipient of action. Usually the indirect object but may also be the direct object if it does not undergo any action but receives something.	Father bought *mother* a bouquet of roses. Our mascot brought *us* good luck. He built a treehouse for his *daughter*. I loved that *movie*.
Temporal	Fulfills the adverbial function of time in response to a *when* question. May also be the subject of a sentence or a complement.	I'll see you *later*. We'll meet at *four o'clock*. *Then*, I'll know. *Tomorrow* is a holiday. *Tuesday* will be our first meeting. It is *time to leave*.
Locative	Fulfills the adverbial function of place in response to a *where* question. May also be the subject of a sentence or a complement	Some of us looked *in the old log*. I knew it was right *here*. *Chicago* is indeed a windy city. *Our house* has three bedrooms.
Manner	Fulfills the adverbial function of manner in response to a *how* question.	We stalked the big cat *carefully*. He worked *with great skill*.
Accompaniment	Fulfills the adverbial function of *with X* in response to *with whom* or *with what* questions.	He swam *with his sister*. She left *with Jim*. He hunted *with his dogs*.
Empty subjects	Serve a grammatical function.	*It* was sunny. *There* may be some rain.

Sources: Adapted from Chafe (1970), Dever (1978), Fillmore (1968)

cannot take a long walk while still indoors. Other examples establish the temporal relationship more clearly, as in "I'm going to the store before I go to the party."

Causal conjoining implies a dependency in which one clause is the result of the other, for example, "I went to the party because I was invited." The preschool child may use *because* alone or at the beginning of a clause, as in "Cause I want to," although true clausal conjoining occurs much later (see Table 4.7).

Finally, in adversive conjoining, one clause contrasts with information in the other, as in "I read the article but I was unimpressed." One clause opposes or negates the other.

Negatives may be expressed in several ways and develop at different stages. Klima and Bellugi (1973) have identified four mature negative forms including: (a) *not* and *-n't*; (b) negative words, such as *nobody* and *nothing*; (c) the determiner *no* used with nouns; and (d) negative adverbs, such as *never* and *nowhere*. Again, the more mature language user should have a variety of forms. Those used by the child can be compared to the developmental data available in Table 4.7.

Prepositions are some of the hardest working and most versatile English words. They can be used to mark location (*in the box*), time (*in a minute*), or manner (*in a hurry*), and to fill adjectival and adverbial functions. These small, often unstressed words may be misinterpreted or misunderstood by language-impaired children. A strategy they use is overreliance on one form. As mentioned previously, the speech-language pathologist examines the sample for the breadth of use. In general, language-impaired children exhibit difficulty interpreting sentences in which the information might possibly be interpreted in a reverse manner (van der Lely & Harris, 1990). For example, a passive sentence, such as "The cat is chased by the dog" might be interpreted incorrectly as "The cat chased the dog" using a subject-verb-object interpretation strategy. Language-impaired children have difficulty interpreting the grammatical functions of words and integrating grammatical and semantic information.

Figurative Language

Nonliteral meanings used for effect are more characteristic of school-age and adult language than of preschool language. Examples include metaphors, similes, idioms, and proverbs. For the purposes of analysis, jokes and puns can also be considered figurative language. The speech-language pathologist considers the range of figurative language used. Some children overrely on well-worn phrases and expressions, with little knowledge of their actual meaning. Such expressions as these can be probed by the speech-language pathologist to determine the child's actual knowledge.

CONCLUSION

The conversational sample is a rich source of data about children's language. Each utterance can be analyzed for a variety of language features within the five aspects of language. Obviously, such analysis is very time consuming. Speech-language pathologists should analyze areas of suspected difficulty for each child rather than attempt a blanket analysis.

Utterance-level analysis is only the first step. Larger units and the devices used to give these units structure and cohesion provide information of a very different nature.

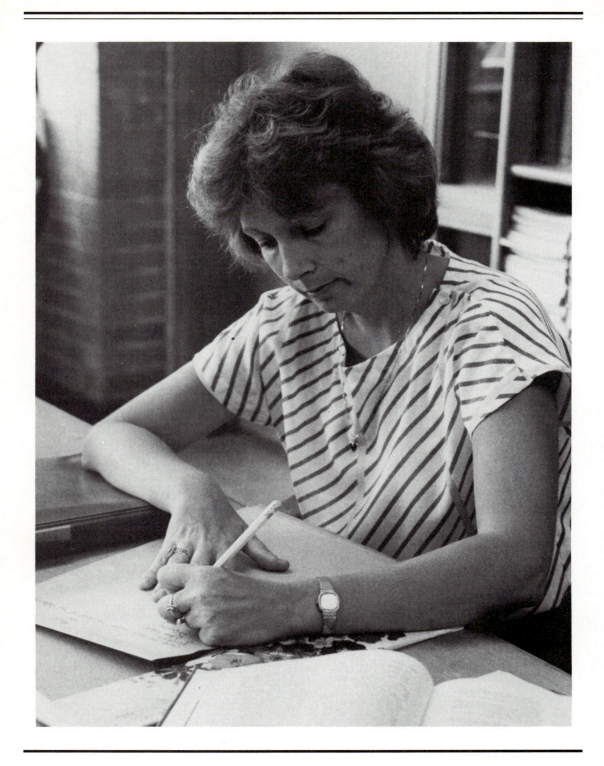

5

Analysis across
Utterances and Partners
and by Communication Event

To analyze language only at the utterance level is to miss many of the child's language skills, especially those aspects that govern cohesion and conversational manipulation. For example, pronoun analysis is very different when analyzing for case or person at the utterance level and when evaluating use of reference and cohesion within a conversation. Only by going beyond individual utterances can the speech-language pathologist gain an understanding of the child's use of the many language skills possessed (Biber, 1986; Scott, 1987). Secondary and tertiary analysis would be across utterances and partners and by communication event.

This chapter explores these levels of analysis, noting the adjustments the speaker must make to meet conversational demands. As in Chapter 4, these analyses are suggested when the speech-language pathologist suspects difficulties. Obviously, the many types of analysis mentioned in this chapter would be too numerous to examine and too time-consuming to analyze with every child. Because little normative information is available on conversational skills, analysis at these levels is largely descriptive. Table 5.1 lists the types of analyses possible across utterances and partners and by communication event.

ACROSS UTTERANCES AND PARTNERS

Analysis at the utterance level reveals much about the child's discrete, finite language skills but may obscure the child's knowledge of the ''big picture,'' the cohesion that threads through conversations. Some linguistic devices serve this co-

TABLE 5.1

Types of analysis across utterance and partners and by communication event

Across partners and utterances
Stylistic variations
   Register
   Channel availability
Referential communication
   Presuppositional skills
     What is coded and how
     Linguistic devices: Deictics, definite and indefinite reference
Cohesive devices
   Reference: Initial mention and following mention
   Ellipsis
   Conjunction
   Contrastive stress

By communication event
Social versus nonsocial
Conversational initiation: Method, frequency, and success rate
Topic initiation: Method, frequency, success rate, and appropriateness
Conversation and topic maintenance
   Frequency and latency of contingency
Duration of topic: Number of turns, informativeness, and sequencing
Turn taking: Density, latency, and duration
   Overlap: Type, frequency, and duration
   Signals
Conversation and topic termination
Contingent queries: Frequency and form
Conversational repair
   Spontaneous versus listener-initiated
   Strategy and success rate

hesive purpose, and larger units than the utterance must be analyzed to assess their development. Other devices vary across whole conversations, and one sample may be very different from another.

Stylistic Variations

The style of talking, whether formal, casual, or varied in other ways for the situation, usually does not change utterance by utterance. Rather, it is a manner of talking with a specific language partner or in a specific situation. Different styles may also be seen in role play. The speech-language pathologist is interested in the different styles used by the child in the various samples collected.

    As early as age 4, children use a different style of talking when they address younger language-learning children. This style resembles *motherese* or *parentese*, the stylistic changes made by parents when they address these same younger children. Mature language users have a variety of styles at their disposal and can switch styles with little effort. Such variation requires the speaker to consider the listener and the situation and the resultant requirements on the speaker.

Register

Code switching, the move from one style to another, must be judged against the age, sex, and language ability of the speaker and listener. Styles differ according to role-taking characteristics, dialectal variations, the amount of politeness, and conversational control.

Conversational roles can be established by the topics chosen, vocabulary (*dear, sir, honey*), pronunciation, and the discourse style selected. Usually, the more dominant partner takes longer turns and asks more questions. The degree of politeness also varies. In general, speakers are more polite when in the less dominant role or when requesting something that belongs to or is controlled by the other partner, who may be unlikely to grant the request. One politeness vehicle is the indirect request that does not directly state the desired consequence. Examples include ''Can you close the window?'' and the more indirect ''Do you think it's cold in here?''

Children with language learning disabilities often fail to use styles based on differing situational variables. Data suggest these children do not adjust to different speakers or may adjust in different ways than non-LLD children. Children with language learning disabilities may fail to recognize the characteristics of different settings. The language-impaired child may not be able to discriminate dominant from nondominant roles and the language form that goes with each. The most frequent problems with register include providing insufficient information for the listener, knowing when to make a statement, asking inappropriate questions, giving insufficient reason for the cause and effect of a situation, and adjusting register to the speaker (Johnson et al., 1984).

It may be especially difficult for the child with a language learning disability to express feelings and emotions. These expressions may be very direct and negative.

The speech-language pathologist studies the sample to determine the stylistic variations present. By now, the value of collecting language samples in two very different but client-appropriate situations is apparent. The speech-language pathologist should look for modifications in politeness, intimacy, and linguistic code based on the age, status, familiarity, cognitive level, linguistic level, and shared past experience of the listener (Roth & Spekman, 1984a). Of interest is the attention the child gives to the listener's characteristics. In addition to noting stylistic variations, the speech-language pathologist looks for inappropriate styles—those that are too casual or include excessive swearing where unnecessary.

Channel Availability

Some individuals enjoy talking on the telephone. I am not among them. In part, this lack of comfort may reflect the pressure placed on the speaker to be very explicit with language in this situation. Nonlinguistic channels are unavailable.

Most children below age 11 experience less communication success when they do not visually share the communication environment (Roth & Spekman, 1984a). As the number of channels decrease, the child with a language impairment should have increasing difficulty communicating. In fact, children with language learning disabilities often have great difficulty if forced to rely solely on the verbal channel.

This situation can be observed in any classroom for LLD children. When the teacher gives directions, the children often observe what others are doing before attempting to follow the instructions.

While gathering the language sample, the speech-language pathologist can manipulate channel availability systematically. During play, the pathologist can look away and then ask the child to describe what he or she is doing. Barrier games or blindfold games with the child in charge may also elicit interesting information. Role playing with the telephone is more realistic.

Referential Communication

Referential communication is the ability of a speaker to select and verbally identify the attributes of an entity in such a way that the listener can accurately identify the entity (Bowman, 1984). To succeed, the speaker must be able to determine what information the listener needs, deliver that information in a specific manner, make comparisons, and use feedback on message adequacy and breakdown.

Referential communication includes directions, explanations, and descriptions. These are three essential aspects of classroom discourse, and their impairment may contribute to the academic difficulties of children with language learning disabilities (Donahue, 1985).

Presuppositional Skills

As noted in Chapter 3, presupposition is the speaker's assumptions about the context and about the listener that modify the manner and content of the speaker's utterance (Johnson et al., 1984). The speaker must take the conversational perspective of the listener(s) and determine what information to communicate and its form.

From early on, informativeness is a characteristic of communication. Even toddlers tend to code information that is maximally informative, thus talking about things that are new, different, and changing. For most children, the receptive and expressive ability to consider a partner's perspective is established by age 10 (Sonnenschein & Whitehurst, 1984). Although both comprehension and production require understanding of the critical features needed, production also requires knowing how and when to provide information. At age 10, children with language learning disabilities have poor referential skills and are less likely to adjust to the listener (Knight-Arest, 1984), more likely to provide ambiguous information (Spekman, 1981), and less likely to supply enough overall information (Noel, 1980). In addition, although LLD children seem to understand directions given by others, they take longer to comply than do age-matched non-LLD children (Feagans & Short, 1986) and have great difficulty giving adequate instructions.

The speech-language pathologist should be alert to the informativeness of the child's utterances and to the social context. The following questions can be applied to the sample (Roth & Spekman, 1984a):

☐ What does the child choose to encode in the situation?

☐ Does the child encode what is novel or merely comment on what is already given?

☐ Does the child encode new information gesturally or linguistically?

☐ Are messages informative, vague, or ambiguous?

☐ Are different referents clearly established?

☐ Does the child talk differently about things present and things not?

What's coded and how.   Conversations usually contain information that is novel and informative. The speech-language pathologist is interested in whether the child adds to the conversation or only comments on what is given. In the following exchange, the child takes a turn but adds nothing of substance to the conversation.

> PARTNER: Wasn't that a great baseball game on TV last night?
> CHILD: Yeah, great game.
> PARTNER: What a great home run in the top of the ninth; I didn't expect Cincinnati to pull it out.
> CHILD: Great home run.
> PARTNER: I think they'll probably go on for the pennant. How about you?
> CHILD: Pennant.

If this sounds like the conversation of someone who doesn't know the topic well enough to comment, that may be partially correct. The child may not be able to identify the topic. Frequent repetition may indicate a semantic (word retrieval), processing, or pragmatic (not sure of the contextual demands) problem. Other language-impaired children may make vague or ambiguous contributions or use empty words, such as *one* and *thing*.

Linguistic devices.   Several linguistic devices are used to mark informativeness, including deictics and direct/indirect reference (Roth & Spekman, 1984a). Both of these devices can be used to note referents internal or external to the conversation; other cohesive devices, listed in Table 5.2 (Halliday & Hasan, 1976), establish relations entirely within the discourse.

Deictics.   As noted in Chapter 3, deictic terms are linguistic elements that must be interpreted from the perspective of the speaker in order to be understood as the speaker intended. The use of deixis is based on the *speaker principle*, in which the referential point shifts as speakers change, and on the distance principle, in which referents are coded by their distance from the speaker.

Words with deictic meanings appear in several word classes, including personal pronouns (*I/me* and *you*), demonstrative adjectives (*this, that, these,* and *those*), adverbs of time (*before, after, now,* and *then*), adverbs of location (*here* and *there*), and verbs (*come* and *go*).

Deixis can be elicited using object-finding tasks in which the child directs the conversational partner toward a hidden object. The child's behavior, especially the errors, should be analyzed to determine confusion or overreliance on one principle or one aspect of a principle.

Definite and indefinite reference.   The mature language user is able to mark specific (definite) and nonspecific (indefinite) referents by manipulation of definite (*the*) and indefinite (*a/an*) articles. The speaker must consider what the listener(s) knows about the topic under discussion.

Article use can be especially difficult for the language-impaired child. In part, this difficulty may reflect the use of articles also to mark new and old information, as mentioned in the following section. There is a tendency for language-impaired children to overuse the definite article.

Cohesive Devices

Conversational *cohesion,* how language hangs together, can be a useful analysis tool (Halliday & Hasan, 1976). Cohesion can be expressed through syntax and vocabulary. For example, *reference* is a device that uses a pronoun or demonstratives, such as *this* or *that,* to refer to the referent, which was identified previously in the conversation. Conjoining, the connection of phrases, clauses, and sentences through the use of such conjunctions as *and, because,* and *if,* is also used for cohesion. The major cohesive devices used in English are listed in Table 5.2.

The most frequent problems of cohesion relate to providing redundant information, deleting necessary information, using unclear and ambiguous reference, sequencing old and new information, and marking old and new information with articles and pronouns (Johnson et al., 1984). In short, errors usually reflect including or excluding too much information or confusing new and old information.

Reference

Reference is a linguistic device used continuously in conversation to keep information flowing and to give it cohesion. In the process, new information is stated clearly, then subsequently implied by the referral to it as old information, one utterance presupposing the other. Some children with language impairments, such as autistic children, have difficulty marking new and old information (McCaleb & Prizant, 1985).

The speech-language pathologist must note the method of introducing new information and the use of following mention. Speakers should ensure that listeners can easily determine noun-pronoun relationships. This investigation requires looking beyond traditional utterance level analysis.

TABLE 5.2
Cohesive devices used in English

Relation	Explanation	Example
Reference	Initially, the entity is named and may use the indefinite article (*a/an*). Subsequent mention may use a pronoun, words such as *this, that,* and *one,* or use the definite article (*the*) with the noun.	*John* went looking for *a car. He found one* in the city. I want to buy *a coat,* but *that one* I saw last night is too expensive.
Ellipsis	Subsequent sentences omit redundant or shared information.	Who *ate all the cookies*? I did. (Eat all the cookies) I would like to *make a phone call.* May I? (Make a phone call)
Conjunction	Conjunctions join clauses to express additive, causal, and other relationships.	We went to the circus, *and* I saw elephants. John's angry *because* I drank his soda.

Source: Adapted from Halliday, M., & Hasan, R. (1976). *Cohesion in English.* London: Longman.

Initial mention.   In initial mention, mature speakers establish mutual reference clearly, especially if the entity mentioned is not present. Generally, the referent name is stressed and preceded by the indefinite article (*a/an*). The referent is often placed at the end of the sentence, the most salient position. The following are examples of the introduction of new information:

> Did you see *John at the party*?
> We went to a *circus* yesterday.

In addition, referents that are present may be pointed to or handled. Young children tend to rely more on these nonlinguistic behaviors to establish new referents.

Children with language learning disabilities or autism have difficulty with new information (McCaleb & Prizant, 1985; Rees & Wollner, 1981). As speakers, they may not identify new information for the listener, assuming that the listener ''just knows'' what the speaker is thinking. As listeners, these children may have difficulty identifying the new information but will ask few questions to clarify. As Dr. Joel Stark notes, ''These children often do not know what they do not know'' and, thus, cannot inquire about it (Stark, 1985). With increasing language skills the child is able to be more specific linguistically.

Children with word-finding difficulties or poor vocabularies may use empty words, such as *that, one,* or *thing,* that do not help to clarify the referent. These children may rely on the immediate context and use pointing to specify the referent that their nonspecific vocabulary failed to identify.

Following mention.   In following mention, previously identified referents are often moved to the initial position in the sentence and may be referred to by the use of the definite article (*the*) or a pronoun. This referral to previously cited information is called *anaphoric reference.* Pronoun use is appropriate when the referent is unambiguous or clearly identified. The pronoun should be in close proximity so there is no confusion as to which noun it refers.

Storytelling and the introduction of new entities into the task are good methods for eliciting referencing skills. The speech-language pathologist is interested in the way the child introduces new information and refers to that information later. Also of interest is any confusion with article and pronoun use. Pronouns and a method of recording the child's use were discussed previously and included in Table 4.6. It is not uncommon for the child with a language learning disability to introduce new information with "She did it," leaving the listener to determine who *she* is and what *it* was.

Ellipsis

Ellipsis is a process in which redundant information is omitted. For example, the response to "What do you want?" is "Cookie," which omits the shared information "I want."

Elliptical fragments are used frequently to keep the conversation moving smoothly and rapidly, but they are missed if linguistic analysis concentrates solely on full sentences. Language-impaired children may not realize that information is shared or may assume that it is shared when it is not. Either assumption interferes with the flow of conversation. For example, the child might repeat "Cookies, cookies, cookies" until someone asks, "What about cookies?" To which the child responds in surprise, "I want some," having assumed that the *I want* was shared.

Conjunction

Conjunctions, such as *and, then, so,* and *therefore,* are used to connect thoughts. Although preschool children have several conjunction-type words in their vocabularies, they rarely use them to join clauses. Even kindergarten children will overrely on *and,* which becomes an all purpose conjunction. In addition, *and* is often used to mean *and then* when giving a sequence of events. A developmental progression for conjunctions is given in Table 4.7.

Just as conjunctions can be analyzed at the utterance level because of their use in linking clauses, conjunctions can also be analyzed across utterances, as in the following exchange.

PARENT: We had a great day at the zoo. I liked the monkeys best.
CHILD: *And* feeding the deer babies.

Analysis at the level of the child's utterance alone would miss the child's considerable skill.

Contrastive Stress

Contrastive stress or emphasis can be used to negate or correct the message of a conversational partner. For example, if one speaker said "Kathy brought cookies," the other might correct "*Mary* brought cookies." Again, the speech-language pathologist must transcend the traditional utterance-level analysis.

COMMUNICATION EVENT

Communication event, a term coined by Roger Brown (1973) and modified by others, can represent an entire conversation or a portion thereof that includes one topic. For purposes of our discussion, we use the larger definition and include within it a conversation that comprises one or more topics.

Usually, there is a shared or negotiated agenda(s) within a conversation. Utterances within the event support this agenda. The teenager who wants to be granted a privilege, such as getting to use the family car, is polite, and each utterance supports this agenda.

Conversations may be too open-ended for some children unfamiliar with the process or unable to decipher the code. The child may be unclear about the purpose of conversation and his or her role in it. Much of this difficulty can be alleviated by using familiar conversational partners and situations and by following the child's lead. Younger children and those with a language impairment may need events with more definite beginnings and ends, such as putting together a puzzle.

The social organization of discourse consists of the two roles of speaker and listener. The effective communicator has the ability to function in and contribute to the conversation by assuming responsibility for both roles. Assessment variables that might measure a child's ability to participate effectively are the amount of socialized speech and the child's adaptive style; conversation and topic initiation, maintenance, and termination and the completeness, relevance, and clarity of the child's behavior; on-topic exchanges and turn taking; and conversational repairs (James, 1989; Lund & Duchan, 1988; Prutting, 1983; Roth & Spekman, 1984a).

There are two levels of analysis, the molar and the molecular (Prutting, 1983). At the molar level, the clinician evaluates each behavior for appropriateness or inappropriateness within the conversational context. Inappropriate behaviors may indicate problem areas for further assessment. At the molecular level, the clinician is interested in the *frequency, latency, duration, density,* and *sequence* of the child's behaviors (Prutting, 1983).

Frequency data will reveal inordinately high- or low-frequency features and information on the range of features. Latency, or the span of time when an individual does not engage in behavior, is also important. Pauses and hesitations may reveal difficulty decoding the preceding utterance or forming a response. Duration is the length of time that the child and partner are engaged in a certain behavior, such as conversational gaze or conversational turns by both partners. Density is the number of behaviors within a certain period of time. Of interest are the density of different conversational topics or specific linguistic structures, such as questions. Sequence includes the order of events within a topic or conversation. The child exhibiting difficulty with sequencing of a conversation may not understand the rules of conversational participation.

Social versus Nonsocial

Social speech is speech addressed explicitly to and adapted for a listener. It is characterized by explicitness and clarity, repairs of breakdowns, and an obligation for the listener to respond. Social communication includes dialogues and social monologues that are addressed to a listener or uttered for the mutual enjoyment of both the speaker and listener, such as rhyming and poetic nonsense. The speaker adapts the explicitness of the message for the listener and repairs breakdowns. The speaker's message is delivered as if the speaker expects a listener response.

In contrast, nonsocial speech is not addressed explicitly to a listener, and the listener has no obligation to respond. Nonsocial communication is usually for the speaker's own enjoyment and often consists of asocial monologues.

Although preschoolers produce many asocial monologues, the amount of time spent in this type of production decreases with age. Nonimpaired school-aged children produce very little nonsocial speech. An important measure of communication would be the percentage of the child's utterances or the amount of total talk time that can be characterized as social (Roth & Spekman, 1984a).

Conversational Initiation

The most efficient way to initiate a conversation is to gain the listener's attention, greet the listener, and clearly state the topic of conversation or some opener, such as ''Guess what happened to me yesterday?'' or ''Where have you been? I haven't seen you in ages.'' Openers set the tone of the conversation and the subsequent turns. Opening and closing a conversation is one of the pragmatic problems most frequently encountered with language-impaired children (Johnson et al., 1984). Children with autism initiate very little conversational behavior—even less than do other children with language impairments (Loveland et al., 1988). Of clinical interest is how the child initiates the conversation and how successful the child is in having the conversation continue (Roth & Spekman, 1984a).

Method
It is best to get the listener's attention before initiating a conversation. This is usually accomplished by eye contact and a greeting. The language-impaired child may begin without any greeting or may interrupt an ongoing conversation with

"Hey." Some children use the same opener repeatedly (e.g., "Guess what?"), whatever the conversational context.

Data may need to be collected over a wide variety of situations to discern a pattern. Role play can be used to determine the child's knowledge of conventional openers.

Frequency and Success Rate

Children who are withdrawn or unsure of the conversational expectations may initiate conversations only rarely. Instead, they adopt a more passive, responsive role. In contrast, other children may interrupt frequently and attempt to initiate conversation indiscriminately. Of interest to the speech-language pathologist is the density of initiations or the number of initiations over a given time. Obviously, this figure will change with the situation. For children, lunchtime, recess, or group projects may be appropriate forums in which to collect such data.

The success rate of children in initiating conversations is also significant. Although children may attempt to begin conversations frequently, they may be ignored or mocked depending on the audiences they choose. Each of us has experienced the "cold shoulder" at least once. Socially inappropriate children may experience more than their share.

Topic Initiation

Once a conversation has been initiated, the participants negotiate the topics that will be discussed. This negotiation process begins with one partner introducing a topic; the other partner(s) agrees to adopt that topic by commenting on it, disagrees by changing the topic, or ends the conversation. Mature language users identify the topic clearly by name and, if in the immediate context, by pointing. Preschool childen and those with language impairments rely more on non-linguistic cues, such as pointing to and holding or shaking objects.

In general, language-impaired children are less adept than both their age-matched and language-age-matched peers in their ability to direct the conversation by introducing topics (Donahue, 1983). This lack of ability might reflect difficulty introducing topics clearly and/or these children's limited lists of potential topics (Bedrosian, 1985; Dollaghan & Miller, 1986).

Method

An effectively initiated topic is identified clearly in order to establish mutual regard. As mentioned, the speaker may point, look at, and/or state the topic. Generally, the speaker provides information the listener needs to identify referents and their relationships. Topics are negotiated between speakers, and even when explicitly stated, topics are based on the shared assumptions of each participant.

In general, the less sure the speaker is that the listener knows the topic, the longer the speaker will take to introduce it. The more mature speaker is adept at presupposing the prior knowledge of the listener(s). In return for the introduction, listeners assure speakers that they understand, or they ask for clarification when they do not understand.

Topics are typically changed by stating a new one. Older elementary school children, adolescents, and adults increasingly use a conversational technique called *shadowing* in which the conversation is steered from one topic to a closely related one. Adult conversations only occasionally contain very disparate topics.

The language-impaired child may not establish topics, preferring to adopt those of others. If the child does introduce topics, there may be little or no background information to aid the listener. The language-impaired child may have a very restricted set of conversational or topic openers or may rely on a stereotypic utterance (e.g., ''Guess what?''). Children with emotional difficulties may continue some internal conversation with the assumption that the listener has been privy to this information. As mentioned previously, children with word-finding difficulties or poor vocabularies may rely on nonspecific nouns, such as *one* or *thing*. Nonspecific verbs, such as *do* and *get*, may also be used frequently.

The child's response to the openers of others may be noncontingent or off topic. The child may not be able to identify the topic or to determine what response is required to the partner's opener.

Both the linguistic and nonlinguistic aspects of the sample should be analyzed. The nonlinguistic aspects regulate the linguistic ones and are significant in the regulation of turn initiation and termination, topic choice, and interruptions (Argyle & Cook, 1976; Craig, 1979; Duncan, 1974; Prutting, 1982; Rosenfeld, 1978).

Frequency and Success Rate

As with conversational initiation, the density and success rate of topic initiation are noteworthy. In general, less dominant speakers will introduce fewer topics and will be less successful in having their topics adopted by their partners. Lack of success may also indicate problems with topicalization, such as establishing and commenting on, marking changes in, and maintaining the topic for a sufficient length of time (Johnson et al., 1984). Related factors to be evaluated are the articulation clarity, degree of completeness, and form of the topic statement; social adaptation of the child's language style; degree of content relevance to the ongoing activity and to listener interests; use of eye contact; and physical proximity (Roth & Spekman, 1984a).

Appropriateness

The appropriateness of a topic is determined by the context. Some topics, such as the weather, are always appropriate, whereas others, such as age, income, or sexual behavior, are appropriate only in limited contexts. Each of us has favorite topics. We tend to talk about what we know.

The speech-language pathologist is interested in determining the child's favorite topics and in assessing their appropriateness in context. Although some topics will work in one context, they are inappropriate for others. Some language-impaired children have only limited topics or perseverate on a few regardless of the context.

Conversation and Topic Maintenance

Once a topic is introduced, speakers comment on that topic, each sentence reflecting the general discourse topic. In effective conversations, the participants seem to adhere to four principles: stay on topic, be truthful, be brief, and be relevant (Roth & Spekman, 1984a).

Each partner depends on the contingency or relatedness of a response to the preceding utterance. Each response should add new information on the topic. The topic must be mentioned frequently enough to enable both participants to recall it as the conversation progresses, because the topic becomes less specific with subsequent reference.

Topic continuance may be signaled by maintenance devices, such as *Now, Well, And then, In any case, Next, So, I* (you, we, they) (did something). Some devices, called *continuants*, maintain the conversation but add little if any new information. Examples of this behavior include *yeah, uh-huh,* and *okay* when used as a signal that the listener is paying attention. Other maintenance devices include repeating a portion or all of the previous utterance.

Children with language impairments tend to engage in fewer and shorter interactions than do nonimpaired children. The most frequent pragmatic problems for language-impaired children include terminating sentences, connecting discourse, listening and responding to the speaker, knowing when to take a turn, and knowing how to ask and answer questions (Johnson et al., 1984).

Although there is little difference between the turn-taking skills of language-impaired and nonimpaired children at the one-word level, a disparity occurs and widens as language becomes increasingly more complex (Foster, 1985; Prelock, Messick, Schwartz, & Terrell, 1981; Reichle, Busch, & Doyle, 1986). Autistic children may not respond to initiations while other language-impaired children may overuse turn-fillers of acknowledgments (*Uh-huh*) to keep the conversation going (Bedrosian, 1988; Brinton & Fujiki, 1989; Dewey & Everard, 1974).

Frequency of Contingency

Contingent or semantically contingent utterances relate to or reflect the meaning of the prior utterance. One example of contingency is the topic of an utterance. Thus, a contingent utterance maintains the topic of the previous utterance and adds to it in some way. For example, in response to the utterance ''We went to Captain Jake's for dinner last night,'' a second speaker might make the contingent remark ''Oh, did you enjoy the food?'' A noncontingent remark would be ''My uncle lives on a farm.''

Assume for a moment that the name of the restaurant in the previous example was Uncle Jake's. In this situation, the child's remark, although off topic, does have some link to the previous sentence. If these links can be identified, there may be a pattern that will reveal the child's processing strategy.

In general, language-impaired children are less reponsive than are their age-matched nonimpaired peers (Rosinski-McClendon & Newhoff, 1987; Siegel, Cunningham, & van der Spuy, 1979). This low level of responsiveness may reflect a history of unsuccessful communication. Often, these children respond to questions with stereotypic acknowledgements (*uh-huh, yeh*) and with nonspecific requests for clarification (*what, huh*) (Fey et al., 1981; Rosinski-McClendon & Newhoff, 1987; Watson, 1977).

The frequency of contingent behaviors by the child and caregiver is of interest. The child who exhibits few contingent utterances may prefer to initiate new topics frequently (Prutting, 1983). The speech-language pathologist notes the percentage of the child's utterances that are on topic, the relevance of the child's questions, and the child's nonverbal responses, such as following directions or looking at something that was mentioned.

A large percentage of off-topic responses may indicate a semantic disorder characterized by difficulty in identifying the topic of discussion. A listener's ability to identify a topic subsequently affects comprehension of comments made about that topic.

The speech-language pathologist should look for underlying contingency that may not be readily obvious. Children with language learning disabilities may assume that their partners know the underlying relationship and, therefore, may only include unshared information.

Of particular interest are the child's responses to questions. Such responses should be appropriate to the question and factually correct. For example, the question "Why is he eating?" might elicit the following responses from different children:

1. Food.
2. Because.
3. He has to.
4. So he won't be hungry.
5. He's hungry.

The first answer is functionally inappropriate although functionally accurate. It does not answer the question but tells what the man is eating. The second and third responses are appropriate but too brief to be accurate. The fourth and fifth answers fulfill appropriateness and accuracy criteria.

If an answer does not fulfill both requirements, it is in error and may indicate any number of possible breakdowns in the communication process. I have seen a severely emotionally disordered client give extremely inappropriate replies to emotional or personal questions, although her responses to factual questions were usually both appropriate and accurate.

A language-impaired child may not understand what the speech-language pathologist or the question requires or may not realize that a reply is required. The question form and the specific *wh-* question type may also be confusing.

In general, recognition and delivery of the general kind of information required develops prior to the ability to respond with the accurate information. Some *wh-* question forms seem easier than others (Parnell & Amerman, 1983; Parnell, Patterson, & Harding, 1984). Three groupings, from easiest to most difficult, are as follows:

Easiest	What + be, which, where
	Who, whose, what + do
Most difficult	When, why, what happened, how

This order suggests a hierarchy for analysis and intervention. In addition, it is easier for children to respond to questions referring to objects, persons, or events within the immediate setting.

Various semantic question prompts can be used to facilitate production of the child's inadequate responses (Blank, Rose, & Berlin, 1978). The child's responses to these prompts can provide useful information for intervention. Table 5.3 shows a procedure for comparing the efficacy of various prompts in eliciting appropriate and accurate responses from the child. A plus sign (+) indicates appropriate or accurate responses; a minus sign indicates inappropriate or inaccurate ones (Parnell et al., 1984).

Latency of Contingency

When the child makes contingent responses, there should be little delay or latency between his or her turn and the preceding speaker's turn. Gaps between the turns of mature speakers are brief or nonexistent (Sacks, Schegloff, & Jefferson, 1974). Research has indicated that the average amount of time needed for two adults to switch from one speaker to the next is a half second or less.

Preschoolers and language-impaired chldren may allow long gaps to develop without any of the apparent embarrassment found among adults when there are long unfilled pauses. A noticeable latency prior to the child's response may indicate word-finding difficulties. Frequently, the linguistically more mature partner will fill in for the child, an act that also violates the rules of turn taking.

Latency is an important measure for both contingent and noncontingent utterances, whether adjacent or nonadjacent. Delay may be evident in the adjacent utterances of a child with word-finding difficulties as well. Adjacent utterances are spoken as sequential behaviors by the same speaker. A nonadjacent utterance crosses conversational turns and is an utterance or turn of one partner followed by an utterance or turn of the other. Definitions and examples of these categories are presented in Table 5.4.

Duration of Topic

A topic is sustained as long as each conversational partner cares to continue and can contribute relevant information. The number of turns taken on a topic is a function of the particular topic and partners involved, the conversational context, and the conversational skill of each participant.

TABLE 5.3
Score form for the efficacy of various question prompts

Prompt Type	Strategy Description	Prompt Effectiveness (+, −)		Comments
		Appropriate	Accurate	
Standard focusing phrase with repetition	*Listen to the question* signals the student that a response was in error. Direct student's attention to the repetition; highlights content			
Model example with related content	Use another adult or child in context to model correct response. Then ask child, same form, new content			
Analogous examples	*What are alligators covered with?*—No response. *Seals are covered with fur. What are alligators covered with?*			
Visualization of relationships	*How are an apple and a cookie alike?* No response. Draw semantic feature chart:			

	bakes	eat	grows on tree
apple	+	+	+
cookie	+	+	−

Prompt Type	Strategy Description	Appropriate	Accurate	Comments
Relevant comparison yes/no	*What does a hockey player need?* No response. *Does a hockey player need skates? Yes. Good. What does he need?*			

The child's inadequate responses can be modified by using question prompts. Successful responses following a prompt are recorded as a + under both the *appropriate* and *accurate* columns.
Source: Moeller, M., Osberger, M., & Eccarius, M. (1986). Cognitively based strategies for use with hearing-impaired students with comprehension deficits. Reprinted from *Topics in Language Disorders*, Vol. 6, No. 4, p. 40, with permission of Aspen Publishers, Inc., © September 1986.

Number of Turns

The speech-language pathologist is interested in the number of turns taken by the child and partner on a given topic and in the manner of changing topic. In general, there will be a greater number of turns in an adult-child conversation if the child rather than the adult initiates the topic. Topics that are sustained longer than others may suggest the child's interest or knowledge, or both.

Below age 3, children rarely maintain a topic for more than two turns (Bloom et al., 1976). In general, preschoolers take very few turns on a single topic unless enacting scenarios, describing events, or solving problems (Schober-Peterson &

TABLE 5.4
Definitions and examples of utterance pairs

Types	Definitions	Examples
Contingent	The utterance of one speaker is based on the content, form, and intent of the other speaker.	S_1: What do you want for lunch? S_2: Peanut butter. S_1: I hope I don't miss my plane. S_2: Don't worry. Every flight is delayed.
Noncontingent	The utterance of one speaker is not based on that of the other.	S_1: What do you want for lunch? S_2: Gran'ma gots a new car.
Adjacent	Utterances spoken sequentially by the same speaker.	We went to the zoo. I saw monkeys and elephants. But my favorite part was petting the sheeps.
Nonadjacent	Utterances spoken sequentially by different speakers. The utterances may be contingent or noncontingent	S_1: Here comes the school bus. S_2: Yukk, I was hoping he'd get a flat tire. (Contingent)

Johnson, 1989). Although the number of turns increases slightly with age, there is not a great increase until midelementary school. More turns will generally be produced when the preschool child is directing the partner through a task or when the child is telling a story.

Informativeness
Each turn should add to the conversation by confirming the topic and contributing additional information. Children who have difficulty identifying the topic or determining what is expected of them conversationally may repeat or paraphrase old information, overuse continuants, or circumlocute. Circumlocution occurs when the child is unable to identify the topic or retrieve needed words and, thus, talks around the topic in a nonspecific manner. The speech-language pathologist can rate each utterance for its contribution to the topic being discussed.

Sequencing
Once a topic is introduced, a sequence of conversational acts follows. In general, more specific information is introduced until there is a natural termination or a change in topic. Answers or replies follow questions, comments or questions follow comments. New information is introduced and later referred to as old information, as mentioned previously. A lack of sequencing may indicate a semantic

disorder or a pragmatic disorder characterized by a lack of presuppositional abilities.

Turn Taking

Turn taking is an excellent vehicle for evaluating the interactional framework of the listener and speaker. The unit of analysis is the dyad and the interaction rather than the individual behaviors of the child (Prutting, 1982).

The rules of turn taking (Sacks, Schegloff, & Jefferson, 1974) specify that if there are only two participants, both have speaking turns. In general, children's conversations consist primarily of this nonsimultaneous talking pattern (Craig & Washington, 1986). If there are more than two, however, no participant is guaranteed a speaking turn. There is usually only one speaker at a time. If two or more speak simultaneously, all but one withdraw. Children with emotional disturbances may interrupt frequently and ask and answer the same question within their single turn.

The listener(s) pays attention to the speaker and demonstrates this behavior by turning toward or looking at the speaker, not interrupting, and/or acknowledging that he or she has heard and understood the speaker. Eye contact among children with language learning disabilities and emotional disturbances is often fleeting or nonexistent.

The minimum number of turns to complete an exchange is three. The person who begins the exchange must have a second turn before an interaction has occurred, for example:

SPEAKER 1: We just returned from Florida.
SPEAKER 2: Oh, did you go to Disney World?
SPEAKER 1: No, we were in Fort Lauderdale.

Each full conversational turn consists of three elements: an acknowledgment of the preceding utterance, a contribution by the present speaker, and an indication that the turn is to be shifted. In the preceding example, the previous turns are acknowledged by *oh* and *no*. Indications of turn allocation may consist of questions (as with speaker 2), intonational markers, and pauses.

Transitions across speakers are orderly, occurring at transition points signaled by the participants. For example, the speaker will look at or address the listener when about to change a turn. The listener may look away, gesture, become restless, or emit an audible sigh when desiring a turn. A really anxious listener may cut off the last few syllables of the speaker's turn without disrupting the topic. Language-impaired children often do not use these subtle turn indicators and miss their signal value when used by others (Rees & Wollner, 1981).

Finally, the speaker who wishes to continue a turn may increase the speed or intensity of talking and continue through the transition point. If overlap occurs and interferes with understanding, the speaker "repairs" the misunderstood portion.

Children with language impairments may fail to follow many of the turn-taking rules. For example, children with emotional handicaps may interrupt the speaker before the turn has ended, may ask and answer their own questions, and may take another speaker's turn (Rees & Wollner, 1981).

The speech-language pathologist marks the transcript as turns 1-2-3 for each exchange. Of particular interest are the location and cause of exchange breakdown, eye contact, and turn allocation signaling. In addition, the frequency, variety or range, and consistency of the child's communication are noted. In other words, the child should initiate, add to, and terminate exchanges. Within each turn, the speech-language pathologist notes the presence or absence of the three aspects of a full turn and the average amount of time spent in a turn (Roth & Spekman, 1984a). The speech-language pathologist can also examine the effects of adult behaviors on the child's conversational turns, and later, can help adults to develop more facilitative styles.

Density

The speech-language pathologist is interested in the density of turns within each conversation and on various topics. A low density may indicate that the child's conversational partner dominated the conversation by taking very long turns, relinquishing them to the child only occasionally, or that the child was very reticent. Children with autism may take relatively few verbal turns, thus leaving the partner to fill the void (Loveland et al., 1988). In contrast, if the child talked for lengthy turns, the density would also be low because the listener would have little chance to reply.

Latency

The speech-language pathologist can summarize the overall contingent and noncontingent latencies of the child. Whereas the average adult-to-adult turn changes within about half a second, the child may be slightly slower to react. Longer periods and/or the continual use of fillers and interjections may indicate difficulties with topic identification or word finding.

Duration of Turns

There is no ideal length for a turn, although most listeners know when a turn has continued for too long. We all know at least one incessant talker who doesn't know when enough has been said. A child who talks incessantly may be a child who is exhibiting a semantic disorder of not knowing what information is needed to close the topic, a pragmatic disorder of not knowing the mechanisms for closing a topic, or a processing problem of not being certain what information was conveyed.

The speech-language pathologist is interested in the average length of the child's and partner's turns. Different situations, partners, and topics may yield clinically significant differences in the length of these turns.

Type of Overlap

Most turns will be nonsimultaneous (Craig & Evans, 1989). However, overlap or simultaneous speech can be very revealing. In general, there are two types of overlap: *internal* and *initial* (Gallagher & Craig, 1982). Sentence internal overlaps are used to complete the other speaker's turn and secure a turn. This ability requires a high level of pragmatic-linguistic knowledge. The child with a language impairment may interrupt internally, but in a way that indicates a lack of understanding of this process. The child may add new information or change the topic rather than complete the other speaker's utterance (Craig & Evans, 1989).

Sentence initial overlaps result when the listener interjects between sentences in order to secure a turn. This may occur when the listener is unsure of the speaker's intention to continue or when the listener wants to gain a turn at speaking. Continual overlaps of this type may indicate a breakdown in turn taking as a result of the behavior of one or both partners. In contrast, a low incidence of interrupting, as noted among specifically language-impaired (SLI) children, may indicate passivity or an inability to initiate a "turn grab" (Craig & Evans, 1989).

Frequency of overlap.   Although it may seem counterintuitive, data indicate that, as a group, children with language impairments exhibit less simultaneous speech in their conversation (Craig & Evans, 1989). Although language-impaired children may be responsive, they tend to be passive in initiating interaction or turn taking (Fey & Leonard, 1983).

Duration of overlap.   The adult rules for turn taking state that when there is an overlap in turns (when two speakers speak at once) one speaker will withdraw. Young children or children with language impairments may continue to talk or try to outshout their partners. Some children withdraw habitually. The speech-language pathologist must determine whether the child in question is more likely to withdraw or to continue talking.

How Signaled?

Changes in turn are signaled very subtly. The language-impaired child may miss such signals. Occasionally, such a child will respond only to questions, knowing that in this situation a response is required. Other children lack a basic understanding of the expectation to reply within a conversation. Still others cannot decipher the language code efficiently enough to respond.

Conversation and Topic Termination

Conversations or topics are ended when no new information is added. In the case of a conversational termination, the topic is not changed. As with the opening of a conversation, there are often adjacency pairs, such as "Bye, see ya"-"Have a nice day" or "Thank you"-"You're welcome."

Preschool or language-impaired children may end the conversation abruptly when they decide that it is over, occasionally just "turning tail" and exiting the conversational context. Children with a language learning disability may not prepare the listener for the termination of the conversation by signaling with body language, for example, becoming restless, looking away, or looking at a watch. In the opposite extreme, children with a language learning disability or emotional disorder may be unable or unwilling to end the conversation and may perseverate or continue to ask questions which have already been answered.

Topics are usually terminated by shifting to another related topic. For more mature language users this process is accomplished by *shadowing,* in which the speakers shift to a closely related topic, as in the following exchange:

SPEAKER 1: I biked along the canal path yesterday.
SPEAKER 2: Oh, I love to bike there at this time of year.
SPEAKER 1: I didn't know you bike. What sort of bike do you have?
SPEAKER 2: I have an inexpensive twelve-speed.
SPEAKER 1: I have a ten-speed . . .

The original topic of the canal bike path slid into the topic of bicycles.

Whether topics are shadowed or changed abruptly, there is some continuity, and the new topic is clearly stated as mentioned previously. When there is little left to discuss on a given topic, the conversation shifts. The speech-language pathologist notes the method the child uses to terminate and change topics and to terminate conversations.

Contingent Queries

Contingent queries or requests for clarification signal the listener's attentiveness or understanding and skill in addressing the point of conversational breakdown. Conversations may be maintained by use of contingent queries or requests for additional information, such as *Huh?, What?,* and *I don't understand.* Contingent queries maintain the conversation by indicating the point of breakdown, obligating the speaker to clarify, and specifying the appropriate form for that clarification.

The type of contingent query varies with the linguistic maturity of the speaker and with the information sought. In general, young children use unspecific requests, such as *Huh?* and *What?* More mature speakers try to specify the information desired, as in the following exchange:

SPEAKER 1: ''We went to the zoo and saw monkeys in big cages.''
SPEAKER 2: ''What was in the cages?'' (Or ''Where were the monkeys?'', ''Where did you go?'')

Appropriate contingent queries and responses by the child demonstrate an awareness of the cooperative nature of conversation. Not only must the child attend to the partner's message, detect misunderstandings, and initiate an appropriate request, but he or she must also possess the knowledge and willingness to use clarification strategies to aid the partner's comprehension (Dollaghan, 1987a; Donahue, 1984).

The child who continually responds with *Huh?* or *What?* may not be attending to the conversation or may have difficulty understanding. In the classroom, such children may rely on routines to make the world understandable. In this case, the child may often look around at the other children for assurance before performing the expected behavior.

The speech-language pathologist is interested in the degree to which the child requests additional information toward maintaining the conversation and in the form of these requests. These conversational mechanisms can be triggered in conversation by garbling or confusing the message. This can be accomplished by mumbling, failing to establish the topic, or providing insufficient information or confusing instructions.

The language-impaired child may be unaware that communication breakdown has occurred. The speech-language pathologist can hypothesize the child's awareness of misunderstanding and confirm the hypothesis through manipulation of utterances addressed to the child. In general, children first gain awareness of breakdowns caused by unintelligible words. The order of awareness to breakdown may be as follows (Dollaghan & Kaston, 1986):

> Unintelligible word
> Impossible command
> Unrealistically long utterance
> Unfamiliar word
> Question or statement without an introduction and ambiguous, inexplicit, and open-ended statements.

Frequency and Form

In general, preschool or language-impaired children, such as those with LLD, tend to blame themselves rather than the speaker for misunderstanding (Meline & Brackin, 1987). Thus, these children use fewer clarification requests than might be expected, especially given the greater likelihood of communication breakdown (Brinton, & Fujiki, 1982; Donahue, 1984; Donahue, Pearl, & Bryan, 1980; Lee, Kamhi, & Nelson, 1983). The requests produced tend to be less specific, reflecting the difficulty encountered with these forms. In short, LLD children do not accept the responsibility of the listener to signal miscomprehension, even when taught the procedures for doing so (Donahue, 1984). Instead, these children assume that the speaker will be unambiguous, informative, and clear.

Children's clarification strategies can be assessed in different contexts, such as familiar topics, unfamiliar topics, and contrived pragmatic violations by the speech-language pathologist (Moeller et al., 1986). The child's attempts to clarify the information can be recorded on a form such as that in Table 5.5. Check marks in the appropriate spaces would signal the child's attempts to repair and clarify.

Although there are no norms for the frequency of clarification requests, there are general guidelines that indicate a change in both the frequency and type of contingent query with age. The earliest requests for clarification are repetitions of the partner's utterance with rising intonation (*Doggie go ride?*) or neutral requests for repetition (*What?*). With age, requests become more specific and increase in frequency, although both vary according to the conversational partner.

TABLE 5.5
Record of clarification requests

Clarification Skills	Familiar Topic	New Topic	Contrived Pragmatic Violation
Fails to seek clarification			

Indicates nonunderstanding
—nonverbally
    puzzled expression
    shrugs shoulders
—verbally
    asks for repetition
    says/signs *What?*
    I don't understand
    I don't remember			

Indicates inability to answer
    I don't remember
    I don't know the word for it
    I can't explain it			

Requests specific clarification
    What did you say about
    the ____?
    What does ____ mean?			

A pattern of clarification requests may evolve as the speech-language pathologist records the number of requests by type and by conversational context of the familiar or new topic, or contrived violation. Contrived errors or violations can be used to elicit requests for clarification.
Source: Moeller, M., Osberger, M., & Eccarius, M. (1986). Cognitively based strategies for use with hearing-impaired students with comprehension deficits. Reprinted from *Topics in Language Disorders*, Vol. 6, No. 4, p. 41, with permission of Aspen Publishers, Inc., 211 September 1986.

With an adult partner, 24- to 36-month-olds use approximately 7 requests an hour, and 54- to 66-month-olds use approximately 14 (Fey & Leonard, 1984; Gallagher, 1981). When the partner is a familiar peer, the mean rate for 36- to 66-month-olds is 30 per hour (Fey & Leonard, 1984; Garvey, 1977). Obviously, there is greater likelihood of misunderstanding when two preschool peers communicate.

Conversational Repair

Conversational repair may be spontaneous or in response to a contingent query. Preschool children spontaneously repair very little. Even in first grade, children spontaneously repair only about one-third of their conversational breakdowns. Young children or children with language impairments often do not attempt to repair communication breakdowns. Children with unintelligible speech may find their repairs as unintelligible as their initial attempts.

Most 10-year-olds are able to determine communication breakdown and repair the damage (Lempers & Elrod, 1983). Although LLD children at that age can identify faulty messages, they do not seem to understand when to use these skills (Donahue et al., 1980).

By age 2, most children respond consistently to neutral requests for clarification (Gallagher, 1977, 1981; Tomasello, Farrar, & Dines, 1984), although they are more likely to respond if the conversational partner is an adult rather than another child. Two-year-olds also tend to overuse "yes" and thus confirm interpretations even when incorrect, possibly because nonconfirmation requires clarification. By age 3 to 5, children respond correctly, even to specific requests, about 80% of the time regardless of the partner (Anselmi, Tomasello, & Acunzo, 1986; Garvey, 1977).

Repair can provide valuable information about communication breakdowns. The speech-language pathologist should note the cause of breakdown, the presence or absence of a repair attempt, the identity of the repair initiator, the repair strategy used, and the outcome (Roth & Spekman, 1984a). Breakdown can occur for a number of reasons, including lack of intelligibility, volume, completeness of information, degree of complexity, inappropriateness, irrelevance, and lack of mutual attention, visual regard, or mutual desire (Garvey, 1975; Keenan & Schieffelin, 1976). In general, children with language impairments experience a greater number of breakdowns than do age-matched non-LLD peers (MacLachlan & Chapman, 1988; Fey, Warr-Leeper, Webber, & Disher, 1988).

Repairs usually focus on the linguistic structure (Clark & Andersen, 1979) or on the content or nature of the information conveyed (Garvey, 1977). They may use extralinguistic signals, such as pointing, to clarify. These strategies are not mutually exclusive. In general, successful outcome is related to the explicitness and appropriateness of the repair strategy chosen.

When the child repairs spontaneously, the nature of the original error and the repair attempts should be noted. The speech-language pathologist scans the transcript for all fillers, repetitions, perseverations, and long pauses. All of these may indicate word-finding difficulties on the child's part. The original error or repair attempt may be based on any number of relationships with the intended word or phrase, as noted in Table 5.6.

Spontaneous versus Listener-Initiated

The speech-language pathologist is interested in the percentage of conversational repairs that are self- or listener-initiated. Usually listeners signal a breakdown with facial expression, body posture, and/or a contingent query.

Strategy

Immature speakers usually respond to listener-initiated requests for clarification by restating the previous utterance. First graders and younger children will repeat only once in response to a request before becoming irritated. By second

TABLE 5.6

Relationship of word-finding errors and repair attempts to the intended word

Association	Example
Definition	*the thing you cook food on* for *stove*
Description	*the long skinny one with no legs* for *snake*
	book holder for *bookend*
	fuzzy for *peach*
Generic (less specific)	*do* for more specific verb
	hat for *cap, bonnet, scarf,*, etc.
	thing or *one* for name of entity
Opposites	*sit* for *stand*
Partial	*ball . . . big ball . . . red ball* for *big red ball*
Semantic category	*stove* for *refrigerator* (both are appliances)
Sound	*toe* for *tie* (initial sound similar)
	goat for *coat* (rhyme)

grade, children are usually willing to repeat twice before becoming angry. Continued requests may also result in children providing additional information, although children with language impairments seem less flexible in the use of this strategy (Brinton, Fujiki, & Sonnenberg, 1988).

More mature speakers usually give additional information or reformulate rather than repeat the utterance. Using their presuppositional skills, such speakers may also hypothesize about the supposed point of breakdown and supply more information on this specific area. When requested to clarify, language-impaired children tend to respond less frequently and with less complex responses than do their nonimpaired peers (Brinton & Fujiki, 1982; Brinton, Fujiki, Winkler, & Loeb, 1986). The responses of language-impaired children lack flexibility and usually consist of repetition with little new information included to aid comprehension. Nonimpaired children seem to have a greater range of repair strategies (Brinton, Fujiki, & Sonnenberg, 1988). The 10-year-old LLD child is more likely to repeat rather than reformulate unsuccessful utterances (Feagans & Short, 1986).

The speech-language pathologist should prepare a list of the various types of contingent queries and use them in conversation with the child. Of interest is the child's rate of responding to various requests and the nature of the child's response (Fey et al., 1988).

Frequency of Success

The speech-language pathologist is interested in how successfully the child identifies breakdowns, repairs them spontaneously, and follows listener requests. In general, language-impaired children make more inappropriate responses to listener requests than do age-matched peers (Brinton et al., 1988). The responses of the listener enable the speech-language pathologist to determine the child's success.

CONVERSATIONAL PARTNER

Language does not occur in a vacuum. Children converse with many conversational partners, both at home and in school. Each partner helps to form a dynamic context in which the child communicates and learns.

Parent-child interactions offer an example of a communication process finely attuned to the language skills of the child (Snow, 1979). Thus, the adult-child dyad represents a highly individualized learning exchange based on the interactional styles and skills of the two communicators (Lieven, 1978).

Variables that affect language learning are complexity, semantic relatedness, redundancy, maternal responsiveness, and reciprocity. In general, maternal linguistic complexity seems to be related to the language learner's level of comprehension.

Semantically related utterances provide a contingency-based language-learning experience. The topic and subsequent content are usually derived from the child. Approximately 68% of the mother's speech is directly related to the child's verbal, vocal, and nonverbal behavior (Cross, 1977; Snow, 1977).

The mother's input tends to be highly redundant because it relates to ongoing contextual occurrences and attempts to explain, clarify, and comment on the child's experiences and behavior. In addition, the caregiver may repeat content several times in different forms.

Consistent maternal responsiveness teaches children that their responses and behavior have a predictable effect (Beckwith, Cohen, Kopp, Parmelee, & Marcy, 1976; Bradley & Caldwell, 1976). One valuable lesson the child learns is that communication and communication partners are predictable.

These caregiver-child exchanges are reciprocal in that the child is treated as a full conversational partner and allowed to gain early conversational experience (Bateson, 1975; Stern, 1971; Stern, Jaffee, Beebe, & Bennett, 1975). Even infants are treated as full conversational partners by their mothers.

There is indication that some mothers of language-impaired children provide input that is not regulated by their children's level of understanding and, thus, it is significantly longer and more complex than their children's level of comprehension (Tiegerman & Siperstein, 1984). The MLU may be near that found in adult-adult communication and may include complex structures, such as indirect directives, embedded constructions, and how/why questions (Buium, Rynders, & Turnure, 1974; Tiegerman & Siperstein, 1982).

The proportion of utterances of mothers of language-impaired children that are semantically related is lower than that reported for mothers of nonimpaired children (Tiegerman & Siperstein, 1984). In addition, the form of these utterances may be highly restricted, providing the child with a limited variety of input. Because few of the maternal utterances are semantically related, there is little redundancy. Instead, mothers discuss events in the past or future and objects or events not present within the immediate shared context.

Language-impaired children may have little effect on the conversational interaction, and their verbal and nonverbal behaviors may be ignored. Mothers may persist in introducing new topics, reflecting this non-child-centered approach. Mothers of language-impaired children may be more dominant in conversations than are mothers of nonimpaired children, and they may initiate conversation and use directives more frequently (Loveland et al., 1988). In short, these interactions often lack the qualities of language-learning conversational exchanges.

Especially when working with preschool children, the speech-language pathologist should observe the conversational behavior of the primary caregiver and determine the language-learning contributions. Utterances can be rated as to semantic relatedness, redundancy, and reciprocity. From these data, the speech-language pathologist can comment on the overall teaching environment provided by the caregiver's utterances and behaviors.

CONCLUSION

A language sample is a rich source of information on the child and conversational partner's language abilities. Analysis may be accomplished at the individual utterance, as in Chapter 4, across utterance and across partner, and by conversational event. Obviously, this entire analysis would not be attempted unless the speech-language pathologist had a thorough description and understanding of the child's language. Then a language sample would be analyzed to examine the portion of that language in question. A conversational sample can be the best example of a child's actual language use in context. If the goal is to train language that works in these contexts, then the speech-language pathologist must first determine how that language is presently working.

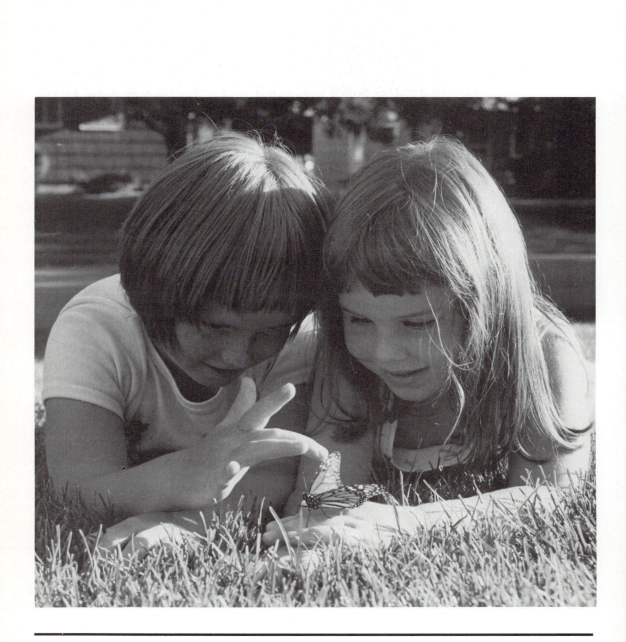

6
Narrative Analysis

Narratives are an important part of the language assessment of older school-aged children, because they provide an uninterrupted sample of the child's language, which the child modifies to capture and hold the listener's interest (Chappell, 1980; Crais & Chapman, 1987; Culatta, Page, & Ellis, 1983; Johnston, 1982; Liles, 1985, 1987; Scott, 1988). Although narration and conversation share many qualities, they also differ in very significant ways. First, narratives are extended units of text. Second, events within narratives are linked to one another temporally or causally in predictable ways. Narratives are organized in a cohesive, predictable, rule-governed manner representing temporal and causal patterns of relating information not found in conversation. Finally, the speaker maintains a social monologue throughout. The speaker must produce language that is relevant to the overall narrative while remaining mindful of the information needed by the listener.

Many professionals incorrectly equate narratives with fictional storytelling. This misunderstanding leads to narrative evaluation consisting of the child recounting fairytales or formulating stories from pictures. For the purposes of language analysis, we consider *oral narration* to include the telling of self-generated stories, storytelling of familiar tales, retelling of movies or television shows, and recounting of personal experiences. Most conversations include narratives of this latter type. How often we begin conversations with ''You'll never believe what happened to me coming to work today'' or ''Let me tell you what it means to get into a hassle.''

Although conversation and narratives share many elements, such as a

sense of purpose, relevant information, clear and orderly exchange of information, repair, and ability to assume the perspective of the listener, they are not the
same thing (Roth, 1986). Conversations are dialogues, whereas narratives are es-
sentially decontextualized monologues.

In decontextualized narratives the language does not center on some ongoing activity but usually communicates some experience not directly shared by the
speaker and listener. In order to share the experience, the speaker must present
an explicit, topic-centered discussion that clearly states sequential and causal relationships.

The major characteristics found in narratives but not in conversation are the
agentive focus and the temporal contingent structure (Longacre, 1983). Narratives are about people, animals, or imaginary characters engaged in events over
time. Other differences include the narrative use of extended units of text, introduction and organizing sequences that lead to a narrative conclusion, and the
relatively passive listener role that provides only minimal informational support
to narratives (Roth, 1986).

The narrative speaker is responsible for ordering and providing all of the
information in an organized whole (Roth & Spekman, 1985). Narratives, therefore, are found more frequently in the communication of more mature speakers
and should be included in an analysis of the language of school-aged children.
Hedberg and Stoel-Gammon (1986) summarize the clinical importance as follows:

> Narrative analysis is one of the most valuable skills a language clinician can possess.
> People of all ages from all cultures experience stories daily . . . in representing events
> in their own lives and in participating in the happenings, both real and imaginary, in
> the lives of others. Knowledge of story structure contributes to people's understand-
> ing of how the world functions, facilitating predictions of actions and consequences,
> causes and effects. (p. 58)

Some studies have failed to find significant differences between the narratives of language-impaired and nonimpaired children (Hedberg & Fink, 1985;
Klecan-Aker, 1985; Ripich & Griffith, 1985; Roth & Spekman, 1989). In general,
though, the narratives of language-impaired and language learning disabled
(LLD) children are shorter and less mature and have less mature episode and sentence structure than those of age-matched nonimpaired peers (Merritt & Liles,
1987, 1990; Roth & Spekman, 1986). Possibly because of the communication demands placed on the child in narration, the narratives of LLD children exhibit a
greater rate of communication breakdown in the form of stalls, repairs, and aban-
doned utterances (MacLachlan & Chapman, 1988). Although language learning
disabled and non-LLD children display similar patterns of cohesion, such as the
use of conjunctions and unambiguous reference, LLD children are less efficient in
their use (Klecan-Aker, 1984; Liles, 1985). In general, children with language
learning disabilities use fewer conjunctions and exhibit more ambiguous reference, often failing to consider the needs of their audience (Liles, 1987). The internal story organization of language-impaired children is also less complete than

that of age-matched peers (Merritt & Liles, 1987). The narratives of language-impaired children contain more statements that are not integrated into the episode structure than do those of nonimpaired children. Usually, such children have difficulty describing and manipulating props and activities (Sleight & Prinz, 1985).

DEVELOPMENT OF NARRATIVES

Before the appearance of first words, children have well-established notions of agents, actions, and objects, and of the relationships these have to each other and to such notions as location and negation (Bates, 1979; Golinkoff, 1981; Robertson & Suci, 1980). They also have some understanding of familiar events and of the positions of some actions at the beginning, middle, and end of sequences (Bruner, 1975; DeLemos, 1981; Ninio & Bruner, 1978; Ratner & Bruner, 1978). Although children by age 2 possess basic ideas, called *scripts*, about familiar events and sequences, they are not able to describe sequences of events until about age 4 (Karmiloff-Smith, 1981; Nelson & Gruendel, 1979; Peterson & McCabe, 1983; Slobin, 1973).

Children begin to tell self-generated, fictional narratives between the ages of 2 and 3 (Sutton-Smith, 1986). These stories may have a vague plot and usually center on certain highlights in the child's life. There is little recognition of the need to introduce, to explore with, or to orient the listener to the story, and these stories usually lack easily identifiable beginnings, middles, and ends. Disquieting events are the theme and are repeated with endless variation. Frequently children repeat phenomena that they find disruptive or extraordinary in their own lives, such as danger, violence, and deprivation (Ames, 1966).

Two-year-olds usually construct additive chains in which one sentence is added to another, as in "This is kittie. This doggie bowl." There is no storyline, no sequencing, and no cause and effect. The sentences may be moved anywhere in the text without changing the meaning of the entire text. Additive chains may describe a scene, as in "There is kittie. Water in doggie bowl. Doggie sleep." Again, there is no temporal structure.

In these early stories, there is a dominance of performance and textual qualities over text (Sutton-Smith, 1986). Sound production and prosody may be used to move the story along at the expense of information (Scollon & Scollon, 1981). Between 3 and 7 years, children's narratives gradually change from prosodic poetry to prose with plots (Sutton-Smith, 1986).

Temporal event sequences emerge between the ages of 3 and 5. Events follow a logical sequence, for example:

> There is this kittie. He runs to door. Then he goes outside to play. He rolls in the grass and then goes to sleep in the sun.

Although there is sequencing, there is no plot and no cause and effect or causality. Temporal chains often exhibit third person pronouns, past tense verbs, and temporal conjunctions (e.g., *and, then,* and *and then*) and have a definite beginning and ending.

Causal chains are infrequent until ages 5 to 7. Causality involves descriptions of intentions and unobservable states, such as emotions and thoughts, and the use of causal connectives. Although 2- and 3-year-olds have mastered some causal expressions, they are unable to construct coherent causal narratives (Kemper & Edwards, 1986). Their stories consist predominantly of actions from which physical and mental states must be inferred. Initiations and motivations are largely absent.

Causality can be seen, however, in the use of agency, connectives, plans, scripts, and descriptions of mental states used by 2- and 3-year-olds to describe their own behavior (Kemper & Edwards, 1986). A plan is a means or series of actions intended to achieve a specified end. As an intention, a plan is a model of causality. Many of the first words of children refer to intentions and consequences, such as *all gone, there, uh-oh,* and *oh dear.* By age 2½, the child has acquired the words to describe perceptions (*see, hear*), physical states (*tired, hungry*), emotions (*love, hate*), needs, thoughts (*know*), and judgments (*naughty*) (Bretherton & Beeghly, 1982).

Scripts form an individual's expectations about event sequences and, as such, are an attempt to impose order on event information (Johnston, 1982). Based on actual events, scripts are not content free as are story grammars that outline narratives. Scripts influence our interpretation and our telling and retelling of events and narratives.

Children's understanding of *agency,* the ability of humans to initiate actions and to respond with mental states, develops gradually between ages 1 and 3. By age 3, children are also able to describe chains of events within familiar activities, such as a birthday party (Nelson, 1981b). These familiar activity sequences or scripts (Nelson, 1981b) are causally and temporally ordered events within routine or high-frequency regularized activities.

"To tell a story, a child must be able to relate the chain of events in such a way as to explain what happened and why" (Kemper & Edwards, 1986, p. 14). The elements of event knowledge are seen in the narratives of 4-year-olds. Underlying every story is an event chain, a chronology of events. Events include actions, physical states (e.g., possession and attribution), and mental states (e.g., emotions, dispositions, thoughts, and intentions) that are causally linked as motivations, enablements, initiations, and resultants in the chain. Causal explanations are a repetitive cycle of these events.

Children gradually learn to link events serially and only later with causal connectives (Hood & Bloom, 1979). Psychological causality, such as motives, is used more frequently than physical causality or the connection between events in the narratives of 4- to 9-year olds (McCabe and Peterson, 1985). Connectives are acquired in the following order: *and, and then, when, because, so, then, if,* and *but* (Bloom, et al., 1980). The fuller adult range of connectives (*therefore, as a result of, however*) is gradually acquired during the school years.

Between ages 2 and 10, the child's stories begin to contain more mental states and more initiation and motivation as causal links (Kemper & Edwards,

1986). Around age 4, children's stories begin to contain more explicit physical and mental states. Agentive actions or natural or social processes influence characters' thoughts and emotions. By age 6, children's stories describe motives for actions.

Generally, it is not until age 6, however, that children's narratives are causally coherent (Kemper, 1984). Narratives require the skill to manipulate content, plot, and causal structure. Although 4- and 5-year-olds have many narrative elements in their conversation, especially about common plans and scripts, they do not have the linguistic skill to weave all the elements into a coherent narrative. Between ages 5 and 7, plots emerge consisting of a problem and some resolution of that problem. Gradually, these simple plots are elaborated into a series of problems and solutions or are embellished from within.

Narratives of 7-year-olds typically involve a beginning, a problem, a plan to overcome the problem, and a resolution. Both adults and children prefer goal-directed stories, such as the overcoming of an obstacle, to non-goal-directed stories (Stein & Policastro, 1984). The plot usually centers around the past actions of a clearly fictional main character, allowing the storyteller greater flexibility. The presentation is manipulated dramatically by performance.

Causal chains may go through stages of development before they emerge as full goal-directed narratives. For example, the narrative may be truncated as in the following:

> And there was a big dragon who stole the princess and burned all the land. So, this little guy with a sword fixed everything up. The end.

In this example, the problem is solved but it is unclear how this occurred. Similarly, the problem may be resolved but not because of the intervention of the principals in the story. An example of this type of story is the very complex and complicated problem that is solved when one character awakens to find that it was all a dream.

By second grade, the child may use not only beginning and ending markers (*once upon a time, lived happily ever after, the end*), but also evaluative markers, such as *that was a good one*. Story length increases, greatly aided by syntactic devices, such as conjunctions (*and, then*), locatives (*in, on, under, next to, in front of*), dialogue, comparatives (*bigger than, almost as big as, littlest*), adjectives, and causal statements. Although disquieting events are still central to the theme, there has been a change from inconsistent to consistent characters and from distinct but similar episodes to a chronology (as yet there is no fully developed plot).

The sense of plot in fictional narratives is increasingly clear after age 8 (Labov, 1972; Peterson & McCabe, 1983; Sutton-Smith, 1981, 1986). Now there is definite resolution of the central problem. The child's presentation relies primarily on language rather than on performance. The child manipulates the text and the audience to maintain attention.

In general, the narratives of older children are characterized by the following (Johnston, 1982):

1. Fewer unresolved problems and unprepared resolutions.
2. Less extraneous detail.
3. More overt marking of changes in time and place.
4. More introduction including setting and character information.
5. Greater concern for motivation and internal reactions.
6. More complex episode structure.
7. Closer adherence to the story grammar model.

Children learn to recognize, anticipate, respond to, tell, and read narratives within their homes and their language community. Because different sociocultural groups provide different learning situations for children, various types of narratives emerge (Heath, 1986b). Although every society allows children to hear and to produce at least four basic narrative types, the distribution, frequency, and degree of elaboration of these types vary greatly. The four genres include three factual types, called *recounts, eventcasts,* and *accounts,* and fictionalized *stories* of animate beings who attempt to realize some goal (Stein, 1982).

The recount, common in school performance, brings to present attention those past experiences the child participated in, read about, or observed. Someone in authority usually asks the child to verbalize this shared experience. This form occurs infrequently outside of middle- and upper-class school-oriented families.

The eventcast is a verbal replay or explanation about some current or future event. A child often uses eventcasts to direct the actions of others in imaginative play or to try to influence others' behavior. Use of eventcasts enables the child to consider and analyze the effect of language on others.

Accounts seem to be the preferred form for children's spontaneous narratives. Within acounts, children share their experience ("You know what?"). Children initiate this narrative form, rather than report information requested by adults. Therefore, accounts are highly individualized.

In contrast, stories have a known and anticipated pattern or structure. Language is used to create the story form, and the listener plays a necessary interpretive function.

In middle- and upper-class school-oriented families, the earliest types of narratives are eventcasts that occur during nurturing activities, play, and reading with children. Caregivers share many accounts and stories, and by age 3, children are expected to appreciate and use all forms of narration. Invitations to give recounts decrease with age.

By the time most children begin school, they are usually familiar with all four forms of narration. This is not true for all children. In a white, working-class Southern community, referred to as Roadville, recounts, tightly controlled by the interrogator, are the predominant form throughout the preschool years. Accounts do not begin until children attend school. Children and young adults also tell few stories, which seem to be the province of older, higher-status adults (Heath, 1983).

In contrast, Southern black working-class children produce mostly accounts or eventcasts and have only minimal experience with recounts because of the difficulty in gaining adult attention. As long as these children remain within their families and communities, their language helps them maintain a positive self-image. These children are at a disadvantage, however, when they encounter the expectations of educational institutions (Heath, 1986a). Likewise, Chinese-American children are encouraged to give accounts within, but not beyond, their families.

Learning-disabled students demonstrate knowledge and use of story grammars but convey and recall less information (Weaver & Dickinson, 1982). In addition, learning-disabled children retrieve less information and make fewer inferences than do non-LD children (Hansen, 1978; Oakhill, 1984). Although the stories of learning-disabled children contain all the elements in the generally appropriate order, they are substantially shorter and contain fewer complete episodes. Episodes are also less likely to be related linguistically (Roth & Spekman, 1985). This paucity of information may reflect a lack of presuppositional skills (Roth, 1986).

COLLECTING NARRATIVES

The quality of the narrative is influenced by the selection of appropriate stimuli and topics based on the age, verbal ability, interests, and gender of the child (Hedberg & Stoel-Gammon, 1986). Stimuli may include objects or pictures used for original constructions and heard or read stories used for retelling. In general, the task used to elicit the narrative influences the speaker's adaptation to the listener.

As only one linguistic form used in communication, narratives should form only a portion of any child language analysis. The results should be compared to the child's other linguistic abilities prior to making judgments on the adequacy of the child's language system.

There are many different types of stories and many different contexts within which to tell them. The story type and context affect the eventual narrative form produced (Scott, 1988). In general, maximally naturalistic topics and contexts elicit the most representative narratives (Peterson & McCabe, 1983). Other variables that may affect the narrative form are the story genre, the child's experiential base, the task in which the narrative is told, the source of the narrative, the topic, the formal or informal atmosphere of the context, and the audio-visual support available (Scott, 1988).

Because the unit of analysis is the entire narrative, several narratives must be collected. The wide variation in narratives that can be produced by a single child within different contexts supports this notion. Prior to collecting, the speech-language pathologist decides on the type of narratives desired and the stimuli to be used in their collection.

In general, fictionalized narratives with a vicarious experiential base may result in incomplete narratives with little emphasis on goals, character's feelings or motivations, and endings. The pace, action orientation, and frequent commercial interruption found in television form a very different base for narratives than does experience or even traditional fables or fairytales (Collins, 1983; Collins, Wellman, Keniston, & Westby, 1978). Pictures tend to constrain the form of the narrative and may lead to the production of additive chains. In contrast, photographs or discussions of familiar events foster temporal chains.

Narrative retelling and recall can be used to determine the child's memory organization (Graybeal, 1981; Lovett, Dennis, & Newman, 1986; Stein, 1983). In narrative retelling, the child listens to a well-formed story and then reconstructs the story orally or in writing.

In general, children with language impairments produce longer and more complete story grammars in retold narratives than in self-generated ones (Merritt & Liles, 1989). Clause length is also greater in retold narratives. Comprehension can be assessed within retold narratives by questioning the child when the retelling is complete. In general, children with language learning disabilities perform much like younger children, recalling less of the stimulus story (Crais & Chapman, 1987).

It is important to consider the amount of structure inherent in the stimulus and its effect on retold story construction. For example, nondescript dolls or puppets or sets of vehicles provide no structure. In contrast, a sequence of related pictures provides maximal structure. In general, the more structure found in the stimuli, the less structure the child must provide. Thus, there is a greater degree of structure in the stories of language-impaired children if this structure is provided by the stimuli (Lemme, Hedberg, & Bottenberg, 1984; Merritt & Liles, 1989). Possibly, the child is better able to use the cognitive schema of story organization within the retold narrative format.

Independent, self-generated narrative production requires the child to use his or her own organizational structure and narrative formulation. Narratives can be classified as fictional, personal-factual, or a combination of the two. Fictional or make-believe stories are good vehicles for preschoolers and may be stimulated by objects or pictures (Roth & Spekman, 1986; Westby, 1984, 1985). The speech-language pathologist should provide a model narrative, begin the story for the child, or ask the child to relate a story about the object or picture beginning with "Once upon a time. . . ." This initial structure usually results in a more literate style.

Personal-factual narratives may be collected from conversation or prompted. This type of narrative is very common in early elementary school, especially in show-and-tell activities. The speech-language pathologist should not try to elicit these narratives with open-ended prompts, such as "What did you do yesterday?"

It may be helpful for the speech-language pathologist to establish some common experience with the child and to share a narrative about this experience as an example for the child. Experiential topics prompted in this fashion usually result in the longest and most complex narratives (Peterson & McCabe, 1983).

The child can also be prompted to relate the scariest or funniest thing that ever happened (Garnett, 1986). In addition, the child might be asked to relate a favorite movie, television show, or story.

The speech-language pathologist should add nothing to the child's narrative other than feedback in the form of *uh-huh, okay, yeah, wow,* or a repetition of the child's previous utterance. The narrative can be resumed or the child prompted to continue by such utterances as "And then what happened?".

In story retelling tasks, the clinician must consider the comprehension skills needed to understand the story, the mode of presentation (oral or written), story length, the child's past experience with the story genre (fairy tale, mystery, etc.), the child's interest in the content, and the degree of story structure (Hedberg & Stoel-Gammon, 1986). In general, more familiar, more interesting, and more structured stories result in more complete, better organized retellings.

Well-formed stories should be chosen for retelling, and these should be modified to enhance clarity and organization (Gordon & Braun, 1983, 1985). Stories should be rewritten to reduce complexity in their oral form and to summarize important sections. Subparts and transitions between parts of the narrative may need to be highlighted. Good narrative models often have repetitive elements, such as those found in myths, fables, and fairytales (Westby, 1985).

Stories are also enhanced by familiarity with the physical setting and with the listener. The speech-language pathologist should decide ahead of time on strategies for terminating rambling stories and for probing to elicit longer ones. A suggested guideline is not to expect children to engage in storytelling unless their MLU is 3.0 or more (Hedberg & Stoel-Gammon, 1986).

NARRATIVE ANALYSIS

Narrative analysis is a portion of an overall language analysis. As with dialogues, narratives can be analyzed in several ways, such as narrative levels, story grammars, and cohesive devices (Johnston, 1982; Lahey & Silliman, 1987; Westby, 1984). Narrative levels are concerned with the structural relationship of the narrative parts to the narrative as a whole. Events may be seemingly unorganized or organized sequentially or by causality.

Narrative levels do not have a goal-based organization, whereas story grammars (what happens in the story) do. Narrative level analysis is most appropriate for the stories of 2- to 5-year olds (Applebee, 1978) and for school-aged children with limited verbal abilities; story grammar analysis is best for those over age 5 (Glenn & Stein, 1980).

Story grammars describe the internal structure of a story, including its components and the rules underlying the relationships of these components (Mandler & Johnson, 1977; Rummelhart, 1975; Stein & Glenn, 1979; Thorndyke, 1977). By serving as a framework, story grammars may facilitate narrative processing (Snyder & Downey, 1983). Ideally, components of a story are told in a way that increases understanding. Story grammars may be used to remember and interpret stories (Christie & Schumacher, 1975; Mandler & Johnson, 1977; Stein & Glenn, 1979; Whaley, 1981) and to anticipate content (Baggett, 1979).

Cohesion analysis (Halliday & Hasan, 1976) describes the linguistic devices used to connect the elements of the text. In narratives, coherence or making sense is conveyed through cohesion. For example, appropriate use of anaphoric reference provides cohesion and indicates topical links across utterances (Newman et al., 1986). Inappropriate or inadequate use of cohesive devices results in a disjointed text that is difficult to comprehend. For example, individuals take longer to comprehend sentences in which a pronoun can refer equally to two previously mentioned nouns (Caramazza, Grober, Garvey, & Yates, 1977).

From the analysis, the speech-language pathologist should address the following questions (Johnston, 1982):

1. Does the narrative contain chains? If so, what type?
2. Does the narrative follow the typical story grammar model? Is the story organized maturely?
3. What are the guiding scripts of the narrator, and what do they reveal about the storyteller's knowledge of events and expectations?
4. What linguistic means are used to create a cohesive unit?

In addition, the speech-language pathologist is interested in the sensitivity of the narrator to the perceived needs of the listener.

Narrative Levels

Children use two strategies for organizing their stories: *centering* and *chaining* (Applebee, 1978). Centering is the linking of attributes or objects to form a story nucleus. The links may be based on similarity or complementarity of features. Similarity links are formed by perceptually observed attributes, such as actions, characteristics, and scenes or situations. Causal links are not present, although sequential ones may be. Complementary links consist of conceptual bonds based on abstract, logical attributes, such as members of a class or events linked by cause-and-effect bonds. *Chaining* consists of a sequence of events that share attributes and lead directly from one to another.

Most stories of 2-year-olds are organized by centering. By age 3, however, nearly half of the children use both centering and chaining. This percentage increases, and by age 5, nearly three-fourths of the children use both strategies.

These organizational strategies can result in six basic developmental stages of story organization (Applebee, 1978), presented here in developmental order:

Heaps are sets of unrelated statements about a central stimulus. The statements identify aspects of the stimulus or provide additional information. The common element may be the similarity of the grammatical structure for there is no overall organizational pattern.

> Dogs wag their tails and bark. Dogs sleep all day. A dog chased a cat.

Sequences include events linked on the basis of similar attributes or events that create a simple but meaningful focus for a story. The organization is additive, and sentences may be moved without altering the narrative.

> I *ate* a hamburger. And Johnny *too*. Mommy *ate* a chicken nuggets. Daddy *ate* a fries and coke.

Primitive temporal narratives are organized around a center with complementary events.

> I go outside and swing. Bobby push swing. I go high and try to stop. I fall. And I start to cry. Bobby pick me up.

Unfocused temporal chains lead directly from one event to another while linking attributes, such as characters, settings, or actions, shift. This is the first level of chaining, and the links are concrete. As a result of the shifting focus, unfocused chains have no centers.

> The man got in his boat. He rowed and fished. He ate his sandwich. (Shift) The fishes swimmed and play. Fishes jump over the water. Fishes go to a big hole in the bottom. (Shift) There's a dog in the boat. He's thirsty. He jump in the water.

Focused temporal or causal chains generally center on a main character who goes through a series of perceptually linked, concrete events.

> This boy, he found a jellybean. And his mother said not to eat it. And he did. And a tree growed out of his head.

Narratives develop the center as the story progresses. Each incident complements the center, develops from the previous incident, forms a chain, and adds some new aspect to the theme. Causal relationships may be concrete or abstract and move forward toward the ending of the initial situation. There is usually a climax.

> There was a boy named Tommy. And he got lost in the woods. He ate plants and trees. And he was friends with all the animals. He builded a tent to live in. One day, he builded a fire, and the policemen found him. They took Tommy home to his mommy and daddy.

Each narrative is divided into episodes that are analyzed according to this scheme. Table 6.1 contains examples of narratives and their analysis by narrative level.

Story Grammars

Story grammars provide an organizational pattern that can aid information processing (Johnston, 1982). The competent storyteller constructs the story and the

TABLE 6.1
Narrative level analysis

Example	Classification
Simple frames Granma lives on a farm. There are horsies and piggies. The cows moo. I can ride on the tire swing in a tree. And the calf licked me. That's all.	Sequence
Once there was two kids, Joey and . . . and Fred. Fred's a funny name. And they was fighting. Their mother said, ''Why are you fighting?'' Joey and Fred doesn't know why. They stop and be friends.	Focused chain
Complex narrative frame with episodic development The kids all went to Burger King on Halloween. Super John—that's me —got a cheeseburger. My sister got a Big Mac. Mommy and daddy got nuggets and salad bar. They were eating when a big ghost came out of my milkshake. He threw milkshake on everyone and got them mad. Super John stuck the ghost with a fork. The ghost got flat. All the air came out. Daddy was so happy that he buyed ice cream cones for all the kids.	Sequence Narrative

flow of information to maximize comprehension. The speech-language patholo-gist should note the story grammar elements present and produce a model of the child's story grammar (Roth, 1986).

A story consists of the setting plus the episode structure (story = setting + episode structure) (Johnston, 1982). Each story begins with an introduction con-tained in the setting, as in ''Once upon a time in a far-off kingdom, there lived a prince who was very sad. . .'' or ''On the way to work this morning, I was cross-ing Main Street. . . .''

An episode consists of an initiating event, an internal response, a plan, an attempt, a consequence, and a reaction. An episode is complete if it contains an initiating event or response to provide a purpose, an attempt, and a direct conse-quence (Stein & Glenn, 1979). Episodes may be linked additively, temporally, causally, or in a mixed fashion. A story may consist of one or more interrelated episodes.

The seven elements of story grammars occur in the following order (Stein and Glenn, 1979):

1. Setting statements (S) that introduce the characters and describe their habitual actions along with the social, physical, and/or temporal con-text and that introduce the protagonist.

2. Initiating events (IE) that induce the character(s) to act through some natural act (e.g., an earthquake), a notion to seek something (e.g., trea-sure), or the action of one of the characters (e.g., arresting someone).

3. Internal responses (IR) that describe the characters' reactions, such as emotional responses, thoughts, or intentions, to the initiating events. Internal responses provide some motivation for the characters.

4. Internal plans (IP) that indicate the characters' strategies for attaining their goal(s). Children rarely include this element.

5. Attempts (A) that describe the overt actions of the characters to bring about some consequence, such as attain their goal(s).

6. Direct consequences (DC) that describe the characters' success or failure at attaining their goal(s) as a result of the attempt.

7. Reactions (R) that describe the characters' emotional responses, thoughts, or actions to the outcome or preceding chain of events.

The two very different stories in Table 6.2 present examples of story grammars.

TABLE 6.2
Story grammar examples

Narrative	Story Grammar Elements
I. Single Episode	
There was this boy, and he got kidnapped by these pirates.	Setting statement (S) Initiating event (IE)
So when they were eating, he cut the ropes and got away.	Attempt (A) Direct consequence (DC)
And he lived on a island and ate parrots.	Reactions (R)
II. Multiple episode	
Once there was this big dog on a farm.	Setting statement (S)
And he got hungry 'cause there wasn't enough food.	Initiating event$_1$ (IE$_1$)
The dog . . . His name was Max . . was sad with no food, so his owner went to find some.	Internal response$_1$ (IR$_1$) Attempt$_1$ (A$_1$)
He met a witch, but she wouldn't give him food 'til he killed a yukky toad.	Initiating event$_2$ (IE$_2$)
He was scared but he decided to build a trap.	Internal response$_2$ (IR$_2$) Internal plan$_2$ (IP$_2$)
He dug a hole and filled it with frog food.	Attempt$_2$ (A$_2$)
The frog wanted to eat the man but got caught.	Direct consequence$_2$ (DC$_2$)
The man went back to the witch and she got some hamburgers for the man and the dog.	Direct consequence$_1$ (DC$_1$)
And the man and Max ate hamburgers and were happy.	Reaction$_1$ (R$_1$)

There appears to be a sequence of stages in the development of story grammars (Glenn and Stein, l980). Certain structural patterns appear early and persist, whereas others are rather late in developing. The apparent developmental sequence is as follows:

Descriptive sequences consist of descriptions of characters, surroundings, and habitual actions. There are no causal or temporal links. The entire story consists of setting statements.

> This is a story about my rabbit. He lives in a cage. He likes to hop around my yard. He eats carrots and grass. The end.

Action sequences have a chronological order for actions but no causal relations. The story consists of a setting statement and various action attempts.

> I had a birthday party.(S) We played games and winned prizes.(A) I opened presents.(A) I got balloons.(A) I blowed out the candles.(A) We ate cake and ice cream.(A) We had fun.(A)

Reaction sequences consist of a series of events in which changes cause other changes with no goal-directed behaviors. The sequence consists of a setting, an initiating event, and action attempts.

> There was a lady petting her cow.(S) And the cow kicked the light.(IE) Then the police came.(A) Then a fire truck came.(A) Then a hook-and-ladder came.(A) And that's the end.(S)

Abbreviated episodes contain an implicit or explicit goal. At this level, the story may contain either an event statement and a consequence or an internal response and a consequence. Although the characters' behavior is purposeful, it is usually not premeditated.

> There was a mommy and two kids.(S) And the kids baked a cake for the mommy's birthday.(S) They forgot to turn on … off the stove and burned the cake.(IE) The kids went to the store and buyed a cake.(C) The end.(S)

Complete episodes contain an entire goal-oriented behavioral sequence consisting of a consequence statement and two of the following: initiating event, internal response, and attempt.

> This man was a doctor.(S) He made a monster.(IE) And it chase him around his house.(IE) He run in his bedroom.(A) He push the monster in the closet.(A) And the monster go away.(C) That's all.(S)

Complex episodes are expansions of the complete episode or contain multiple episodes.

> Once there was this Luke Skywalker.(S) And he had to fight Darf Invader.(S/IE) They fighted with swords.(A) And he killed him.(C) And he got in his rocket to blow up these kind of horse robots.(IE) And he shot them.(A) Then all the bad soldiers were killed.(C)

Interactive episodes contain two characters who have separate goals and actions that influence each other's behavior.

> Sally never helped her mom with the dishes.(S) She got mad and said that Sally had to do it.(IE) So, Sally washed the dishes but she was mad.(IR) Then Sally dropped some dishes.(A) Then she dropped more.(A) And her mom said that she didn't have to do any more dishes.(C) And Sally watched TV every night after dinner.(S)

Specific structural properties associated with each structural pattern are listed in Table 6.3.

Language learning disabled children produce fewer mature episodes than do their non-LLD age-matched peers. LLD children make less complete setting statements and are less likely to include response, attempt, and plan statements

TABLE 6.3
Structural properties of narratives

Structural Pattern	Structural Properties	Structural Pattern	Structural Properties
Descriptive sequence	Setting statements (S) (S) (S)	Complex episode	Multiple episodes Setting statement (S) 2 of the following: Initiating event (IE$_1$) Internal response (IR$_1$) Attempt (A$_1$) Direct consequence (DC$_1$) 2 of the following: Initiating event (IE$_2$) Internal response (IR$_2$) Attempt (A$_2$) Direct consequence (DC$_2$)
Action sequence	Setting statement (S) Attempts (A) (A) (A)		
Reaction sequence	Setting statement (S) Initiating event (IE) Attempts (A) (A) (A)		
Abbreviated episode	Setting statement (S) Initiating event (IE) or Internal response (IR) Direct consequence (DC)		
Complete episode	Setting statement (S) 2 of the following: Initiating event (IE) Internal response (IR) Attempt (A) Direct consequence (DC)		Expanded complete episode Setting statement (S) Initiating event (IE) Internal response (IR) Internal plan (IP) Attempt (A) Direct consequence (DC) Reaction (R)
		Interactive episode	Two separate but parallel episodes that influence each other

in their narratives (Roth & Spekman, 1986). Interepisodic relations are also weaker in the narratives of LLD children.

Unfortunately, there is very little normative data for clinical use. In general, nonimpaired children produce all the elements of story grammar by age 9. Children's narratives can be used, however, to approximate their functioning level and to determine which structural elements are present (Hedberg & Stoel-Gammon, 1986). Table 6.4 contains several narratives analyzed by story grammar structural pattern and narrative level.

Cohesive Devices

Text consists of the linguistic properties of a narrative, not the form of individual sentences (Johnston, 1982). Of interest in the text are cohesive devices that lin-

TABLE 6.4
Story grammar analysis

Narrative	Story Grammar Elements	Structural Pattern	Narrative Level
I.			
We went to a farm.	(S)		Unfocused temporal chain
I got to feed chickens.	(S)		
Then I saw cows in the barn.	(S)		
Cows give milk.	(S)	Descriptive sequence	
Cows stay in the field all day and eat grass.	(S)		
At night they come in.	(S)		
II.			
There was this boy who lived in a city.	(S)		Focused temporal chain
And one day a giant bug got out of this place where they keep bugs.	(IE)	Reaction sequence	
And the boy got in an airplane and shot it.	(A)		
III.			
Once there was two boys.	(S)		Narrative
One boy fell into a big hole	(IE_1)		
with rats and he was scared.	(IR_1)		
His brother got a ladder but	(A_1)	Complex episodes	
the rats ate it.	(DC_1/IE_2)		
So, he threw his lunch in the hole.	(A_2)		
The rats ate it, too, and the	(DC_2)		
boy climbed up a rope and was safe	(R)		

Even though the third narrative possesses advanced structural properties, it demonstrates some pronoun confusion. The relationship of the boys is not established until the third utterance.

guistically connect the components. In short, any sentence element that sends the listener outside of the sentence for a referent is a cohesive device. For example, a pronoun may require referral to the previous sentence in order to determine the referent. The five types of cohesive relations are reference, substitution, ellipsis, conjunction, and lexical items (Halliday & Hasan, 1976). Of these, lexical cohesion may be the most difficult to assess reliably (Liles, 1990).

Language-impaired children and children with poor reading abilities exhibit some difficulty communicating well-organized, coherent narratives (Norris & Bruning, 1988). In general, they produce event and sentential relationships more poorly than do their age-matched peers (Johnston, 1982; Liles, 1985; Merritt & Liles, 1985). The most common cohesive errors among language-impaired children are an *incomplete tie,* in which the child references an entity or event not introduced previously, and an *ambiguous reference,* in which the child does not identify to which of two or more referents he or she is referring (Liles, 1990).

Because there is little normative data on the development of these relations, descriptive anlysis is the best diagnostic approach. In general, mature story grammar develops prior to mature use of cohesive devices. It is possible, therefore, to have good episodes but poor cohesion. The two are related but not dependent. There is a metalinguistic quality about cohesion in that the speaker must pay attention to the text apart from the story itself. Cohesive relations are discussed in Chapter 5 and are reviewed only briefly in this section.

Reference

Reference devices, which refer to something else in the text for their interpretation, consist of pronouns, definite articles, demonstratives, and comparatives. The link with the referent should be clear and unambiguous. Clarity is often a problem when the child changes the story narrator frequently, uses dialogue, or includes several characters. Pronouns and definite articles are used to refer to referents previously identified in the narrative.

In contrast, demonstratives locate referents on a continuum of proximity. Nominals, such as *this, that, these,* and *those,* refer to a person or thing; adverbs, such as *here, there, now,* and *then,* refer to a place or time. Use of *now* and *then* is usually restricted to referring to the time just mentioned. In addition, *now* and *then* can also serve as conjunctions.

Finally, comparatives are both general, referring to similarities and differences without reference to a particular property, and specific, referring to some specific quantity or quality. General comparatives include such words as *another, same, different(ly), equal(ly), unequal, identical, similar(ly),* and *else.* Specific quantity words include *more, less, so many, as few as, second, further,* and *fewer than.* Quality words and terms consist of *worse than, as good as, equally bad, better, better than, more happy than,* and *most happy/happiest.*

Substitution and Ellipsis

Substitution and ellipsis both refer to information within the narrative that is supposedly shared by the listener and speaker. In substitution, another word is used in place of the shared information. The words *one(s)* and *same* can be substituted for nouns, as in "Make mine the *same*" or "I'll take *one*, too." Such words as *do* can be substituted for main verbs, as when we emphasize "I *did* already." Finally, such words as *that, so,* and *not* can be substituted for whole phrases or clauses, as in "I think *not*" or "Mother won't like *that*."

Ellipsis differs from substitution in that shared information is simply omitted. Whole phrases and clauses may experience ellipsis. Any portion of the noun phrase may be omitted, as in the following examples:

> I have *four of her brightly wrapped red gifts*. Which is *yours*? Would you like *two*? Do you have *green*?

Verbal material may also be omitted, as in the response "He can't" to the question "Will John attend the concert tonight?" Clausal ellipsis may be demonstrated with the same question when the answer is "Probably."

Conjunction

As noted in Chapter 5, the four types of conjunctive relations are additive, temporal, causal, and adversative. Whereas additive relationships are usually represented by *and,* temporal ones may be signaled with a variety of words, such as *then, next, after, before, at the same time, finally, first, secondly, an hour later,* and so on. Causal conjunctive relationships may also be expressed with a variety of terms, such as *because, as a result of, in that case, for,* and *so* to name a few. Finally, adversative conjunctions include *but* and others, such as *however, although, on the other hand, on the contrary, except,* and *nevertheless.*

Conjunction use may be independent of the specific clausal structure linked (Halliday & Hasan, 1976). In other words, conjunctions link the underlying semantic concepts and, thus, represent the relationship of these units, which many differ from the syntactic units. The way episode parts are linked may reflect the child's underlying episodic organization. We would expect, therefore, that conjunctive relationships between episodic elements would be more complex and difficult than those between sentences. This seems to be true for both language-impaired and nonimpaired children (Liles, 1987).

Lexical Items

Words themselves express relationships by the morphological endings used. For example, the present progressive *-ing* ending is used to express actions taking place at the present time. The following example demonstrates a clear understanding of the relationship of the process to the product:

> He *had been writing* for several months. When the book was finally *written* he celebrated for days. He swore never *to write* another novel.

Categorical relationships can also be expressed and demonstrate convergent and divergent organizational patterns. Convergent thought goes from the members to the category, as in "She had *petunias, dahlias, roses, and pansies* in her garden, but she could never have enough *flowers*." Divergent thought goes from the category to the members, as in "She liked several kinds of *sports*, but was best at *soccer, rugby, and lacrosse.*"

Finally, words can express relationships, such as opposition or part-to-whole. In a narrative, the speech-language pathologist can look for antonyms, synonyms, ordered series, and part-whole or part-part relationships. Ordered series include memorized sequences, such as the days of the week, or hierarchies, such as instructor-assistant professor-associate professor-full professor. Part-whole relationships are expressed by entities that form a portion of the whole, as in rudder-boat, pedal-bike, and January-year. Finally, part-part relations contain parts of the same whole, as in nose-chin, finger-thumb, and rudder-sail.

CONCLUSION

In general, the more mature the narrative, the more complete the structure and the story grammar. In addition to causal chains, more mature narratives contain greater cohesion to aid the listener in interpretation. Mature narratives are structurally cohesive and proceed from one event to another in a logical fashion that demonstrates the narrator's attempt to guide the listener.

More mature narratives also include more insight into the thoughts and feelings of the central characters and greater use of devices for expressing time and place. There are fewer extraneous details and loose ends.

The speech-language pathologist should be cautious when evaluating children from cultures whose narratives do not closely follow the literary pattern described in this chapter. Children from some Spanish-speaking and some Native American cultures may have less experience with story narratives. To varying degrees, these cultures may make extensive use of more descriptive narratives. The use of pictures and elicitation techniques, such as "Tell me a story about this picture," may evoke a very different narrative than what is sought.

The near universal use of some form of narrative suggests, however, its importance in communication. As in dialogue analysis, it is important to analyze narratives simultaneously at several levels. Although there is little normative data on narrative development against which to compare a child's performance in any culture, the speech-language pathologist can use the model described in this chapter to analyze and describe a child's performance.

THREE
Intervention

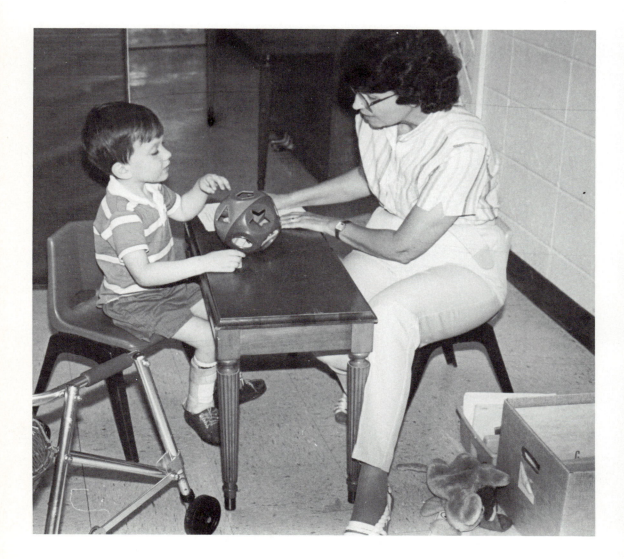

7

A Functional Intervention Model

Traditional language intervention does not consider either the integrated nature of language or the context of language use. Language is viewed as a hierarchically organized set of rules rather than as a wholistic set of variable context-sensitive rules (Rice, 1986). Thus, traditional language intervention usually focuses on isolated linguistic constructs without considering the interrelationship of these units (Gullo & Gullo, 1984). Although the focus may include form, content, and use, the overall design is usually additive rather than integrative (Craig, 1983). Often, the stated goal is to learn specific language units, not enhance communication. Language methods that emphasize very specific skills seem to have very specific, limited effects (Leonard, 1981). Although structured approaches may generalize to situations that differ in one or two respects from the teaching environment, there is little evidence that newly acquired forms will generalize to everyday conversational use (Leonard, 1981; Mulac & Tomlinson, 1977; Stokes & Baer, 1977; Warren & Rogers-Warren, 1980; Welch, 1981; Zwitman & Sonderman, 1979).

Clinical intervention should be a well-integrated whole in which the various aspects of language combine to enhance communication (Snow et al., 1984). The purposes of intervention should be (a) to teach a generative repertoire of linguistic features that can be used to communicate in socially appropriate ways and (b) to stimulate overall language development (Warren & Kaiser, 1986a).

As discussed in Chapter 1, a functional language intervention model attempts to target language features that the child uses in the everyday context, such as the home or classroom, and to adapt that context so that it facilitates the learning of language. Table 7.1 compares the traditional language intervention model with a more functional integrated approach.

The functional approach recognizes a need to orient language training toward the inclusion of family members and teachers as language facilitators and toward the use of everyday activities for encouraging functional communication (Mahoney & Weller, 1980). Therefore, routines within the home, school, and community are used with an array of language facilitators (Rice, 1986). In this way, aspects of language can be trained as they relate to one another within the context of a meaningful experience. As a result, the intervention experience more closely approximates patterns of nonimpaired language development. Content is based on common experiences.

This functional approach, with its integrative and interactive aspects, changes the nature of the clinical interaction and the role of the speech-language pathologist (McDermott & Hood, 1982; Shultz, Florio, & Erickson, 1982). The clinician becomes a consultant for the other language facilitators, who interact more frequently with the child, training them to modify the contexts within which language can occur and to elicit and modify the child's language.

Functional language intervention, however, requires more than just the

TABLE 7.1
Comparison of traditional and functional intervention models

Traditional Model	Functional Model
Individual or small group setting using artificial situations.	Individual or small or large group setting within contextually appropriate setting.
Isolated linguistic constructs with little attention to the interrelationship of linguistic skills.	Relationship of aspects of communication stressed through spontaneous conversational paradigm.
Intervention stresses modeling imitation, practice, and drill.	Conversational techniques stress message transmission and communication.
Little attention to the use of language as a social tool during intervention sessions.	The use of language to communicate is optimized during intervention sessions.
Little chance or opportunity to develop linguistic constructs not targeted for intervention.	Increased opportunity to develop a wide range of language structures and communication skills through spontaneous conversation and social interaction.
Little opportunity to interact verbally with others during intervention.	Increased opportunity to develop communication skills by interacting with a wide variety of partners.

Source: Adapted from Gullo, D., & Gullo, J. (1984). An ecological language intervention approach with mentally retarded adolescents. *Language, Speech, and Hearing Services in Schools, 15*, 182–191.

adoption of a conversational style. Concern for generalization is foremost and governs the overall intervention approach because the goal is to train language useful in the everyday context. Planning by the speech-language pathologist along with the language facilitators is essential. Implementation and generalization may be hampered or impeded by any number of factors, such as the targets selected, the intervention setting, the training methods used, and caseload and scheduling considerations.

Intervention should begin with a generalization plan (Stremel-Campbell & Campbell, 1985) that identifies features of the child's communication environment relevant to generalization. All too often, generalization is the last step in the intervention planning process rather than the overall organizing aspect.

Once the appropriate generalization variables have been identified, the speech-language pathologist can begin to design intervention strategies. The relevant features of the communication environment that have been identified can now be enlisted. Ideally, such intervention enables the speech-language pathologist to develop linguistic constructs at the child's developmental functioning level, taking into account the strategies children normally use when acquiring language; to integrate all linguistic areas within the communication framework; and to provide meaningful and age-appropriate contexts (Gullo & Gullo, 1984).

This chapter discusses principles of intervention of the functional approach and an overall model for intervention, focusing on the variables that affect generalization.

PRINCIPLES

Use of a functional approach to language intervention requires the speech-language pathologist to change some methods and to be mindful of certain principles that aid communication with and learning for the child. It is important to engage the child in a meaningful dialogue or in some other communication event, and this event must become the vehicle for learning and generalization.

The following section includes some of the most important principles of the functional approach. Undoubtedly, some important ones have been omitted that the reader will want to include in his or her repertoire.

The Language Facilitator as Reinforcer

As communicators, we continue to interact with individuals who provide positive feedback and reinforcement. Each of us avoids communicating with certain individuals who are nonresponsive, caustic, or overly critical. Children avoid certain potential conversational partners for many of the same reasons. If speech-language pathologists want children to communicate with them, then they must be people with whom children want to communicate.

The way the speech-language pathologist approaches children is very important for future communication. By reducing the authority figure persona, demonstrating an attentiveness and a willingness to adopt the child's topics, and remaining accepting while providing evaluative feedback, the speech-language pathologist can send a message of acceptance of the child as a partner. Most children will respond in kind.

Children respond most readily to adults who convey a genuine caring and respect for them. These attitudes are conveyed by the adult who tries to meet the child halfway. Adults who desire to be effective conversational partners must appreciate the world from a child's perspective. Events easily understood by an adult may be quite incomprehensible to a young child. It may help to recall that for children the world is full of wonder and delight, full of things that cannot be explained, and full of magic.

Adults demonstrate concern for children when they are willing to attend to children, to listen, and to accept their topics. As much as possible, intervention should be nonintrusive, with facilitators providing supportive evaluative feedback to the child.

An important question in the intervention setting is, What sense is the child making of this situation? The child's sense of things will influence behavior and language within that situation (Duchan, 1986a). An activity that seems very concrete to the facilitator, such as looking at pictures, might be very abstract for the preschool child.

Few child linguistic responses are totally wrong. Even seemingly incorrect utterances demonstrate the child's understanding of the situation and of the underlying relationships. Acceptance of the child includes acceptance of these utterances. Usually, some portion of the utterance can be reinforced.

> CHILD: I need ear-gloves.
> PATHOLOGIST: That's right, they are like little gloves for your ears. We
> call them ear*muffs*. Here, let me help you put on your earmuffs.

The pathologist has accepted the child's utterance, recognized the child's understanding of the situation, corrected the utterance, and left the child's ego in tact.

The intervention setting itself should "create and sustain an atmosphere containing fun, surprise, interest, ease, invitation, laughter, and spontaneity" (Cochrane, 1983, p. 160). In such an atmosphere, children will be eager to participate. One of my best lessons on verbal sequencing used mime, complete with whiteface. The children enacted familiar everyday event sequences, such as making breakfast, while other students tried to guess the name of the sequence. After the correct guess was given, the actor stated each event in the sequence while performing it. Finally, each actor attempted to reconstruct the sequence verbally. The lesson was messy, fun, enjoyable, and thoroughly successful.

Children also respond favorably if the facilitator occasionally plays the clown or buffoon. I may wear a cooking pot on my head in order to evoke a response. On other occasions, I purposely make incorrect verbalizations or actions. These behaviors add to the magic of the communication situation and encourage children to communicate in an accepting atmosphere.

Closely Approximate Natural Learning

Language intervention strategies should closely approximate the natural process of language acquisition. The strategy should be communicative in nature and should use language as it naturally occurs (Mahoney & Weller, 1980). Teaching language devoid of its communicative function deprives the child of intrinsic motivation and of one essential element of generalization.

Natural language models—parents, teachers, aides, and others—should be the principal resources for implementation of language intervention (Mahoney & Weller, 1980). These individuals serve as language models with or without the speech-language pathologist's input. Their potential as language facilitators can be best exploited, however, when they are guided in content selection and trained in facilitative techniques. When using these language facilitators within the child's everyday situations, the role of the speech-language pathologist changes to that of consultant (Lyngaas, Nyberg, Hoekenga, & Gruenewald, 1983).

Follow Developmental Guidelines

The language development of nonimpaired children can guide the selection of training targets. As a group, nonimpaired children develop language in a similar, albeit individualistic, manner. Generally, language form is preceded by function, with easier, less complex structures being learned first. Children use the language they possess to accomplish language goals or uses. These uses are the framework within which new forms develop. The overall result is hierarchy that suggests steps for training language.

Of course, no speech-language pathologist would ever adopt a language intervention hierarchy without some personal adaptations. Slavish adherence to a developmental hierarchy is inappropriate for two reasons. First, the developing child's hypothesis testing of language rules occasionally results in nonproductive strategies. For example, young children learn a few irregular past tense verbs early in their language development. Upon learning the regular past tense -ed rule, these children apply it to the previously learned irregular verbs. This results in such delightful forms as *eated* and *sitted*. No speech-language pathologist would wish to adopt these forms as training targets, although they appear in the language of nonimpaired children.

Second, good teaching may suggest alternative hierarchical teaching patterns. For example, nonhandicapped children develop the verb *to be* as both an auxiliary verb and as a main verb or copula. In intervention, therefore, these forms might be targeted separately. Our knowledge of carryover might suggest, however, that we train them together, making little distinction between the forms.

Developmental hierarchies can act as guides for intervention. These hierarchies suggest several subprinciples:

1. Language evolves from nonverbal communication means.
2. Social and cognitive prerequisites are necessary in order for the child to use language in certain ways.
3. Simple rules are acquired before more difficult ones.
4. Development is not uniform across all aspects of language.
5. At different levels of development, children act differently.

Each subprinciple has several implications for intervention.

Because language has evolved as a sophisticated communication means from a nonverbal communication system, intervention with low-functioning children should begin with less sophisticated systems and progress toward symbol use (Mahoney & Weller, 1980). In addition, the speech-language pathologist needs to be mindful of the many ways in which a message may be sent by any communicator and to note development within the nonlinguistic and paralinguistic realms as well as within the linguistic.

Although social and communicative prerequisites are important prior to the appearance of first words, these prerequisites cannot be overlooked with later development. The speech-language pathologist should be aware of the prerequisites for successful communicative behaviors at the functioning level of the child (Rieke & Lewis, 1984). The child learning plurals need not be able to count but must have a notion of one and more than one. Likewise, successful use of *why* questions and answers requires an ability to reconstruct events in reverse. These cognitive skills may need to be taught prior to attempting the linguistic manner for noting this knowledge.

Similarly, the child needs to understand the requirements and demands of different communication situations to communicate effectively within them. For example, the requirements of classroom give-and-take are very different from having a face-to-face conversation or from talking on the telephone.

As with much learning, simple rules are combined and modified or enlarged to form higher order rules. By carefully analyzing each new training target and monitoring progress, the speech-language pathologist can ensure that the child possesses the appropriate rules for new learning. It is best not to change too many aspects of the training situation at one time. For example, there may be too much new information to absorb if the child is learning new words while being taught different sentence types in which to use these words. Words used frequently by the child should be selected to train longer utterances.

Language-impaired children will not present textbook examples of language development hierarchies. They may have splinter skills or be more proficient in one aspect of language than in others. This situation is not unlike that found in nonimpaired children. Language development and impairment can be very individualistic and may not follow the dictates of a developmental hierarchy. Aspects of language will develop at rates influenced by perception and cognition, opportunity, needs, and training. Of more importance for intervention is the designation of training targets that help the child function more effectively within the everyday environment.

Finally, the language rules observed by most children at each level of development are valid for those children at that time. For example, young children say such things as "Mommy eat" and "More juice" that demonstrate adherence to simple word sequencing rules based on semantics. "Mommy eat" is not a defective form of some longer adult sentence. Children demonstrate rules appropriate to their level of linguistic competence. Requiring adult rule use negates the uniqueness of children and dismisses the importance of child rules as a step in the acquisition process.

At various levels of intervention, it is appropriate to target child rules rather than the more difficult adult ones that, hopefully, will be trained later. These rules provide excellent training targets for language-impaired children who also are beginning to form two-word utterances. Likewise, the language-impaired child who is forming negatives, such as no + noun + verb, should make a logical progression to noun + no + verb rather than to the adult rule with full auxiliary verb. To require language-impaired children to use adult sentence forms seems ridiculous, especially when we do not require such behavior from nonimpaired children. As adults, we sometimes think that the adult way of doing things is the only way.

Even the expectation that a child will use a new or adult-like language rule or feature following brief periods of intervention may be unrealistic (Fey, 1988). Nonimpaired children learn and extend or retract their language rules gradually after many encounters and trials. Over time, these rules come to resemble those of adults. Therefore, it is probably inappropriate to expect near perfect performance from language-impaired children shortly after a target is introduced. Rule learning is complicated and time consuming. In addition, language-impaired children may form rules very different from those intended by speech-language pathologists.

As the child progresses, the language training should be modified accordingly. In other words, the speech-language pathologist ups the ante (MacDonald, 1985) or requires performance just above the child's current functioning level.

Follow the Child's Lead

Often, the expectation that a child will not communicate effectively becomes self-fulfilling. If facilitators expect the child to communicate and plan for it, the child will. At that time, it is essential that the facilitator give full attention to the child.

It is equally important that the facilitator attend to the content and intent of each child utterance and respond appropriately to that content and intent. "Training techniques in which teachers follow the child's lead . . . should be most effective because teaching occurs when the child is attending and because the language being taught to the child is a positive consequence" (Warren & Rogers-Warren, 1985, p. 7).

Language facilitators can either direct and maintain the child's attention or attend to what interests the child. The former is a trainer-oriented approach (Fey, 1986) that gives the trainer virtual control of the entire interaction.

A more child-centered approach guarantees joint or shared reference, enhances semantic contingency, and reduces noncompliance by the child (McDade & Varnedoe, 1987). With semantic contingency, the adult comments on the child's topic or previous utterance, thus facilitating processing by the child.

The child's behavior should be interpreted in terms of intention rather than viewed as inappropriate or incorrect. In other words, a request is still a request even though the form may be wrong, the item desired misnamed, and so on.

When the adult has an agenda different from that of the child, the interaction is diminished. Such interactions are at cross purposes and are faulty (Duchan, 1984).

Children signal those things in which they are most interested by their actions or through verbalizations. This gauge can be used to keep child interest and motivation high in the intervention setting. Often, I will say to a child, ''What toy do you want to play with?'' Although the topic is open-ended, the technique is very specific—as we see later—permitting a flexible choice of topic.

When the child initiates an interaction and is responded to accordingly, the value for learning is greater than when the child's initiation is ignored or penalized (Duchan, 1984). Ignoring or penalizing the child will result in a decrease in future initiations.

While observing a lesson in a training apartment in preparation for the client's move to his own apartment, I overheard the following exchange:

PATHOLOGIST: What are you doing?
CLIENT: Dusting furniture. (Matter-of-factly)
PATHOLOGIST: Good. What else are you doing?
CLIENT: You live in apartment?
PATHOLOGIST: You didn't answer my question. What . . .

The client was obviously interested in living arrangements and would have joined such a conversation willingly if the speech-language pathologist had followed his lead. The speech-language pathologist should follow the client's content and manipulate the conversation to encourage the desired language features. Continued use of directive responses by this speech-language pathologist will diminish the client's initiating behavior.

Actively Involve the Child

Normal language acquisition occurs with the active participation of the learner. Language learning is not a passive process (Mahoney & Weller, 1980).

In like fashion, more rapid learning occurs when the language-impaired child is actively participating in some event. In general, the more actively involved the child, the greater and more stable the generalization (Spiegel, 1983).

Ideally, intervention should consist of motivating participatory activities with the potential for a variety of language use contexts (Kunze et al., 1983).

Language is Heavily Influenced by Context

Context can be a big determiner of what is said and how it is said. Language is a socially based cultural form whose use reflects an individual's linguistic, interpersonal, and cultural competence within a given contextual situation (Rice, 1986). The individual's knowledge of the event or situation influences the way he or she uses language in that situation.

Language intervention should occur within the contexts of everyday events and within the context of conversational give-and-take or of other communication events. The language facilitator needs to create a rich context in which the language-impaired child can experience a variety of linguistic and nonlinguistic stimuli. The integration of talking and listening within conversations should be emphasized (Kunze et al., 1983).

The content for these dialogues is the common experience of the intervention setting. Ideally, this setting reflects or is a part of the child's everyday environment. The child and facilitator talk about the focus of the activities used in training. The skillful facilitator can manipulate both the linguistic and nonlinguistic context to attain desired targets from the child.

Design a Generalization Plan First

Considerations of generalization are essential to treatment program design and should be identified prior to beginning training. Table 7.2 is a suggested generalization plan format. In designing such a plan, the speech-language pathologist considers the individual needs of the child and environment and the relevant variables that will affect generalization.

GENERALIZATION VARIABLES

To ensure generalization to the everyday environment of the child, the speech-language pathologist must manipulate the generalization variables most likely to result in that outcome. As noted in Chapter 1, the variables that affect generalization can be grouped as content and context variables (Table 1.1). Content variables include the training targets and training items. Context variables include the method of training, language facilitators, cues, contingencies, and location of training. Each of these variables and considerations for intervention as they relate to a functional model are discussed in this section.

Training Targets

As mentioned previously, teaching the complex process of language use as discrete bits of language can actually retard growth (Cazden, 1972). Language inter-

TABLE 7.2
Possible generalization plan format

Training targets

Identify settings, situations, and persons in each across which training can occur.

S e t t i n g s

	Situation	Situation	Situation	Situation	Situation	Situation	Situation	Situation
P								
e								
r								
s								
o								
n								
s								

Cues:

Consequences:

vention should be relevant to the particular needs of the child within the communication environment and should target the language use process rather than language products or units. Therefore, intervention must answer two questions (Warren, 1985):

1. What will be the function of the forms and content we are teaching?
2. Are the forms and content being trained in the context of communication events in which the intended function can actually be acomplished?

In general, more frequently used targets are more relevant to the child's world and, therefore, are more likely to generalize. Communicative utterances observed to occur in the home, albeit incorrectly, can be introduced in therapy as natural outcomes of the context. Once introduced, they can be modified by the facilitator.

Language "is often acquired more rapidly and used more effectively if the skill called 'communicative interaction' is established first." (Rieke & Lewis, 1984, p. 44) Language targets need to be those that increase the effectiveness of the child as a communicative partner (Snow et al., 1984).

The first goal of intervention should be successful communication by the child at the present level of functioning. Language goals that are too taxing may result in a lessening of successful communication and decreased initiation by the child. Through observation and language sampling, the speech-language pathologist notes communication breakdowns as a source for identifying possible training targets.

Developmental guidelines can aid target selection but should be followed cautiously. Unfortunately, "all too frequently clinicians take a 'description' of normal acquisition as a 'prescription' for the way language must be taught" (deVilliers & deVilliers, 1978, p. 270).

A review by Bryen and Joyce (1985) of 43 published language intervention studies, however, found that those that used goals approximating a developmental sequence were more successful that those that did not. In general, most earlier emerging forms can be learned in fewer trials and prior to later emerging forms. In addition, earlier emerging forms seem to generalize more readily into the child's use system and at a higher level of use (Dyer, Santarcangelo, & Luce, 1987).

A functional model would suggest teaching forms useful in the natural setting while attending to the developmental order of these forms (Dyer et al., 1987). As mentioned previously, the development of nonimpaired children can serve as a general guideline rather than as a curricular hierarchy. The overriding criteria for target selection should be to aid the children in communicating what is necessary in the contexts in which they most frequently communicate. Chapter 9 offers some guidelines for modifying a developmental hierarchy of intervention.

The best way to determine need is through environmental observation. If, for example, the child frequently requests items in the environment but is generally ineffective, then requesting might be chosen as a target. When there is very little opportunity for a possible training target to occur, it might be best to identify other content for training.

Infrequent opportunity for possible training targets to occur may be the result of low environmental expectations or requirements for the child to produce these forms or functions. For example, there may be few opportunities for children to ask questions when there is little expectation that they will do so. In such cases, low expectations can become self-fulfilling. The communication environment may need to be restructured to facilitate use of newly acquired communication skills. The speech-language pathologist is an invaluable expert in facilitating such language use.

The speech-language pathologist should identify both targets and everyday situations in which the target is likely to occur and in which its use will be affected by and, in turn, affect the context. For example, questions should be trained in situations in which they make sense and in which they perform their intended function of gaining information. Speech-language pathologist instructions, such as "I'm coloring a picture. Ask me what I'm doing," violate the function of questions. Usually, we do not ask questions for which we already have the answer. Similarly, the clinician's attempt to elicit an answer with the instruction "What am I doing?" also violates the function of questions and answers. Although we might wonder about the mental capacity of speech-language pathologists who don't know what they're doing, we can modify the situation and cue to gain this feature more appropriately. For example, the speech-language pathologist might sit behind a screen, give clues, and ask the child "Can you guess what I'm doing?"

Training Items

The speech-language pathologist should plan to train enough examples of the feature being targeted to enable the child to generalize to untrained members (Stremel-Campbell & Campbell, 1985). For example, it is neither desirable nor possible to train all noun-verb combinations. The goal should be to train enough examples from the noun class in combination with examples of the verb class so that the child will generalize the rule noun + verb to all members of these two classes. Obviously, this process is being simplified in this discussion, and more planning and thought are required. Not all nouns and verbs can be combined. For example, the combination "Desk eat" is unacceptable.

In addition, a sufficient number of items must be trained so that the child can determine both the relevant and irrelevant aspects of the communication context. For example, words or phrases such as *yesterday, last week,* or *in the past,* are relevant to use of the past tense. The child forms a hypothesis that states, "In the presence of *yesterday, last week,* or *in the past* use the past tense." Other aspects may be irrelevant, such as the specific nouns, pronouns, or verbs used. For example, the pronoun *I* is irrelevant and can be used with any tense. If the child is trained to use the form *Yesterday, I . . ., Last week, I . . .,* and *In the past, I . . .,* the resultant incorrect hypothesis might be ''In the presence of *I* use the past tense.'' Knowledge of both the relevant and irrelevant aspects of the context are essential for learning.

Initially, training response classes should be similar so as to limit irrelevant dimensions. For example, the child may first learn to use regular past tense with *yesterday.* Such words as *today* do not signal the tense as clearly and should be introduced later. Gradually, more irrelevant dimensions are introduced.

Not all word classes require the use of all training targets. For example, nouns do not require the past tense *-ed* marker and *tomorrow* does not require a past tense verb. The child needs to learn those response classes in which the target is required and those in which it is not.

When a particular syntactic form or function is being targeted, it is especially important to select content words or utterances already in the child's repertoire. With the targeting and introduction of new topic words, the wise speech-language pathologist will select familiar structural frames. MacDonald (1984) labels this principle ''new forms-old content/old forms-new content.''

Processing constraints found in all human beings reflect the limited capacity of the brain to process information. When these boundaries are reached, there must be performance sacrifices or trade-offs in one area because of demands in another. For example, children omit more grammatical markers in longer, more complex sentences than in shorter, less complex ones (Nakayama, 1987). Language-impaired children are particularly susceptible to these constraints because the automatization of linguistic processing takes longer (Kamhi, Catts, & Davis, 1984). Training items that exceed the information-processing constraints of these children may result in inadequate learning and poor generalization (Johnston, 1988).

Often a behavior fails to generalize because the child has not learned the rules or conditions that govern the use of the behavior. Within the typical intervention model, the child learns imitative responses followed by elicited ones. Thus, the child internalizes this unique relationship between the communication variables.

Because the child often lacks metalinguistic awareness, rule explanation is not a viable clinical tool (deVilliers & deVilliers, 1978). The speech-language pathologist must structure the environment so that linguistic regularities are obvious.

Contrast training is one method of overcoming generalization problems (Connell, 1982). In contrast training, the child learns those structures and situations that obligate use from those that do not. For example, the use of the third person *-s* marker is required with singular nouns and third person singular pronouns. The child must also recognize that plural nouns and other pronouns do not require this marker. ''By contrasting sentences which obligate a target form with minimally different sentences which do not . . . the learner can recognize which parts of sentences occur regardless of the presence or absence of the target form'' (Connell, 1982, p. 235).

Conversational use requires recognition of the linguistic contexts within which the training target does or does not appear. The identification of other contexts, such as events, facilitators, and settings, should also be accomplished. Using several different contexts ensures that the child does not identify the speech-language pathologist and the therapy setting as the only contexts in which to use the language being trained.

Ideally, functional training uses multiple exemplars (Stremel-Campbell & Campbell, 1985) or examples, such as the several different categories of linguistic response classes or training items, several facilitators, and several settings. This feature is essential for generalization.

Method of Training

In the past language was taught much as one would teach any other complex behavior, and intervention centered on individual discrete behaviors. The goal was to increase the frequency of these behaviors (Guess et al., 1974). Language, however, is a set of rules that allow a person to use language elements in communication contexts to express intentions (Wilbur, 1983).

A rule is an abstraction that describes similarities in behavior. Language is a rule-governed behavior. Thus, the goal of intervention should be to learn the abstract rules rather than the behaviors that reflect these rules (Connell, 1982; Fey, 1986; Johnston, 1983; Leonard, 1981). Current methods of teaching language do not reflect this goal (Connell, 1987b). There is a discrepancy between the goals and the methods of teaching.

It is not practical with most children and most intervention targets simply to explain the language rule being trained. Instead, training needs to be limited to observations of the rule being applied within situations that contrast the critical conditions that apply to the rule (Connell, 1987b).

The speech-language pathologist's role is to provide organized language data to the child as an illustration of rule use (Johnston, 1983). Thus, the child would be presented with paired minimally different situations that do and do not invoke the rule (Connell, 1987b). For example, these situations could be sentences in which the use of a form, such as pronouns, is alternately appropriate and inappropriate.

By presenting these contrasting situations and encouraging the child to practice, the speech-language pathologist helps the child amass the data necessary to identify the critical elements of the rule. Once the child is aware of the critical elements, the speech-language pathologist has the flexibility to present these elements in any communication situation. In contrast, a behavior-teaching approach would contain none of these systematic alterations of form and function.

The strength of the rule-teaching approach is in the way it simplifies the learning task by condensing relevant input and highlighting critical conditions (Connell, 1987b). Unfortunately, not every form has a direct link to some function

(Bates & MacWhinney, 1982). The passive voice, for example, does not have a clear function and may be used to answer, comment, reply, declare, and so on. Forms that do not have a clear direct function are more difficult to teach. Rules based on abstract grammatical categories are also difficult.

Theoretically, functional techniques should be effective because they incorporate behavioral principles and also use the context of naturally occurring conversations that can be systematically modified by the language facilitator. Generalization is more likely than with more structured approaches, because the cues used resemble the varied ones found in communication events. In addition, the child's attention is focused on objects and events in the environment while the child is receiving linguistic input about those objects and events (Warren & Kaiser, 1986a).

A functional model provides a dynamic context for teaching language. Language training that works for the child in communication events should generalize to those events. "Language programs . . . must be based on communicative needs and must be planned with these functions in mind" (Rieke & Lewis, 1984, p. 48). Training is oriented toward communication rather than toward discrete bits of language. In general, functional intervention, sometimes called *incidental teaching* (Hart & Risley, 1986; Warren & Kaiser, 1986a), in combination with more structured remediation, facilitates both acquisition and generalization of language targets to usage within natural environment situations.

The functional or incidental approach involves (a) selecting appropriate language targets for the child and environment, (b) arranging the environment to increase the likelihood that the child will initiate, (c) responding to the child's initiations with requests for elaboration of the target forms, and (d) reinforcing the child's attempts with attention and access to objects in which the child has expressed interest (Warren & Kaiser, 1986b). Interactions between adults and children arise naturally in unstructured situations, such as play, and can be used systematically by the adult to give the child practice in communication (Warren & Kaiser, 1986b, p. 291).

The child signals a topic by demonstrating interest or requesting assistance. Thus, the child provides the topic and the opportunity for the facilitator to teach the language form (Duchan, 1986b). The child is more likely to talk and more interested in the content of this talk if the topic has been established by the child.

Within these contexts, the speech-language pathologist models the responses that fulfill the child's communication goals. Because the purpose of language is already established in the natural environment, form and content may be more easily learned (Spinelli & Terrell, 1984). The speech-language pathologist also models behaviors for the caregivers in order to facilitate training and increase the likelihood that situations will occur in which the child is successful.

When the desired interactions do not occur, the speech-language pathologist can manipulate the environment to enhance its language-training potential (Norris & Hoffman, 1990). Both linguistic and nonlinguist aspects of the context can be altered to elicit the desired communication.

Activities can be planned around communication contexts that are highly likely to occur for the child. Training outside of the normal environment should be as close to that environment in materials, situations, and persons as possible. Activities should include the child's usual reasons for talking and typical topics, rely on previous experiences and introduce new ones, use familiar focuses of communication, and include the child's normal communication partners (Spinelli & Terrell, 1984).

The speech-language pathologist must recognize that events within the child's everyday environments will differ in the amount of structure provided by the event itself (Duchan, 1986a). Some contexts are highly planned and scripted or routinized, such as bathing or eating, whereas others are relatively free and open, such as playing. The communication demands and the expectations on the child vary accordingly. Language intervention must recognize what the child brings to each context and what is demanded in return. The speech-language pathologist must attend to the child and to his or her understanding of the situation. New information should be organized to meet the functioning level of the child (Norris & Hoffman, 1990).

Routines may provide the best vehicle for training the noninteractive child. The child can ease into participating through repeated exposure to a routine in which the facilitator models actions and communication. Because the event is prescribed and expectations are known, there is some security for the child. Likewise, discussions of familiar events, such as a birthday party, provide a script for communicating.

"Language treatment based on play and daily life experiences with an adult who provides modeling and expansion of the child's forms and meaning is similar to normal language learning processes" (Kunze et al., 1983). For example, children at a 0–36 months functioning level learn through play and interaction with adults. Intervention with children functioning at this level should reflect this reality.

By considering why and how children use words and gestures, the speech-language pathologist increases her or his ability to provide the most natural and optimal situations for eliciting and teaching communication. "This combination of appropriate context as well as specifically targeted behaviors facilitates maximum carryover and generalization of language skills outside the clinical environment" (Kunze et al., 1983, p. 81).

Data from a number of studies indicate that functional intervention (a) teaches target skills effectively, (b) aids generalization across settings, times, and persons, and (c) improves both the formal and functional aspects of language (Warren & Kaiser, 1986b). Functional, conversational techniques have been used effectively to enhance vocabulary growth and grammatical complexity and to increase the frequency of language use (Hart & Risley, 1980; Rogers-Warren & Warren, 1980; Warren et al., 1984).

The technique works well with a number of age groups and specific language-impaired populations and with a variety of specific language responses. Language training generalizes to classroom and home settings and to teachers and parents (Alpert & Rogers-Warren, 1984; Halle et al., 1981; McGee et al., 1983). In addition, the general effects of the technique are beneficial to the overall language learning and functioning of the child (Alpert & Rogers-Warren, 1984, Rogers-Warren & Warren, 1980).

Language Facilitators

If the goal is language use within the child's everyday context, then clearly, the speech-language pathologist is limited as to what can be accomplished (Snow et al., 1984). The brevity of child-clinician contact necessitates the use of a wider variety of social contexts, including various communication partners.

"Obviously, adults who are with the child throughout the day are the individuals who are most able to effect an increase in the frequency of initiated communication and lay the groundwork for the continuing emergence of language behaviors" (Rieke & Lewis, 1984, p. 47). The appropriate partners to be used in training will vary with the age and circumstance of the child. Whereas parents may be appropriate for preschool children, they may have only limited interaction with their school-aged children. Successful use of the behaviors taught in language intervention programs depends, in part, on the expectations of these significant others in the child's environment.

The child must have the opportunity to communicate, thus the facilitator must be attentive and responsive. Communication partners, such as teachers and parents, can be an effective part of an intervention team if they are trained and monitored thoroughly (Jimenez & Iseyama, 1987). Such training can be accomplished in several ways, including direct training and modeling, inservice training, and the use of written and illustrated instructions.

Children with significant communication impairments accompanying autism and mental retardation usually have serious problems with conversational interactions, primarily due to the complex nature of such interactions (Higginbotham & Yoder, 1982). In general, these individuals have difficulty organizing, coordinating, and monitoring all of the various elements that comprise these interactions, such as topic initiation and maintenance, presupposition, turn taking, conversational repair, and the like (Mirenda & Donnellan, 1986).

It is often difficult for retarded toddlers and their parents to establish mutually rewarding interactional patterns (Rieke & Lewis, 1984). Such children are less likely to succeed in a preschool setting. Their experience level and their success in communicative interaction are often minimal, and they may exhibit poor listening skills. Children who are not successful in communication often become resistant or negative and develop attention-getting behaviors.

According to the interactional view, the difficulties experienced by these children reflect their everyday contexts more than their so-called disorder. If this is so, then conversational partners must assume some of the responsibility for the communication failures of these children. For example, the quality and quantity of spontaneous conversational behavior of language-disordered children are inversely related to the number of verbal initiations and directives by their adult conversational partners (Prizant & Rentschler, 1983; Semmel, Peck, Haring, & Theimer, 1984).

Partially in response to these children's language deficits, adults modify their own language to include more imitations, semantic expansions, directives, and questions (Goldberg, 1977; Marshall, Hegrenes, & Goldstein, 1973; Nakamura & Newhoff, 1982; Scherer & Owings, 1982). The frequency of parental self-repetitions is negatively correlated with the rate of language growth. Mothers of language-impaired children repeat more than do mothers of nonimpaired children. Most of these maternal repetitions are imperatives (demands) or directives (commands), which also correlate negatively. "A highly directive interaction style is certain to provide the child with minimal opportunity for immediate comparisons between his or her own utterances and those of the caretaker since there is no necessary connection between the use of a directive and any utterance of the child" (Lieven, 1984, p. 16). In turn, the children's contributions are determined by the complex contribution of social, environmental, and cultural factors (Mishler, 1979).

Adult verbal control of interactions seems to affect adversely the verbal output of language-disordered children. For example, although the question-answer style of adult communication may aid children functioning around age 2 to maintain a conversational topic, it can discourage children from commenting outside of the topics initiated by the adults (Bloom et al., 1976; Mirenda & Donnellan, 1986; Moerk, 1977). As both handicapped and nonhandicapped children move beyond this developmental level, the use of a question-answer strategy is counterproductive to the goal of spontaneous conversational behavior.

The use of an adult facilitative style of conversation can increase language-impaired children's use of topic initiations, questions, and topic comments (Mirenda & Donnellan, 1986). An adult facilitative style (a) allows the child to control and initiate conversational topics, (b) follows the child's conversational lead, and (c) encourages the child to participate in various ways.

In contrast, an adult directive style includes verbal conversational behaviors that (a) control and initiate conversational topics, (b) lead the conversation, and (c) structure the nature of the child's contribution (Mirenda & Donnellan, 1986). These behaviors ensure a cohesive and fluent conversation at the expense of the child's spontaneous initiations.

The facilitative adult is less interested in conversational flow than in providing an opportunity for the child to participate and to assume control of the conversation. Specific behaviors that define each style are given in Table 7.3 (Duchan, 1983a; McDonald & Pien, 1982; Olsen-Fulero, 1982).

Several conversationally based parent-training programs have demonstrated an increase in parent responsiveness and a decrease in directiveness toward their preschool language-impaired children (Cheseldine & McConkey, 1979; Mahoney & Powell, 1986; McConkey & O'Connor, 1982; Price, 1984; Seitz, 1975; Weistuch & Lewis, 1986). Other changes include increased willingness to follow their child's lead, more equality in turn balancing, shorter parental MLU, and fewer questions.

TABLE 7.3
Characteristics of the directive and facilitative styles

Directive	Facilitative
Initiate at least half of the topics of conversation.	Initiate fewer than half of the topics of conversation.
Use direct questions to initiate most topics.	Use indirect questions or embedded imperatives to initiate most topics.
Use primarily direct questions and occasional imitations or expansions to maintain topics.	Use primarily direct statements, encouragements, imitations, expansions, or expansion questions and occasional direct questions to maintain topics.
Do not ask for clarification directly, relying instead on encouragement, imitation, and expansion strategies.	Use direct clarification questions or statements when necessary and appropriate.
Do not allow lapses in turn taking to occur, but use direct questions to require the child to respond.	Allow lapses between turns to occur and after a short wait, initiate topics as noted above.

Mothers who receive facilitative training are more responsive to and less directive of the children's behavior than are untrained mothers (Girolametto, 1988; Tiegerman & Siperstein, 1984). These changes in parental behavior are causally related to such child language changes as increased MLU, increased number of utterances, increased lexicon, and improved standardized test scores. Children whose parents receive training initiate more topics, are more responsive, use more verbal turns, and have a more diverse vocabulary. These results suggest that the effect of parental conversational strategies may be greater on semantics and pragmatics than on linguistic form.

An increase in the percentage of semantically related utterances can, in turn, provide greater opportunity for topic maintenance and turn taking (Tiegerman & Siperstein, 1984). With more opportunity to participate, the child gains more control over both the adult's behavior and the exchange process.

There is an ongoing debate, however, on the form of language to be addressed to language-impaired children. Parents of nonimpaired language learners use child-directed language patterns. These differ in syntactic completeness from the language employed in many teaching programs. Language directed at nonimpaired children in natural settings consists of reduced, syntactically complete utterances (deVilliers & deVilliers, 1978). In contrast, language used in teaching programs is often syntactically incomplete (Page & Horn, 1987).

Language-impaired children differ in comprehension of different language styles according to their linguistic stage (Page & Horn, 1987). Early stage I children use a semantically based comprehension strategy, especially agent + action and action + object, rather than one based on syntax (Miller & Yoder, 1974). In addition, these reduced adult forms facilitate the production of two-word semantic relations for some language-impaired children (Nestheide & Culatta, 1980). The use of either adult forms or reduced forms does not seem to affect the comprehension or production of stage II language-impaired children (Page & Horner, 1987).

Children's spontaneous verbalizations can also be enhanced when adult facilitators provide a high level of verbal feedback coupled with little verbal directing (Woods, 1984). Examples are given in Table 7.4. Data from several studies suggest that children's conversational abilities can be increased by adult behaviors that are highly responsive to the children's spontaneous communicative behaviors.

One effective technique that can be used to increase verbalizations is a time delay procedure (Halle et al., 1981; Halle, Marshall, & Spradlin, 1979; McLean & Snyder-McLean, 1988; Snell & Gast, 1981). First, the child is trained to produce verbal requests for a desired reinforcer in response to a direct verbal cue, such as ''What do you want?'' Later, the facilitator withholds the cue while waiting for the child to vocalize or verbalize spontaneously. Gradually, the child learns to respond to the naturally occurring stimulus rather than to the adult verbalization. Other techniques are discussed in following sections.

Language facilitators plan their role in the communication event and their communication turns to maximize the learning opportunity for the child. Within

TABLE 7.4
Examples of minimally-directive verbal feedback to children

CHILD:	I went to the zoo, yesterday.
PARTNER:	Oh, that's one of my favorite spots. I love the monkeys best.
CHILD:	I have a birthday party, tomorrow.
PARTNER:	Oh, that should be fun. What do you want for your birthday?
CHILD:	We went whale watching on vacation.
PARTNER:	I've always wanted to do that. Bet it was exciting. Tell me about it.
CHILD:	My picture is a cowboy.
PARTNER:	A big cowboy on a spotted horse.
CHILD:	I'm gonna be a ghost for Halloween.
PARTNER:	Don't come to my house; I'm afraid of ghosts. I think I'll be a witch and scare your ghost.

In each of these five exchanges, the adult followed the child's lead by commenting on the child's topic and then cueing the child to provide more information or waiting for a reply.

each turn, the facilitator responds to the child while trouble-shooting the child's previous utterance, maintains the conversation by taking a meaningful turn, and provides an opportunity for the child to respond (see Table 7.4) (Craig, 1983).

Speech-language pathologists should be mindful of the differing expectations and desires of various ethnic and racial minorities. The role of parents and the expectations for children within a minority population should be thoroughly understood prior to intervention. Children are viewed quite differently across Asian, Hispanic, and African-American cultures. Likewise, the speech-language pathologist's conversational style may have a great effect on future involvement with members of that community (Matsuda, 1989).

Training Cues

If one accepts the premise that pragmatics is the governing aspect of language, then the clinician must be concerned with the context within which training occurs. Certain linguistic and nonlinguistic contexts require or provide an expectation of certain linguistic units.

In part, the problem of lack of success in generalization is due to *response programs* "in which children are taught specific responses to specific, often carefully worded, directions or questions" (Rieke & Lewis, 1984, p. 49). The child's everyday world lacks this careful control. The everyday context contains many irrelevant stimuli that do not and cannot elicit trained communication behaviors.

Relevant common stimuli within the everyday communication context can serve, however, to elicit the child's new language targets if these stimuli are included in the training (Stremel-Campbell & Campbell, 1985). Targets can be trained across several behaviors, facilitators, and settings to ensure generalization. For example, the child's toys or everyday items and daily routines are used in the training.

The systematic introduction of increasingly more irrelevant stimuli from the communication environment into the training context has been termed "loose" training (Stremel-Campbell & Campbell, 1985). The overall goals are for the newly trained behavior to be emitted in response to a variety of stimuli and for a single stimuli to result in a variety of responses. These goals can be achieved by using concurrent behaviors, response variations, and linguistic and nonlinguistic cue variations. In concurrent behavior training, relevant and irrelevant stimuli are presented together so the child learns which ones affect the newly learned behavior.

Response variation teaches the child that several responses can be used to achieve the same communication goal. For example, a drink can be attained by saying "Want drink," "Drink please," "May I have a drink?," "I'm thirsty," and "Are you as thirsty as I am?"

Verbal and nonverbal cues also can be varied to ensure that the child does not become dependent on one stereotypic stimulus. Too often, the traditional approach has relied on very narrow and somewhat stilted cues unlike those found in conversation. The use of these traditional cues, such as "Tell me the whole thing,'' may result in training characterized as apragmatic pseudoconversational drills (Cochran, 1983). Pragmatically, the cues do not make sense, for example, asking a question to which the speaker already knows the answer. As a result, the conversations within which training occurs are little more than drill with a conversational veneer.

Use of a functional conversational approach requires the speech-language pathologist to assess thoroughly the effects of certain cues and to explore the possibilities of eliciting language with a variety of linguistic and nonlinguistic cues (Constable, 1983). Those speech-language pathologists who rely on traditional cues are unaware of the rich variety of cues available for creating contexts in which language targets can occur.

Contingencies

Once the language facilitator has elicited language from the child in a conversational manner or the child has initiated language, the facilitator can begin to modify that language if necessary. In short, the child's utterance is the stimulus to which the facilitator responds. These responses or contingencies help to form the context for the child's utterance.

Children learn language within the context of several different and individualistic interactional contexts. Nonetheless, several particular aspects of parent-child communication affect the rate of language acquisition. Overall, the amount of parental speech is correlated positively with language growth. Mothers of language-impaired children communicate less with their children and in a much less intelligible fashion than do mothers of nonimpaired children (Grimm, 1982; Schodorf, 1982).

Natural maintaining consequences should be identified prior to beginning training. As much as possible, these consequences should be directly related to the response. Such consequences as "Very good" and "Good talking" should be avoided (Stremel-Campbell & Campbell, 1985). When the child message ("I saw monkeys") and the consequence ("Good talking") are unrelated, the child's language fails to retain its communicative value. Instead, communication behaviors can be maintained by conversational responses ("Oh, I think monkeys are funny. What did they do?"). Often, simply attending to the child is sufficient to maintain the child's participation.

As much as possible, conversational consequences should be semantically and pragmatically contingent and should serve to acknowledge the child's utterance. *Semantic contingency,* the relatedness of a parent's or facilitator's response to the content or topic of a child's previous utterance, has a positive effect on the rate of language development (Barnes et al., 1983; Cross, 1978, 1981; Ellis & Wells, 1980; Nelson, 1981c; Nelson & Denninger, 1977; Newport, Gleitman, & Gleitman, 1977).

Adult speech that is semantically contingent on the child's immediate utterances decreases the amount of processing the child has to do to understand and analyze the structure and meaning of the adult's utterances (Shatz, 1978). The sharing of a conversational topic and common vocabulary decreases the child's memory load for processing and increases the ease of immediate language production. The facilitator's utterance provides a prop or scaffolding (Scollon, 1979) for the child's own analysis and production. In contrast, frequent topic changing or refocusing of the child's attention by the adult impedes the child's language acquisition (Snow et al., 1984).

It is not enough, however, just to comment on the child's topic. In the following example, the facilitator's response is semantically contingent but lacks *pragmatic contingency.*

> CHILD: I want cookie, please.
> FACILITATOR: Johnny wants a cookie.

The facilitator's response should make sense within the conversational framework. In this example, more appropriate responses would be ''What kind of cookie do you want?,'' ''Okay, but just one,'' ''Help yourself,'' or ''No cookies until after lunch.'' This example shows that such contingencies as ''Good talking'' violate pragmatic contingency and do not help to continue the interchange. The child's language is more naturally reinforced when its purpose and intention are met (Arwood, 1983; McCormick & Goldman, 1984; Sprodlin & Siegel, 1982).

In brief, as noted previously, parental behaviors that attempt to increase the child's participation in the interaction, that is, a child-centered interactional style, enhance the child's language skills (Lieven, 1984; McDonald & Pien, 1982). By relinquishing some control and adopting the child's topics, language facilitators can ensure more child participation and interest. This interactive, child-centered style can be the therapeutic model for language-impaired children (Lieven, 1984; Wood, 1983).

As a group, parents of language-impaired children are less positive and accepting of their children's utterances than are the parents of age-matched or language level-matched peers. In other words, parents of language-impaired children acknowledge their childrens' utterances less frequently (Ellis & Wells, 1980; Furrow, Nelson, & Benedict, 1979).

It is possible that we have a cycle in which the child responds to the adult's language infrequently, causing the adult to interact less. This, in turn, provides less reinforcement for the child, so the child communicates less and the process begins again. We have no idea which participant begins the cycle, but it probably evolves as an interactional pattern for each dyad over a lengthy period of time.

Overall, in the clinical setting, it is important that facilitators accept a child's utterance as representative of the child's understanding of the world and of the requirements being asked. Answers considered wrong by the adult may, in fact, represent the child's somewhat different perspective. The child's response meaning can be negotiated by the facilitator and child as the conversation continues. This degree of acceptance translates into indirect acceptance of the child.

Location

Location of training may include both the physical location in which training occurs and the conversational context formed by the child and facilitator. In many ways, the conversational context is more important for generalization because it does not depend on physical setting and transcends the clinic, classroom, and home (Johnston, 1988). Given the flexibility of these natural communication sequences, training is more a matter of *how* than *where* (Craig, 1983).

Physical Location

When possible, training should occur wherever the child is likely to use the newly trained language skill. Most communication takes place within familiar events that influence the way the participants communicate. For example, storytelling, conversation, and classroom participation have different rules for participation that affect the language used. Therefore, language intervention should take place within these types of discourse events as they occur in the child's everyday physical locations.

Obviously, parents and teachers will need to be trained for their new roles as language facilitators. Parents may come to the clinic or school to be trained. If this is not possible, evening group sessions or written guidelines can be used. Even if the parents only modify their expectations for the child, this will help with the generalization of language training.

Conversational Context

Behavior must be evaluated and trained within some dynamic context in order to make sense. Language and communication are heavily influenced by the context of what precedes and follows (linguistically and nonlinguistically) and by the expectations for participation with that specific context. For example, the expectations for storytelling are different from those for conversation. Ordering at a fast-food restaurant presents different expectations than chatting with a friend on the phone. Each event follows certain scripts. Chapter 8 addresses the linguistic and nonlinguistic contexts and their manipulation by the language facilitators.

Sentences trained out of context are, therefore, more difficult for the child to learn. The speech-language pathologist is not training static forms but a generative, versatile system. The contextual expectations and scripts must be examined prior to beginning intervention within each context.

Conversations provide a dynamic context in which language serves a purpose or function. Although these conversational sequences may mirror natural sequences, the speech-language pathologist and other language facilitators are mindful of the teaching situation and the facilitator-child model (Craig, 1983). Communication strategies can be provided to the child as needed (Spinelli & Terrell, 1984). Teaching approaches used previously can be adapted to this setting to more closely approximate conversational exchange.

CONCLUSION

By carefully considering the variables that affect generalization, the speech-language pathologist can modify training to maximize this effect. Targets and design decisions can be made on the basis of the likely effect on generalization and on ultimate use within the events and situations of the child's everyday environment. Language can be elicited, modified, and consequated using techniques that mirror the conversational style used by the child's usual partners within these contexts. Motivation is provided by the child's desire to participate in enjoyable activities with responsive and attentive adults.

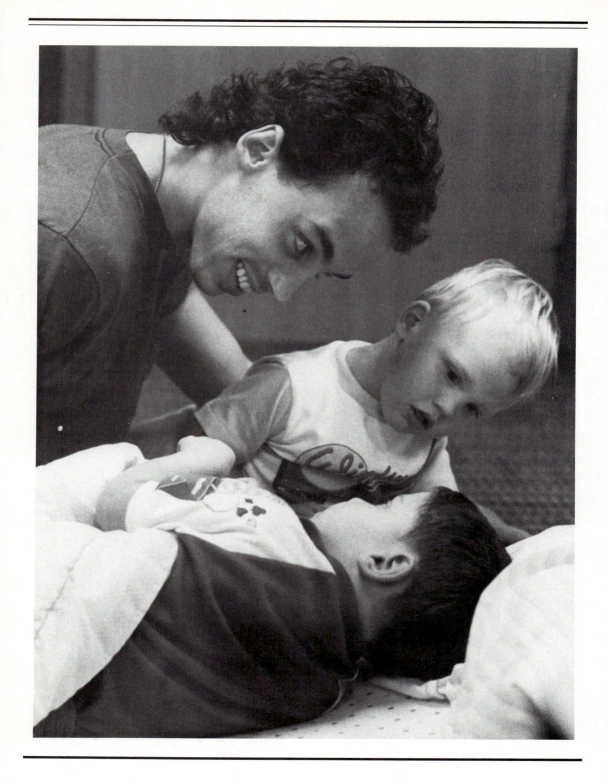

8
Manipulating Context

Language is pragmatically based in that the demands of the nonlinguistic and linguistic context give rise to both the form and content of the language expressed (Bates, 1976; Cole, 1982; Gallagher & Prutting, 1983, Prutting, 1982). Therefore, a primary goal of language intervention should be for the child to learn the appropriate language skills to function effectively within everyday communication contexts or environments.

Within each activity, the facilitator strives to provide an active experience with language use. It seems appropriate, then, that the speech-language pathologist and other language facilitators learn to manipulate these contexts to provide the child the maximum learning possible. The facilitator's role "is to accept the child's spontaneously occurring verbal or nonverbal behavior as meaningful communication, interpret it in a manner that is contextually appropriate, and become a collaborator with the child in communicating the message more effectively" (Norris & Hoffman, 1990, p. 78).

When language can be used to achieve goals within everyday communication contexts, the chances of generalization to these contexts increases. Language acquires a purpose or function. The training becomes functional in nature.

This chapter explores various strategies that can be used to manipulate the nonlinguistic and linguistic contexts in which language occurs. These strategies can be used within the everyday activities of the child and, thus, become a part of that natural environment. As much as possible, natural and conversational strategies are recommended. But the reader should be forewarned that there may be even better, more interactional ways to train children than are those presented here.

NONLINGUISTIC CONTEXTS

Speech-language pathology is so oriented toward linguistic forms of communication that it is easy to overlook the nonlinguistic aspects. Yet, the nonlinguistic context—what happens in the environment—offers a rich source for eliciting language. The speech-language pathologist can manipulate the nonlinguistic contextual cues to elicit desired language and to ensure that the child initiates language. All too often, the language-impaired child's training paradigm allows the child little control. Therefore, the child assumes a passive, responsive role to the clinician's linguistic cues.

Certain nonlinguistic contexts naturally elicit more language than do others. For most adults, cocktail parties are more likely to elicit language than are theater engagements. Inherent in the theater experience is the necessity to remain silent during the performance.

Some situations also dictate the type of language used. Most adults do not question and challenge sermons—at least not while the sermon is being delivered. In contrast, learning situations, such as a classroom, are supposed to encourage questioning. Fast-food establishments are likely to elicit demands or requests.

If targets have been selected to help the child communicate better, then the speech-language pathologist has already identified the contexts in which the child attempts these targets. In other words, the nonlinguistic contexts that are highly likely to elicit the target are known. Although the child is expected to perform, the speech-language pathologist believes that the performance will be in error, because the target was chosen from aspects of language with which the child has experienced difficulty.

Likewise, the speech-language pathologist has some control of the topics the child will discuss. The facilitator's "role is not to change the topic, once the child has chosen it, but to determine through environmental arrangement what topics the child will choose" (Hart, 1985, p. 80).

Ideally, the nonlinguistic context serves to elicit the target language behavior; the clinician can then help the child modify the target into a correct form for that situation. In theory, the child who makes a meaningful response in context will be interested in that response and motivated to change it in the desired manner. This corrected response should more easily generalize to everyday use because it is being trained within the context of everyday events and conversations.

Table 8.1 contains a sample of nonlinguistic contexts and the type of language each may elicit. Small group projects or tasks usually elicit lots of language from children. For younger children, role play and dress-up are good contexts for language. Routines can also be established within the home or classroom for asking for desired objects or privileges.

Within these nonlinguistic contexts, language may be elicited through the

TABLE 8.1
Nonlinguistic contexts and language elicitation

═══

Turn taking and requesting objects:
Provide only one plastic knife for children to share as they make a fruit salad.
Provide one highly desirable outfit in the dress-up corner of the class.
Provide only enough art supplies for half of the children and request that children share equipment.

Following directions and directing others:
While working in a group, recreate a construction paper collage of the teacher. The teacher should be careful not to supply precut paper or to help children with the color tints. The goal is to get the children to ask for help and to direct others and themselves.
In groups of two, duplicate a cake decoration previously completed by the teacher.
As a group, plant seeds in cups as the teacher has previously done. A more involved project might involve planting a garden, keeping the different crops straight and making signs.
Bake while following a written or pictured recipe.
Put together a model following written or oral directions.
Play dumb. By making lots of mistakes, the teacher can have children direct or correct the behavior.
Have a child explain how to do something known by only that child.
Have children direct each other through activities blindfolded.
Have the child be the teacher.

Requesting information:
Give only partial directions for completing a task.
Put objects that the children need for a task in an unusual location so that they will need to ask for the location.
Introduce visually interesting items but do not name them or explain their function to the children.

Giving information:
Explain class projects to children from another class.
Explain class projects to parents at a special event or Parents' Night.
Have children tell about events they experienced, for example, summer vacation, a weekend trip, a birthday party. This task and explaining how something is accomplished are excellent vehicles for sequencing.
Have children request information from children who need to improve their ability to give information.
Have children tell make-believe stories.

Reasoning:
Have children try to float or submerge objects in water. Include objects that float and those that do not so that the children must find various combinations.
Build a suspension bridge from straws, string, toothpicks, and tongue depressors.
Design a city with transportation, schools, recreation facilities, and residential, industrial, and business areas.
Play initiative games in which groups of children must solve a common problem.
Make large projects in connection with class projects. For example, children might

(continued)

TABLE 8.1 *(continued)*

design the ''perfect'' world, make montages that demonstrate male and female roles, or design a board game, such as On the Way to Your Birthday that illustrates stages of fetal development.

Requesting help:

Pose problems that children cannot solve themselves.

Sabotage activities, such as holes in paper cups, dried markers and paints, glue bottles glued shut, not enough chairs, missing gloves and hats, and so on. The list is endless.

Imagining and projecting:

Set up a drama or dress-up center.Set up a puppet stage with a variety of characters.

Set up simulated shops and stores or a housekeeping center.

Role play. (Role play can elicit a variety of intentions.)

Protesting:

Play dumb, as in forgetting to give children peanut butter and jelly with which to make sandwiches.

Miss a child's turn or withhold needed objects.

Violate a routine or an object function by using objects in novel or nonsensical ways.

Give a child too much of something or more than is needed.

Put away objects before the child is finished using them.

Ask a child to do something that is not physically possible (but safe).

Initiations:

Pose problems and *wait* for children to initiate communication.

Ask children to talk to lonely animals for you.

Sources: Author's experience, Constable (1983), Kunze et al. (1983), Staab (1983).

use of delays, introduction of novel elements, oversight, and sabotage (McLean & Snyder-McLean, 1988). Delaying or waiting for the child to initiate communication is often a very effective strategy, especially after the child has mastered a desired behavior (Hart, 1985). Too frequently, adults do not expect the child to communicate, and this expectation becomes self-fulfilling when the adult communicates for the child.

The language facilitator waits for the child to initiate the interaction. The facilitator may sit near the child and look questioningly or display some interesting item while looking at the child (Hart, 1985). When the child looks at the adult, the adult does not speak for a specified period of time unless the child does. If the child does not verbalize, the adult models or prompts the desired verbalization. Upon successful completion, the child is given the desired item.

If the item is edible, it should be small and quickly consumed. In a camp situation, I was able to maintain a small autistic child's communication initiations over 8 days with two large sugar cookies, crumbled into very small pieces. Nonedible items may be used for specific, limited tasks, such as gluing one piece of colored paper to another, and then returned to the facilitator.

Novel or unexpected events can be introduced into the situation to evoke communication. Most individuals will notice and remark on such events. For example, a kitten, guinea pig, or bright toy might be found in an unexpected spot. Even children functioning at the single-word level will comment on elements in the situation that are novel, different, or changing.

Oversight or forgetting by the facilitator will also elicit language from the child eager to become the teacher. I often play dumb, forgetting object locations or children's turns. Needed objects, such as glue or scissors, can be omitted or used in unusual ways.

Finally, sabotage of activities or routines involves taking actions or introducing elements that will not permit the activity to continue or to be completed (Constable, 1983; Lucas, 1980). My favorite example is the classroom teacher and aide who would buckle the children's boots together and turn their coats inside out sometime during the day. One can imagine the chaos at the end of the day and all of the language elicited as children requested assistance.

LINGUISTIC CONTEXTS

The goal of language use within a conversational context necessitates a thorough evaluation of the linguistic cues used with children in the training situation. Cues, such as ''What do we say?'' and ''Now, tell me the whole thing,'' are examples of pseudoconversational cues mentioned previously.

Eliciting language through constant prodding or interrogation can be unpleasant and result in less talking by the child. Such communication is one-sided, with the child assuming the role of receiver or occasional reluctant speaker (McDade & Varnedoe, 1987).

Linguistic contexts can be divided into those that model language with or without a child's response, those that directly and indirectly cue certain behaviors, and those that do not cue these behaviors. A particular utterance will cue one type of behavior but not others and, thus, can be used in contrast training to teach contextual discrimination.

Modeling

In comparative studies, the efficacy of the modeling approach has been demonstrated repeatedly (Courtright & Courtright, 1976, 1979; Prelock & Panagos, 1980; Wilcox & Leonard, 1978). Modeling is a procedure in which the clinician produces a rule-governed utterance at appropriate junctures in conversation or activities but does not ask the child to imitate. The technique compares favorably with more active techniques, such as question-answer, that require responses by the child (Weismer & Murray-Branch, 1989).

Modeling can be used in any of the following ways:

1. as a high-frequency response in very structured situations (Connell, Gardner-Gletty, Dejewski, & Parks-Reinick, 1981; Courtright &

Courtright, 1976, 1979; Culatta & Horn, 1982; Leonard, 1975; Leonard, Schwartz, Chapman, Rowan, Prelock, Terrell, Weiss, & Messick, 1982; Schwartz et al., 1985; Wilcox & Leonard, 1978).

2. as general language stimulation containing a number of language targets simultaneously (Cooper, Moodley, & Reynell, 1978, 1979; Evesham, 1977; Lee, Koenigsknecht, & Mulhern, 1975).

3. as an element in comprehension training in which the child points to pictures that illustrate the utterance modeled (Paluszek & Feintuch, 1979; Ruder, Smith, & Hermann, 1974; Winitz, 1973).

In general, modeling closely approximates the language-learning environment of nonimpaired children and is an effective language-learning strategy for the language-impaired (Lucas, 1980).

It is expected that the child will acquire some aspect of the language behavior of the facilitator and use it in a similar context later. Unlike direct instruction techniques, interactive modeling considers the child to be an active learner who abstracts the rules used in forming utterances and associates these utterances with events and stimuli in the environment (Leonard, 1981).

It is best to model the training target for the child prior to attempting to elicit the target. Within such *focused stimulation*, the speech-language pathologist produces a high density of the targets in meaningful contexts without requiring the child to respond. Two varieties of this stimulation are *self-talk* and *parallel talk*. In self-talk, the speech-language pathologist talks about what he or she is doing, whereas in parallel talk, discussion centers on the child's actions. Obviously, activities have to be chosen carefully to provide sufficient opportunities for the target to occur.

Once a target has been modeled thoroughly, the speech-language pathologist asks the child to respond in a manner similar to the model. Young, low-functioning, or delayed children may need imitation training with a complete model presented immediately before their response. Imitation is a procedure in which the child repeats the language behavior of a facilitator with the expectation that the child will acquire some aspect of the facilitator's language.

Imitation can be used as a first step in programs to teach specific language targets (Connell, 1987a, 1987b; Courtright & Courtright, 1976; Gottesleben, Tyack & Buschini, 1974; Hegde, 1980; Hegde, Noll, & Pecora, 1979; Zwitman & Sonderman, 1979) or as a correction procedure when the child fails to respond or responds incorrectly (Hester & Hendrickson, 1977; Lee et al., 1975; Warren et al., 1984). By monitoring the child's progress, the speech-language pathologist can provide varied cues, including partial models and/or delayed imitation.

The child may also respond to questions for which the speech-language pathologist has modeled the answers. Initially, the modeled answer may follow the question, but this format can be altered so that the answer precedes the question, is given partially, or precedes the question by increasingly longer periods of time.

Although the modeling procedure seems stilted in writing, it can be applied very flexibly and works well with groups of children. In small groups, children who have acquired a certain target can serve as models for those who have not. By varying turns, the speech-language pathologist ensures that sufficient models are provided for different children with different targets. In a reversal of roles, the speech-language pathologist can also serve as a model for the child, while the child cues the speech-language pathologist.

Some studies have found modeling to be less effective than other more structured methods (Cole & Dale, 1986; Connell, 1987a; Connell et al., 1981; Friedman & Friedman, 1980). Whereas modeling is effective in changing the behavior of nonimpaired children, it is less effective than imitation with the language-impaired child (Connell, 1987a). More structured approaches include imitation, elicitation in the form of fill-ins, stimulation, and comprehension training.

Direct Linguistic Cues

Linguistic cues for certain targets can be direct or indirect. Direct elicitation techniques might include the following target questions:

To elicit. . .	*Use. . .*
Verbs	"What is he doing (are you doing)?" Use any tense. A benefit is that the question contains the target tense.
Noun subjects	"Who/what is verbing?" Again, the tense can be altered for the situation.
Noun objects	"What is he/she verbing?" Tense can be altered for the situation. Obviously verbs that do not take objects should not be used.
Adverbs or adverbial phrases	"When/where/how is he/she verbing?" Tense can be altered. How questions can also be used to elicit process answers, as in "How did you make the airplane?"
Adjectives or adjectival phrases	"Which one . . .?" Tense can be altered. There should be an obvious contrast between choices for the response, such as *big* and *little*. These differences might be noted prior to questioning. Responses of a particular type can be modeled, as in "Which one ate the cookie, the littlest bear, the middle-size bear, or the biggest bear?" To keep the child from responding "That one," the clinician may want to cover her or his eyes or use some barrier.
Specific words	Completion sentences, as in "She is playing in the ____." Rising intonation after the last spoken word will signal the child to respond. If the clinician plays dumb or acts forgetful, this behavior makes more sense conversationally.

Substitution requests can also be used. For example, pronouns can be substituted for old information. The facilitator might make a statement, such as giving one descriptor ("The dog is little"), then ask the child to make a comment ("What can you tell me about the dog?"). This procedure can take the form of a guessing game, as in "Is the dog little? Well, if the dog isn't little, what can we say?"

Although these linguistic cues are conversational in nature, they will seem very nonconversational if used in nonlinguistic contexts in which they make no sense pragmatically. Questions should be used when the facilitator really desires the answer and when the child is interested in the topic of discussion.

The speech-language pathologist can model a response prior to asking the child a question, for example, "I think I want the yellow one. What about you?" This type of cue is more likely to elicit a longer utterance and is more conversational in tone.

One variation of the direct linguistic cue is a *mand-model* (Hart, 1985; Rogers-Warren & Warren, 1980). This procedure follows a routine that is established prior to beginning any activity. The routine serves as a chain in which one stimulus cues the next.

Access to desired items is through the teacher, who determines the criterion for acceptability. In this way, the teacher, not the object, becomes the stimulus for talking. According to this procedure, "it is likely to be not so much what the teachers do—the forms of language they model—as the interactional context in which the adults' models occur that facilitates children's progress in language learning" (Hart, 1985, p. 81).

In the four-step training sequence, the teacher first attracts the child's attention by providing a variety of attractive materials. This may not be necessary if the child already displays an interest. Thus, the teacher establishes joint attention with the child. In the second step, after the child has expressed interest, the teacher (de)mands, "Tell me about this" or "Tell me what you want," requesting a behavior trained previously. If there is no response, the teacher moves to step three and prompts a response or provides a model to be imitated. In the final step, the teacher praises the child for an appropriate response and gives the child the desired item.

Indirect Linguistic Cues

Indirect linguistic cues are more conversational and situational in nature. For example, when attempting to elicit questions, the speech-language pathologist might use unfamiliar objects hidden in boxes to set the nonlinguistic context. Beginning with "Boy, is this neat," the facilitator peeks into the box. An exchange might continue as follows:

> CHILD: What's in there?
> FACILITATOR: This. (Takes the object out. Waits.)
> CHILD: What is it?
> FACILITATOR: A flibbity-jibbit, it does everything.
> CHILD: What it do?

It is easy to see the interplay of nonlinguistic and linguistic cuing.

Another indirect linguistic technique requires the language facilitator to make purposefully wrong statements. A child's clothing can serve as the focus of this conversation, a technique I've dubbed "The emperor's new clothes."

FACILITATOR: (Touching child's red sweater.) What a nice blue blouse.
CHILD: This no blue blouse.

In both examples, the child has given a response that may be something less than what is desired. The speech-language pathologist can now respond and begin to shape the child's previous utterance into an acceptable form.

These examples are only a very few of many indirect techniques. Others are listed in Appendix F.

Contingencies

Conversational consequences can be divided roughly into those that do not require a child's response and those that do. Each type provides some feedback to the child, and each differs with the functioning level and degree of learning exhibited by the child.

Contingencies Requiring No Response

Contingencies that require no response from the child are nonevaluative or accepting in nature and can be used to increase correct production or highlight incorrect production for self-correction. When the child initiates or responds to some cue, the facilitator focuses full attention on the child, creating joint focus on the child's topic. Because the child has established the topic, it now acts as a reinforcer for the child and can be used to modify the child's language. Techniques used to modify the child's response include *fulfilling the intention, use of a continuant, imitation, expansion, extension* or *expiation, breakdowns* and *buildups,* and *recast sentences.*

By fulfilling the intention of the child's utterance, such as handing the child a requested item, the facilitator signals the child that the message was acceptable as received. No verbal response is required.

A continuant is a signal that a message has been received and acknowledged. These signals usually consist of head nods or verbalizations, such as *uh-huh* and *Okay.* Continuants fill the speaker's turn by agreeing with the previous utterance.

In imitation, the facilitator repeats the child's utterance in whole or in part but makes no evaluative remarks. Rising intonation, signifying a question, is not present. Again, this behavior acknowleges the child's previous utterance. Imitation is especially helpful to the child when correctly produced features of interest are emphasized ("She *is* riding the bike"). Imitations might also be preceded by phrases such as *That's right* ("That's right, she *is* riding the bike").

In contrast to imitation, expansion is a more mature or more correct version of the child's utterance that maintains the child's word order, for example:

CHILD: It got stolen by the crook.
FACILITATOR: Uh-huh, it *was* stolen by the crook.

The use of expansion as a teaching tool is very limited for children functioning above about 30 months of age. A more appropriate variety of expansion for older children is a reformulation in which two or more child utterances are combined into one utterance that includes the concepts of each, as in the following:

CHILD: The dog bit the man. The man ran away.
FACILITATOR: Oh, the dog bit the man, who then ran away.

For older children, extension is a more appropriate response. Extension is a reply to the content of the child's utterance that provides additional information on the topic, as in the following:

CHILD: It got stolen by the crook.
FACILITATOR: Oh, I wonder if the crook stole anything else.

Much of our behavior in conversations consists of replies to the content of the other speaker, and these contents can be used effectively regardless of the age or functioning level of the child. Extensions signal the child that the facilitator is attentive and interested.

Breakdowns and buildups consist of dividing the child's utterances into shorter units, then combining them and expanding on the child's original utterance. I use this strategy as my hearing-impaired and senile great-uncle used to do to aid the processing of information, mulling it over before commenting.

CHILD: It got stolen by the crook.
FACILITATOR: (Emotional, disbelieving) It was. (Hmmm) It was stolen. Stolen by the crook. (Disgusted) By the crook. (Finally) It was stolen by the crook.

This strategy works well, especially if the clinician plays dumb or uses a silly puppet who just doesn't seem to get things right. The child may shake his or her head or say ''Uh-huh'' in agreement between the facilitator's utterances.

Finally, recast sentences are a changed form of the child's utterance that maintains the same relations as the original, as in the following.

CHILD: It got stolen by the crook.
FACILITATOR: Was it stolen by the crook?
                            OR
                    It was stolen by the crook, wasn't it?
                            OR
                    The crook stole it.
                            OR
                    Did the crook steal it?

These sentences can be recast in whatever form the speech-language pathologist has targeted.

Contingencies Requiring a Response

Contingencies that require a response are used when the child is able to produce the target reliably but has failed to do so or has produced the target inaccurately in conversation. A skilled use of both nonlinguistic and linguistic contextual cues should set the stage for production of the target in a situation in which it makes good pragmatic sense. As a fully participating conversational partner, the child has an interest in the conversation and in his or her own utterance. Thus, the child is motivated to modify production in order to maintain the conversation and receive the adult's attention.

Most of these contingencies note the child's error, or require the child to find the error, and request that the child produce the target more correctly. A second contingency type requests repetition or a correct or expanded utterance to strengthen correct production. A hierarchy of both types, ranging from contingencies used in initial training to those used when the target is learned, would be *correction model/request, incomplete correction model/request, reduced error repetition/request, error repetition/request, self-correction request, contingent query, repetition request, expansion request,* and *turnabouts* (Duchan & Weitzner-Lin, 1987; Lee et al., 1975; Muma, 1978).

In a correction model/request, the facilitator repeats the child's entire utterance, adding or correcting the target that was omitted or produced incorrectly, for example:

CHILD: I *builded* a big tower out of blocks.
FACILITATOR: I *built* a big tower out of blocks. Now you say it.

The child is gently requested to repeat the facilitator's model.

Initially, the target may be emphasized to aid the child in locating the corrected unit. Later training, except that involving person markers on the verb, might restate the child's utterance as a question, as in ''You *built* a big tower out of blocks?''

Because the entire utterance is desired in the child's response, the facilitator should act confused to maintain the conversational nature of the interaction.

FACILITATOR: You *built* a tower out of big blocks? No, you *built* a big tower out of blocks? Oh, I'm confused, tell me again.

In a correction model/request, the child is provided with a complete or only slightly altered model of the correct utterance.

The facilitator should require the child to produce correctly only those units that are currently in the child's repertoire. It is difficult for facilitators to reinforce utterances even when they contain errors, as in the following example:

CHILD: I *builted* the most biggest tower out of blocks.
FACILITATOR: You *built* the biggest tower out of blocks?

CHILD: Yeah, I *built* the most biggest tower out of blocks.
FACILITATOR: Uh-huh, how big was it?
OR
What kind of blocks did you use?
OR
Where is the tower now?

A conversational approach requires the language facilitator to remain focused on the target and on the hierarchy of teaching strategies being used.

In contrast to a complete correction model/request, an incomplete correction model/request provides only the corrected target. The child must provide the rest of the utterance, as follows:

CHILD: I *builded* a big tower with blocks.
FACILITATOR: *Built.*
CHILD: I *built* a big tower with blocks.

Initially, the child will need a cue to repeat the utterance with the corrected target.

Once the child has learned the target reliably within more structured situations, the language facilitator can use other techniques that require the child to supply the missing or correct target. With reduced error repetition/request, the facilitator repeats only the incorrect structure with rising intonation, thus forming a question. This contingency informs the child that the language unit in question is incorrect and must be corrected, for example:

CHILD: I *builded* a big tower with blocks.
FACILITATOR: *Builded?*
CHILD: *Built.*

The facilitator's question is more conversational than the cue found in correction model/requests and is less disruptive to the flow of conversation. If the child fails to recognize the error, the facilitator can provide a corrected model using an incomplete correction model/request.

With error repetition/request, the facilitator repeats the entire utterance with rising intonation. The child must locate the error or omission and correct it, as in the following:

CHILD: I builded a big tower with blocks.
FACILITATOR: I *builded* a big tower with blocks?

The emphasis on the error can be increased or decreased as needed. For example, increased emphasis might be used to aid the child in finding the error. If this technique is unsuccessful, the facilitator might provide a reduced error repetition/request.

Once the child's target knowledge is reasonably stable, the facilitator can use the error repetition/request contingency even when the child is correct. This procedure helps children to scan their productions spontaneously and to self-correct.

A self-correction request does not provide the child with a repetition of the previous utterance. Instead, the facilitator asks the child to consider the correctness of that utterance from memory, for example, "Is/was that right/correct?" and "Did you say that correctly?" If the child is unsure, the facilitator can provide an error repetition/request.

In contrast to the somewhat stilted tone of the self-correction request, the contingent query is very conversational. It is concerned more with comprehension of the message being sent than with specific targets. Nonetheless, this technique can be used effectively to signal the child that something may be amiss with the production. The child is left to scan recent memory to determine where communication breakdown occurred.

Use of contingent queries should be limited because they can disrupt communication and frustrate the speaker who is continually asked to repeat. Young school-aged children dislike having to repeat more than once or twice.

Contingent queries may be specific or general depending on the abilities of the child. In response to the sentence "I *builded* a big tower with blocks," the facilitator might respond "What did you do with blocks?," "What did you do?," or simply "What?" If the child falsely assumes that his or her production was correct and merely repeats the error or omission, the facilitator might use a self-correction request.

Correct productions of the target can be reinforced by asking the child to repeat. With a repetition request, the facilitator simply says, "Tell me that again" or "Could you say that again." This technique can also be used conversationally, implying that the listener missed some portion of the transmission, not that the transmission was in error.

If the child produces the target correctly but in a smaller unit than desired, such as a one-word response following a reduced error repetition/request, the facilitator can use an expansion request. The typical cue "Tell me the whole thing" is not conversational in tone. It is better for the facilitator to fake confusion and ask for a total restatement, as in the following example:

FACILITATOR: *Built?* What was *built?* Who *built* it? I get so confused. You
    better tell me again.

The advantages of using this routine to elicit language from children were previously discussed.

Turnabouts may be more effective than repetition requests and are more conversational in nature. In a turnabout, the facilitator acknowledges the child's utterance and asks for more, as in "Uh-huh, and then what did you do?" or "Wow, what will you do next?"

Several relational terms may also be used in open-ended utterances to aid the child in providing more information of a specific nature. For example, the facilitator might repeat the child's utterance with the addition of *but* to elicit contrary or adversative information, or *and* to elicit complimentary information.

> CHILD: We played games at the party.
> FACILITATOR: What fun. You played games at the party *and* . . .
> CHILD: And we had cake and ice cream.

TABLE 8.2

Hierarchy of conversational contingencies

For the examples, the child's utterance is "I sawed two puppies." The facilitator should use the contingency farthest down on the list that ensures the child's success with minimal input.

Conversational Contingency	Example
Correction model/Request	I *saw* two puppies. Can you tell me again? (The cue to say it again is optional, unless the child does not repeat spontaneously.)
Incomplete correction model/Request	*Saw.* Can you tell me again? (Again the cue is optional.)
Reduced error repetition/Request	*Sawed?*
Error repetition/Request	I *sawed* two puppies?
Self-correction Request	Was that right?
Contingent query	I didn't understand you. Say it again, please. (Other options include Huh? and What? or in this case What did you do?)
Expansion request	Tell me the whole thing again.
*Repetition request	Tell me again.
*Turnabout	You did; I love puppies. What did they look like?

Example of hierarchy in use:

CHILD:	I sawed two puppies.
PARTNER:	Was that right? (Self-correction request)
CHILD:	Uh-huh.
PARTNER:	I sawed two puppies? (Error repetition/request)
CHILD:	Yeah.
PARTNER:	Sawed? (Reduced error repetition request)
CHILD:	Saw. I saw two puppies.
PARTNER:	Uh-huh, tell me again. (Repetition request)
CHILD:	I saw two puppies.
PARTNER:	I think I love puppies more than kittens. Where did you see them? (Turnabout)

*Used with complete, correct responses.

Other types of relationships and terms are as follows (Norris & Hoffman, 1990, pp. 78–79):

□ Temporal   *and then, first, next, before, after, when, while*

□ Causal   *because, so, so that, in order to*

□ Adversative   *but, except, however, except that*

□ Conditional   *if, unless, or, in case*

□ Spatial   *in, on, next to, between, etc.*

These contingencies can be arranged in a hierarchy similar to that in Table 8.2. This arrangement will differ with the language unit being targeted. The facilitator who is familiar with this hierarchy can respond to the child's utterances in a manner that enhances language stimulation and facilitates language learning.

CONCLUSION

Both the nonlinguistic and linguistic contexts can be manipulated by the speech-language pathologist and other language facilitators to teach language to the child and to encourage use of structures recently acquired. By using the various techniques described in this chapter, the facilitators can maximize interactions with the language-impaired child. Although it would be ideal if facilitators used the full range of techniques, even the adaptation of some would help to make learning more conversational in nature.

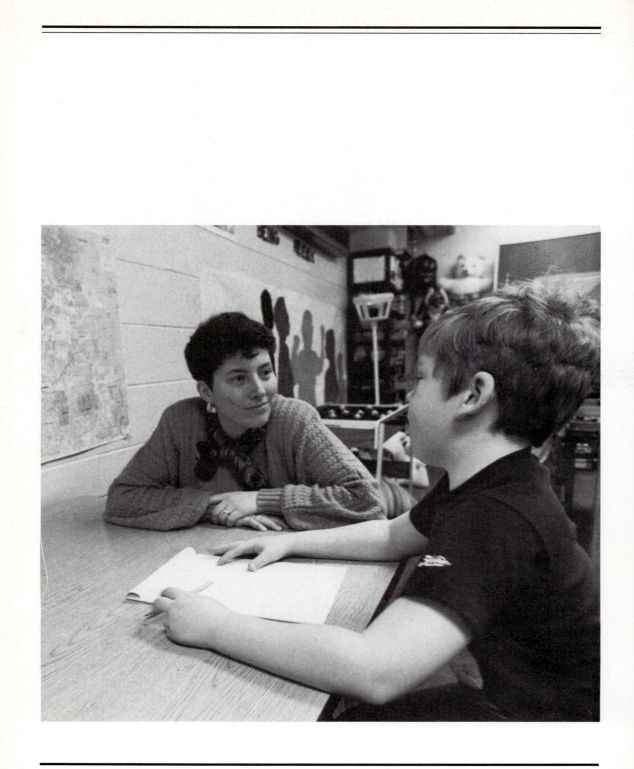

9
Specific
Intervention Techniques

A number of training approaches effectively teach the use of linguistic features to children with language impairments. The success of intervention varies with the particular linguistic feature trained, the manner and duration of the training, and the characteristics of the individual child (Leonard, 1981).

Prior to beginning intervention, the speech-language pathologist should examine all deficit areas for a given child and apply a "So what" criterion. In short, the speech-language pathologist is concerned with the importance of individual deficits on the child's overall communication. Each deficit should be evaluated to the extent that it contributes to the child's communicative functioning. Deficits that greatly affect functioning should be targeted first for intervention.

It is important that the speech-language pathologist consider generalization at the beginning of intervention and make crucial training decisions on the basis of generalization to the use environment. Even in a direct teaching approach, at least a portion of each lesson should involve the conversational context. Intervention that focuses solely on linguistic form can result in limited progress and lack of generalization (Goetz & Sailor, 1988; Halle, 1988). Preferable are specific situations in which language form skills are necessary, such as ordering in a fast-food restaurant or using the telephone (Mire & Chisholm, 1990).

This chapter explores some proven and some promising techniques for intervention within the five aspects of language: pragmatics, semantics, syntax, morphology, and phonology. We discuss hierarchies for training and techniques that lend themselves well to each area. The final portion of the chapter deals with the special needs of bilingual and bidialectal children.

In general, we present a developmental hierarchy of intervention, modified where appropriate by sound teaching principles. It is important to remember that development is a gradual process with much overlap between structures. Development is also not "domain-specific" (Kamhi & Nelson, 1988). Rather, changes in one area of language can affect other areas just as overall developmental changes can affect language. When possible, we use the functional approach explained throughout this text. At all levels of instruction, some elements of the functional intervention model can be used.

Intervention should be fun and challenging, using real conversational exchanges between the child and partners wherever possible. Thus, both partners are actively involved in the process. "The child must be an active speaker who engages in communicative behavior that is effective at changing the attitudes, beliefs, or behavior of the hearer" (Lucas, 1980, p. 31).

For clarity, the chapter is divided into the five aspects of language. The best intervention presents language holistically so that the child can experience newly acquired language as it is used in communication. Some speech-language pathologists accomplish this goal by targeting skills in more than one area of language or by using a stage approach as Prutting suggests (1979). The holistic aspect of intervention is discussed at the end of the next section, and suggested activities are presented in Appendix G.

PRAGMATICS

As children mature, they gain increasingly more complex categorizational or word-associational strategies and increasingly more complex organizational word and structure systems. The most appropriate and effective way of expressing oneself depends on a number of variables that are stylistic, socio-emotional, personal, and contextual. In other words, linguistic variation is the result of skills in pragmatics or language use.

Many children do not use language as an effective tool for learning about their environment. They do not ask questions or request materials. Making mistakes and being corrected is easier for them than asking questions. They wait for the environment to act in some way, and then they respond. Often, adults in the child's world lose their expectation that the child will initiate communication.

Language intervention goals, however, are usually product rather than process oriented (Wilkinson & Milosky, 1987). In other words, language forms are targeted whereas language use is ignored. Although there has been a theoretical shift toward pragmatic models of language, treatment programs continue to emphasize syntax and semantics (Connell, 1982; Fujiki & Brinton, 1984; Goldstein, 1984; Tyack, 1981). In general, communicative context is used only to create fun or as an afterthought relative to generalization (Culatta & Horn, 1982).

Children can acquire very complex forms without totally comprehending them. It is essential, however, that they understand the functional qualities or use of the form (Snow & Goldfield, 1983). Thus, the effect of communicative need overrides the effect of syntactic complexity. We might do better to identify and train pragmatic behaviors and to teach the appropriate contexts in which to use these behaviors. When targeting pragmatics, form errors should be ignored unless they interfere with the intended purpose of the child's utterance.

When appropriate, however, forms can and should be targeted within a functional context. For example, the speech-language pathologist might teach requesting behaviors as a function of the goal of gaining information, action, or materials. She may help children to identify the goal first and then the form that goes with each goal. Subsequently, she may teach children the alternative forms for such requests.

Through role playing and the use of videotaped interactions, the speech-language pathologist can teach the child to identify situations in which the desired information, action, or material was requested inadequately, inaccurately, or inappropriately (Lloyd, Baker, & Dunn, 1984). She can also train reattempts or requests for clarification. Likewise, she can help the child to identify the requested goal of another speaker and to respond appropriately.

The speech-language pathologist may target a number of pragmatic skills within a single lesson, and may use many everyday events and play activities to teach a single pragmatic skill (Johnson, Johnston, & Weinrich, 1981). For example, telephone conversations teach acknowledgment of the interaction, opening and closing conversations, maintaining topic, and referential communication. The use of situational cards and different voices on the other end of the phone can help the child adapt to differing situations. Pretending that you are lost or cannot see can teach requesting and giving assistance and information, roles, and following directions.

Construction toys, such as Legos®, clay, Play-Doh®, or construction paper, used to copy a model can teach requesting assistance, referential communication, giving and following directions, and topic maintenance. More difficult tasks will require more assistance.

Several children's stories can be enacted to help the child learn roles. Recitation of stories or nursery rhymes to different audiences will aid growth of register. The use of several different puppets or dolls or different costumes will aid the learning of role taking.

Finally, the speech-language pathologist can use any number of activities for referential communication. Children can describe objects seen in Viewmasters or through periscopes, felt in paper bags, or hidden. Such activities as I Spy or Twenty Questions also aid referential communication growth and foster requesting and giving information.

If we ''provide the child with the tools and an opportunity to be a successful communicator . . . the child has been given a purpose to maintain linguistic communication'' (Lucas, 1980, p. 201). These tools might take the form of speech acts or conversational abilities.

Speech Acts

Children select and acquire utterances that are communicatively most useful (Snow et al., 1984). This explains why request forms and words that mark the initiation of favorite activities are acquired before labels and descriptive terms (Nelson, 1981a). In training, however, the speech-language pathologist is concerned with the breadth of illocutionary functions that the child is able to express.

The following section addresses the training of several different illocutionary functions (Bedrosian, 1985, 1988; Constable, 1983). Chapter 10 discusses some methods to be used in the classroom. Appendix F also provides several indirect linguistic cues useful for eliciting different functions.

Calling for Attention

Calling for someone's attention requires the presence of a person whose attention the child seeks or who is essential to completion of a task. In general, children seek attention from adults who provide it. Adults or facilitators might give the child an object within a situation and ask him or her to take it to an adult who, for the purpose of training, initially ignores the child. The child might also be asked to relay a message to someone else.

Adults or facilitators should attend to the child as soon as the child requests attention. If the child continually demands attention or uses inappropriate behavior to get attention, the facilitator will have to set some limits, such as only responding in certain situations and never responding to inappropriate behavior.

The form is usually the child calling the facilitator by name or gaining attention by some other means, such as tapping the listener's shoulder, moving into the visual field of the listener, leaning in the direction of the listener, or using eye contact. The child may also specify how the facilitator should respond.

Requests for Action

Requests for action can be trained at mealtime, within small group projects, or during almost any physically challenging task. Again, the child assumes that the facilitator can provide what is requested.

The facilitator will need to design situations in which children require assistance to complete the task. To encourage requesting, she can use initiative games in which children must solve problems. Tasks may also be sabotaged (see Table 8.1). As in requests for objects, attention is gained first, and the form of the utterance is interrogative or imperative.

Requests for Information

Language-impaired children often do not see other persons as sources of information and may produce few such requests. Although the environment can be manipulated to encourage requests for objects and actions, it is not as easy to encourage or increase the child's need and desire to seek information.

Requests for information require that the facilitator omit essential information for some novel or unfamiliar task, such as an art project, a new game, or some challenging academic task. Objects unknown to the child may be introduced without being named or their purpose explained. The child can be gently prodded to ask questions if this does not occur spontaneously.

The child must recognize both the need for this information and that another person possesses the knowledge. Recognition of need is often the most difficult aspect of this training. Confrontational naming tasks, with objects known and unknown to the child, may encourage initial requesting for information. The form of requests for information is either a *wh-* or *yes/no* interrogative with rising intonation.

The facilitator might also encourage the child to ask questions if questioned about other people's feelings or actions of which the child has little knowledge. The child can then be cued with ''Why don't you ask (name).''

The child should be expected to ask questions that reflect the form the child is capable of producing. The facilitator's verbal responses discussed in Chapter 8 can be used to help the child modify incorrect, inappropriate, or immature responses.

Requests for Objects

The facilitator can easily train requests for objects within art tasks, group projects, snack time, job training, or daily living skills training, such as dressing and hygiene. It is essential that the child desire the object requested and that the facilitator can provide it.

The facilitator can change the environment to increase both the opportunities for requesting and the caregiver behaviors that direct the child's attention to these opportunities (Olswang, Kriegsmann, & Mastergeorge, 1982). Many situations, especially those with groups of children, provide an opportunity for overlooking a child's turn, thus encouraging requesting. Of particular importance is a coordinated program designed to teach requesting for the everyday environment by approximating that environment and training those within it to model and elicit requests. Table 9.1 includes general guidelines for caregiver elicitation techniques.

The speech act usually begins with eye contact or some attention-getting behavior, such as using a name. The form, usually accompanied by a reaching gesture, is interrogative or imperative and specifies the desired object. Form training can occur within the actual need situation.

Responding to Requests

Responses may take the form of an answer to a question or a reply to a remark. These forms are very different and require different skills.

In responding to questions, children must recognize that they possess the answer and that they are required to reply. Initial training should disregard the correctness of the answer in favor of reinforcing answering in general. At this stage, teaching *wh-* question responses should reflect the appropriateness-before-accuracy pattern found in early question development (Parnell et al., 1986). In a situation in which the facilitator asks about objects known to the child,

TABLE 9.1
Caregiver guidelines for elicitation of requests

Make statements throughout the day about objects that the child might prefer. Wait for a response.

Use elicitation behaviors to accompany high-interest activities and play. These behaviors include the following:

Modeling with an imitative prompt. Facilitator provides a model of a request and asks the child to imitate.

Direct questioning. Facilitator asks ''What do you want?'' or ''What do you need?''

Indirect modeling. Facilitator provides a partial model followed by an indirect elicitation request, such as ''If you want more *X,* let me know (or ''ask me for it'') or ''Would you like to *X* or *Y*?''

Obstacle presentation. Facilitator requests that the child accomplish some task but provides an obstacle to accomplishment.

''Please get me the chalk over there.'' (There is no chalk.)

''Pour everyone some juice.'' (The container is empty.)

General statement. Facilitator makes a verbal comment about some activity or object that the child might want to request. The facilitator entices the child.

''We could play Candyland® if you want to.''

''I have some Play-Doh® on that high shelf.''

Set up specific situations to elicit requesting.

Provide direct and indirect models as often as possible whithout requiring the child to imitate.

Provide a model at appropriate times when the child appears to need assistance or is looking quizzical.

Have the child attempt difficult tasks in which help is occasionally needed.

Respond *immediately* and *naturally* to any verbal request.

Source: Adapted from Olswang, L., Kriegsmann, E., and Mastergeorge, A. (1982). Facilitating functional requesting in pragmatically impaired children. *Language, Speech, and Hearing Services in Schools, 13,* 202–222.

it is fairly certain that the child will give the appropriate answer. The information requested can gradually expand to conform to the child's ability to respond.

Replying is more difficult to teach because a response is expected but not required. The child's response may be in the form of nonlinguistic compliance or a linguistic response. Children's comprehension of different requests will vary with age (Ervin-Tripp, 1977). Table 3.5 contains the ages at which different types of requests are understood.

The child's ability to reply may be hindered by an inability to determine the topic or to formulate a response. The facilitator may enhance linguistic processing by having the child repeat the request. Over time she can modify this procedure to whispered imitation, mouthing, and silent repetition until the process is internalized. She can help children in identifying important information in requests and in formulating responses.

The speech-language pathologist can elicit denials by giving the child something other than what the child requested or by giving the child something undesirable. The child can reject either an action or proposal. The speaker uses emphatic stress, and the utterance is in a negative form.

Statements

Show and tell, discussions, or current event activities help children state information. During discussions of high interest topics, such as dating, holidays, pets, or competitive games, the facilitator can encourage children to offer their opinions. She also can use mock radio and television broadcasts. With a little cutting and some paint, she can convert a large appliance box into a console television from within which children can deliver daily newscasts.

The facilitator may either know the information the child is sharing or not. In the first instance, the child is recalling a shared event; in the latter, the child is presenting new information and can assume that the facilitator has very limited information. Each situation has different informational needs and requires some presuppositional skill to determine the necessary amount of information to convey.

The form is declarative. Initially, the child must secure the listener's attention and state the discussion topic. Statements can be expanded into narratives whose purpose is also to convey information.

Conversational Abilities

More than other areas of language intervention, the training of conversational abilities requires the use of actual conversational situations. Several clinical programs are commercially available that teach conversational skills in actual or role-played situations (Blank & Marquis, 1987; Carson, 1987; Hoskins, 1987; Larson & McKinley, 1987; Schwartz & McKinley, 1984; Weinrich, Glaser, & Johnston, 1987; Wiig, 1982). The following section presents methods for training selected conversational abilities.

Presupposition

The speaker's semantic decisions are based on his or her knowledge of the referents and the situation and on presuppositions or social knowledge of the listener's needs. The speaker needs to provide information that is as unambiguous as possible. In other words, the speaker and listener need to share the same linguistic context.

Often, children with language impairments are unaware of their audience's needs. There can be significant effect, however, from training speakers to be aware of listener needs (Shantz & Wilson, 1972).

The two aspects of this training are what information to relay and how much. The first can be trained with descriptive or directive tasks in which the child is the speaker. The listener tries to guess or draw the described object or follow the directions. The facilitator can use barrier games, in which she places an opaque barrier between the speaker and listener, for teaching speakers to be aware of their listeners' needs (Muma, 1978; Wallach, 1980). Some clinical materials are available commercially (McKinley & Schwartz, 1987). Because the speaker and listener do not share the same nonlinguistic context, the bulk of the information must be carried by the linguistic element in a clear, unambiguous manner if the listener is to comprehend.

When the child is the listener, the speech-language pathologist can send ambiguous or incomplete messages or directions to give the child an opportunity to identify the missing semantic elements. Obstacle courses are also a good vehicle through which the child can be directed or direct others.

Training the correct amount of information to transmit may be more difficult. Of course, giving insufficient information in the tasks mentioned in the last paragraph would make the directions difficult to follow. The speech-language pathologist can train children to give more as well as more accurate information. For the child who gives too much information, these tasks may be initially trained one descriptor or one step at a time. These can then be grouped into multidescriptor or command steps so that the child experiences offering more information. The relating of very discrete or limited events, such as drawing a picture or washing your face, can control the amount of information to be relayed.

The speech pathologist can also help the child to monitor his or her own production to know when redundancy occurs. She can gently remind the child that certain information was relayed previously. In subsequent training, she can quiz the child about the novelty of information presented.

Referential Skills

Referential skills include identifying novel content and describing this content for the listener. Children with language-learning disabilities have been successfully trained to use referential skills through the use of barrier games (Bunce, 1989). The description of physical attributes is somewhat easier to teach than are relational terms, such as location.

It may be best to pair an LLD child with another child rather than an adult, because the child may assume that the adult partner intuitively knows the object or is pretending not to know. Thus, the child may provide less information to an adult partner.

Topic

Topic performance is an important intervention target for the following reasons (Bedrosian & Willis, 1987):

1. Its use is one means of coordinating conversations and actions, thereby fostering development of interpersonal relations.
2. It regulates the sequence of a conversation.

3. It involves the initiation of conversation.

4. It requires listening and comprehension to maintain the flow of conversation.

5. It provides a framework for making relevant contributions. (Grice, 1975)

In short, topic offers an encompassing framework for considering other language skills.

Topic initiation. Initiation is the verbal introduction of a topic not currently being discussed. Children often do not understand the purpose of conversations or are reluctant to introduce topics for discussion. Topic initiation, a form of conversational manipulation, implies an active conversational strategy. The language-impaired child may not be adept at introducing topics clearly or may have very limited topics (Dollaghan & Miller, 1986).

Adolescents with moderate-to-severe mental retardation have been taught to initiate a topic through the use of waiting and through training in the purpose of conversation (Downing, 1987). In the first step of training, the facilitator maintains eye contact for 10 seconds but does not speak. Planned delay can be an effective strategy for prompting clients to initiate conversation (Halle et al., 1981).

If the child does not initiate the conversation during this wait, the facilitator can explain the purpose of conversation and the enjoyment that can result (Downing, 1987). She can also describe the roles of speaker and listener. Then the facilitator returns to the waiting strategy. If the child still does not respond, the facilitator can suggest that the child find something of interest to discuss by looking through a magazine. The facilitator then returns to the waiting strategy. If the child fails to initiate again, the facilitator can model a topic initiation.

Some children fail to initiate conversations and topics because of a history of failure. It is important that the facilitator focus fully on the child when the child initiates and follow the child's lead. The facilitator should try not to interrupt the child (DeMaio, 1984).

She might first teach the child to gain the listener's attention. When the child inadequately introduces a topic, the facilitator can request further information to identify the topic. Focused activities, such as describing pictures or a shared event or following directions, will show the child the need to share the referent with the listener.

The facilitator can initially tolerate inappropriate topics to give the child some success. Gradually, she can discuss the inappropriateness of these topics and gently steer the conversation to more appropriate ground. She can suggest topics ("Maybe you'll tell me about . . .") and leave it for the child to initiate. She can also train the child to ask other people about their likes and dislikes, favorite foods, sports, TV shows, or exciting trips or vacations in order to include other-oriented topics in the child's repertoire.

Traditional therapy often centers on the immediate context and may inhibit generalization by failing to incorporate displacement or nonimmediate contexts

(Spradlin & Siegel, 1982). In part, the discussion of the immediate context is related to the stimulus items used with children. To increase the frequency of memory-related topics, the facilitator can encourage the child to talk about feelings or activities engaged in prior to the conversation (Bedrosian and Willis, 1987). Elicitation can be direct (''What did you do yesterday?'') or indirect (''I wonder what you did yesterday''). She can encourage the child to ask the same information of the language facilitator. In addition, she can engage the child in activities and then ask the child to discuss what was done. The speech-language pathologist can provide feedback in the form of expansions of the child's utterances. Future-related topic initiations are similar, such as discussing what the child will do next. The use of such conversationally based strategies can increase nonimmediate topic initiations as well as the general level of syntactic performance (Bedrosian & Willis, 1987).

Topic maintenance.   The speech-language pathologist can continue the conversation by commenting on the topic the child initiated and by cuing the child to respond (Downing, 1987). She can use turnabouts—usually a comment followed by a cue for the child to respond, such as a question—to keep the conversation flowing and on topic. Questions should make pragmatic sense, that is, the facilitator should not know the answer prior to asking. Table 9.2 lists various turnabouts.

Off-topic responding may indicate that the child is inattentive or cannot identify the referent or topic presented. Inattentive children may be easily dis-

TABLE 9.2
Variety of turnabouts

Type	Example
Tag	Child: Baby's panties. Mother: It's the baby's diaper, *isn't it?*
Clarification (contingent query)	*Huh?* *What?*
Specific request	*What's that?*
Confirmation	*Horse?* *Is that a hippopotamus?* (Hand object to partner and give quizzical glance)

Expansions
    Suggestions
    Corrections
    Behavior comment
	
	I want one.
	No, it's a zebra! (Expectant tone)
	You can't sit on that.

Expansive question for sustaining conversation	*What would the policeman do then?*

Source: Drawn from K. Kaye and R. Charney, ''Conversational Asymmetry between Mothers and Children,'' *Journal of Child Language.* 1981, *8*, 35–49.

tracted and need help determining the focus of their attention. The facilitator can help the child who cannot sort through the information to identify the referent or topic through the use of questions that highlight those semantic cues of importance to the child. She can also keep the child on topic with such cues as "Anything else you can tell me about (topic)?" or "Tell me more about (topic)." Later, she can use contingent queries to keep the child on topic.

Specific words may confuse the child. The speech-language pathologist must be careful to limit the use of words, such as *what,* that can be used to obtain specific nominative information ("What is this?") and explanations ("What happened at the zoo?").

When the adult and child have shared the same experience, the adult can act as a guide to keep the child on topic. The adult can also help the child sequence events through the use of questions (e.g., "Then what happened?") or probes (e.g., "Are you sure that happened next?").

The facilitator should avoid dead-end conversational bids. Dead-end bids result in a short response that ends the interaction. A common dead-end bid is the overused "What did you do today?" to which every child knows the answer "Nothing."

Duration of topic.   The facilitator may help the incessant talker by using very limited topics with definite boundaries, such as "What animals did you see at the zoo?" If the child strays beyond the topic, the facilitator should interrupt. She can then remind the child of the topic and gently bring the child back to it.

The facilitator should also alert the child when the child has provided enough information or is redundant. Such phrases as "You've already told me about *X*" or "I'll only answer that question one more time" help the child establish boundaries.

Children who provide too little information can be encouraged to provide more with "Tell me more." The speech-language pathologist can also play dumb with such utterances as "Well, I guess it was pretty boring if that's all that happened." In general, children remain on topic longer when they are enacting scenarios, describing, or problem solving (Schober-Peterson & Johnson, 1989).

Turn Taking

It is important not to initiate turn-taking training while also attempting to train topic maintenance. Too many new training targets may confuse the child. The facilitator may have to tolerate off-topic comments initially to correct inappropriate turn taking.

Turn taking can begin at a nonverbal, physical level. The facilitator and child can pass items back and forth as they use them. The item can then become the symbol for talking. Many structured games also require turn taking. The facilitator can also provide a turn-taking model by imitating the child. She can use verbal games and motion songs with groups of children. Later, she can use turnabouts or a question-answer technique to help the child take verbal turns. Nonlinguistic cues, such as eye contact and nodding, can signal the child to take a turn. She can decrease questioning gradually in favor of these nonlinguistic cues and wait for the child to take a turn. She can teach the child attention-getting devices, such as increased speaking volume, to gain a turn. She can also change conversational partners for those with whom the child is more assertive and initiates more frequently. Games in which the child directs other people are highly motivating.

Turn taking is appropriate if it does not interrupt others. The overly assertive child who continually interrupts may need to be reminded not to do so. The facilitator might focus instruction on identifying when speakers have completed their turns. She also should explain appropriate interruptions, as in emergencies. Structured exchanges using an intercom or CB radio may help children understand the importance of turn allocation. Structured games, such as Twenty Questions, also foster turn-allocation learning.

Conversational Repair

Through monitoring, each conversational partner detects and reacts to conversational breakdowns by other people when he or she is speaking and alone when a partner is speaking (Markman, 1981). Language-impaired children often seem unaware of the distinction between understanding and failure to understand and rarely act even when they do not comprehend.

The speech-language pathologist may modify comprehension monitoring through the use of audiotaped language samples in the following training sequence (Dollaghan & Kaston, 1986):

1. Identification, labeling, and demonstration of active listening.
2. Detection of and reaction to inadequate signals.
3. Detection of and reaction to inadequate content.
4. Identification of and reaction to comprehension breakdown.

Although this sequence can be easily trained in an audiotaped mode with first graders, generalization to actual conversational use should not be neglected. The introduction of puppets, dolls, or role playing at each step can facilitate this generalization. Written scripts may be used with older children.

Comprehension monitoring can be facilitated when the child takes an active role in the process. The child is first taught to identify, label, and demonstrate active orientation to listening behaviors, such as sitting, looking at the speaker, and thinking about what the speaker says (Dollaghen & Kaston, 1986). After learning to distinguish successful and unsuccessful performance of the three active listening behaviors, the child labels and demonstrates each. The child might also repeat the previous speaker's utterance or reply to such questions as ''What did (name) just say?''

Next, the child is taught to detect and react to *signal inadequacies,* such as insufficient loudness, excessive rate, or competing noise. These concrete obstructions that prevent representation of the message are relatively easy to identify and enable the child to learn the difference between understanding and not understanding (Dollaghen & Kaston, 1986).

Within everyday activities, the facilitator can encourage contingent queries from the child by mumbling or talking too fast. This works especially well when giving directions needed to complete some fun task. The facilitator can occasionally ask the child, "What did I say? How can we find out?"

Once able to identify signal inadequacies, the child can be taught a variety of responses for requesting clarification. Requests may include general appeals, such as "Pardon?" (or "What?"), "I can't hear you," and "Wait . . . Now say it again" (or "Again please"), or more specific requests, such as "Talk louder please" (or "Louder"), "Could you talk more slowly?" (or "Slow down"), and "Did you say _____?" It is best to begin with more general requests and then move to more specific ones. The request form should reflect the child's overall syntactic level.

Next, the child can be taught to detect and react to *content inadequacies,* such as inexplicit, ambiguous, and physically impossible commands. For example, because inadequate content may not always be obvious, the speech pathologist can ask the child to repeat the message to himself or herself and/or to the speaker and to attempt the task demanded (Dollaghen & Kaston, 1986). Again, the child is taught various methods for requesting clarification of inadequate content. Requests may include "What do you mean?," "Which one?," "Where?," "I can't do that" (or "I can't"), "Do you mean _____?," and "That doesn't make sense."

This part of the training can be great fun, with the facilitator making outrageous statements and ridiculous demands of the child. She can insert intentional content inadequacies into any number of daily activities.

Finally, she can teach the child to identify and react to messages that exceed his or her comprehension capacity by the presence of unfamiliar lexical items, excessive length, and excessive syntactic complexity. This level of comprehension breakdown may be the most difficult to detect because of the often abstract nature of the breakdown.

The child can practice identification and reaction in the form of clarification requests in real-life situations in which these difficulties are likely to occur. Most novel activities include unusual jargon that the facilitator can use to confuse the message. For example, cooking offers such words as *ladle, simmer,* and *skillet.*

Requests for clarification might include "Say those one at a time" (or "One at a time"), "That was too long for me," "I don't know that word" (or "I don't know"), "Can you tell me a different way?," "What does _____ mean?" (or "What do you mean?"), and "Can you show me?" (or "Show me"). As training progresses, the child should identify the point of actual breakdown for the speaker.

Comprehension

Comprehension training should begin with recall from pictures or items and progress to literal recall of one or more details from verbal sources (Cole & Cole, 1981). Gradually, the speech-language pathologist can require the child to recall more details. Later, the child can detail these in sequence, possibly using sequential pictures, photographs of past events, or comic books as aids. Daily events can provide a script to aid comprehension. Next, she can require the child to relate cause and effect from familiar or recently read stories. Once able to reconstruct these relationships, the child can begin to make inferences, draw conclusions, and predict outcomes from stories, riddles, and jokes. Finally, the child can learn to synthesize information and create subjective summaries of the meanings of stories, TV shows, or movies.

To assist comprehension, the speech-language pathologist can manipulate the semantic content, complexity, context, and function to shape question-response strategies (Parnell & Amerman, 1983). The therapy process moves from simple, context-embedded questions to the use of questions in more abstract contexts, while controlling the length of the questions to highlight semantic content (Moeller et al., 1986). In the first stage, the facilitator attempts to build awareness and enhance emerging skills by using topics of high interest as the question contexts. She concentrates on establishing repeatable responses to yes/no questions by using a second adult as a model, multiple choice alternatives (''Do you want a cookie? Yes or no?''), visual cues to signal that a response is desired, and the child's natural, everyday contexts.

In stage two, early developing *wh-* question forms become the targets, and yes/no questions are used to highlight the semantic content desired. Take, for example, the question ''What is the girl wearing on her head?'' A nonresponse, an inappropriate response, or an inaccurate response might be followed by ''Is she wearing a shoe on her head?'' If the child responds negatively, the prompt would be ''That's right, what is she wearing on her head?'' Print, pictures, or signs can be used to highlight the *wh-* words and, thus, emphasize the information desired. These prompts can be gradually faded. In the third stage, new *wh-* forms are added systematically. In the final stages, stimulus content is gradually shifted from concrete, predictable, factually based academic topics to more abstract, less predictable conversational ones.

Narration

Young children use a script-based knowledge organization system (McCartney & Nelson, 1981; Wimmer, 1979). Although older children and adults retain this system, they also use taxonomic or categoric knowledge for processing (Lange, 1978; Mistry & Lange, 1985).

Scripts are sequences of events that form unified wholes. When this event sequence is placed in linguistic form, it is called a *text*, the basis of narratives. Narratives are generally organized by a story grammar consisting of an initiating event, a reaction by the main characters to the event, an attempt to respond to the event, a consequence or outcome to the event, and an ending (Johnston, 1982; Stein & Glenn, 1979).

Knowledge of episode structure forms a framework within which the child can interpret complex events and unfamiliar content. The speech-language pathologist can facilitate development of internalized narrative schemes or story grammars through the following (Nelson, 1986b):

1. Involve children in organized activities, such as daily routines, to help them organize their own real-life scripts.
2. Read and tell real-life stories with clear scripts.
3. Help children transfer from activities to linguistic organization by telling them fairy tales with clearly structured story grammars and then having them dramatize the stories (Moeller & McConkey, 1984).

These exercises can also be written.

The speech pathologist can facilitate production of event descriptions by having children describe familiar events as they occur or as recalled from slides, pictures, or videotape (Duchan, 1986b; Lewis, Duchan, & Lubinski, 1985). Children can role play and describe familiar events as they occur. One of my favorite language lessons included mime and the acting out of familiar situations. Later, these events were described without role playing.

Pictures of familiar events as the child draws them can be used for sequencing. The facilitator can help the child to identify the setting and characters by asking him or her to describe the picture; for example:

FACILITATOR: Well, what do we have here?
CHILD: This is me in the kitchen, and I'm making breakfast.
FACILITATOR: So, we might say, ''This morning, I was in the kitchen making breakfast.'' What did you do first? (Or Then what happened? or What's this next picture?)

After completing a step-by-step description, she can encourage the child to tell the entire narrative.

Children can then progress to fairy tales or their own stories. The facilitator can use questions to move children to more sophisticated ways of organizing and expressing concepts and relationships.

Narrative discourse is the next logical step. Children should have the opportunity to practice forms of narration within a variety of role-playing situations (Heath, 1986b). Narratives can be cued by statements, such as ''Tell me what you did at . . .'' or ''Tell me how you did. . . .''

It is unclear whether cohesion can be directly taught. Increased organization may reflect maturation of children's cognitive-social-linguistic knowledge system (Nelson, 1985; Rice, 1984). Contextualized training can provide the structure needed to foster the development of cohesion in children's communication.

SEMANTICS

Semantic intervention consists of several different but related levels of intervention. Word meanings form relationships with other words that help to categorize and organize not only the language system but also cognitive processes, particularly for older children. For this reason, semantic intervention involves a variety of interrelated intervention strategies much more complex than simply training vocabulary words.

At its core, word meaning consists of concepts or knowledge of the world. Words do not name things, but rather refer to these concepts (Olson, 1970). These conceptual complexes are formed from many experiences with the actual referents.

The process of forming and organizing concepts may reflect general cognitive organization and, in turn, influence that organization (Nelson, 1986b). Semantic training must recognize the importance of these underlying concepts and include cognitive aspects of concept formation. Several commercial resources are available for training cognitive skills essential for conceptualization (Cimorell, 1983).

Inadequate Vocabulary

Reference or meaning is the relationship of the sign or word to the underlying concept. Different strategies are used by different children and by the same child at different developmental times to construct meanings.

Children with language disorders often use one strategy exclusively or predominantly. For example, the meanings of autistic children seem to be unanalyzed, experience-based chunks that are very situationally related (Fay & Schuler, 1980; Prizant, 1983b). Retarded children are often deficient in their ability to form conceptual complexes. Other children may have more conventional concepts but experience difficulty relating these underlying concepts to linguistic signs.

The speech-language pathologist may assist with the building and extending of individual reference systems by providing situations in which children encounter the physical and social world. Dynamic events seem to encourage early concept development better than do static ones (Nelson, 1986b). Therefore, feature learning can be enhanced by focus on movement, contrast, and change.

The experiential base is important, especially for the child below age 7. The child should have the opportunity to have meaningful, real experiences. Children can describe experiences in many different ways. Groups of children on a field trip might touch, smell, and even taste an old log and describe the sensation. Language facilitators can encode features of events and entities to which children attend (Nelson, 1986). Instead of naming unfamiliar entities, such as types of leaves, children can be encouraged to stretch their existing language and give descriptive names, such as five-pointed leaf tree. Older elementary school children can learn from the experiences of others, much as adults do (Lucas, 1980).

Facilitators can also target words used frequently at home and school in everyday activities and events. Such words should be trained along with others that mean the same (synonyms), sound the same (homonyms), or are opposites (antonyms). This training will help the child to organize language for easy storage and retrieval of information. Prefixes and suffixes are also important, as is syllabication.

No one likes to give verbatim definitions. Learning benefits if the child and facilitator can use the word to discuss a relevant topic in context.

The facilitator should not expect dictionary definitions from children below age 12. By that age, however, the child should be able to define words, draw conclusions, and make inferences.

Examples should be prototypes or best exemplars, as these will enhance learning of salient features (Lucas, 1980). In addition, the facilitator should expose children to multiple examples of events and things in familiar contexts in order to perceive these features of events and entities. Language facilitators can act as mediators framing, focusing, and providing salient features of experiences for the child (Nelson, 1986).

Child and adult definitions, especially categorical ones, seem to be organized around a prototype or best exemplar. Understanding and training should progress from these general meanings to more specific ones. It is important for the language-impaired child to expand meanings beyond the often obvious best exemplars. Training should also proceed from more contextual meanings, as in ''hit the ball,'' to less contextual, more figurative meanings, such as ''hit the roof.''

Materials should provide for adequate semantic development. Pictures are too abstract for some children; single examples too limited. ''Materials that isolate word meanings from the total concept are too abstract'' (Lucas, 1980, p. 21). Referents should be presented in a variety of ways to build a total concept. Varying contexts provide for maximum usage and exposure.

Semantic Categories and Relational Words

Meaning extends beyond the word level. As children develop beyond the single-word level, they are able to encode meaning in the form of the utterances produced. Words with the same referent can fulfill different semantic roles or cases that specify the relationships among those referents. Table 4.14 lists the most common cases or semantic classes. Thus, the child forming a sentence must keep in mind both the referent and the semantic role.

Words and phrases also modify the meaning of basic syntactic elements by indicating qualities, such as perceptual attributes, manner, and temporal aspects, and relationships between larger sentential units, such as additive (*and*) or causal (*because*). As a listener, the child can only comprehend other people to the extent that he or she understands the various relationships underlying their utterances (Creaghead & Donnelly, 1982).

Semantic Classes

The speech-language pathologist can teach words to children and place them in different semantic classes. A portion of word definition is the semantic class into which a word can be placed. She also can teach other word types that relate to that class. Language-impaired children may find it difficult to identify and use semantic classes of words.

The agent function found in the subject position of a sentence offers a unique example of semantic category training (Connell, 1986). English is a subject-prominent language in which a large number of morphosyntactic and transformational elements are associated with the subject of the sentence (Cole, Harbert, Herman, & Sridhar, 1980; Keenan, 1976; Li & Thompson, 1976). These elements include subject-verb agreement as with the verb *to be* and the third person singular, present tense marker; pronouns; and auxiliary verb inversions in questions. These elements are not critical to the content of a sentence, and they can be omitted without greatly affecting the understanding of the sentence.

The speech pathologist may facilitate teaching these elements by teaching the concept of *subjecthood* (Connell, 1986). She can accomplish this using a functional approach in which she teaches the child the purpose of subject.

The function of a sentence's subject, represented by a noun phrase, is to designate the perspective used in the sentence (Dik, 1980). In contrast, the topic designates the focus of discourse. If there is action in the sentence, the agent designates the actor. In the sentence "John ate the salami" (Connell, 1986, p. 482) all three elements are the same. In "John was arrested by the police" (ibid.), "John" is the topic and the subject, but "police" is the agent.

Subjects can be identified by the pronouns used with them. Subjects take nominative case pronouns whereas topics and agents may take different types. Subjects also agree with predicates whereas topics and agents need not.

The speech-language pathologist can train children to identify the topic and the subject using the following forms (Connell, 1986):

1. Objecive   nominative   verb/
   case   +   case   +   *be*   +   adjective/
   pronoun   pronoun   adverb/noun

   (Him,   he   is   running)

2. Nominative case prononun + *be* + verb/adjective/adverb/noun

   (He   is   running)

The first is taught in response to "Which one is. . .?" type of question, and the second in response to a "What is the man doing?" or "Who is. . .?" type of question. Children can induce the function of the subject and its separateness from the topic by the varying sentential contexts in which they are used.

Children can learn each sentence form by imitation and then in response to questions within ongoing activities. Training should begin with the second sentence type because it is included within the first. Once children have learned the formats, the questions can be alternated. Later, the habitual or simple present form of the verb, such as *eat* or *drink,* can be introduced to teach children subject-verb agreement within the same subject-highlighted format.

Other semantic classes may be taught in a similar manner. Table 9.3 presents suggestions for training.

TABLE 9.3
Suggestions for training semantic classes

Instrument
Initially, this class can be trained in the final position of the sentence preceded by the word *by,* as in ''The wood was split *by his axe.*'' Position and the preposition *by* act as signals for this class. This class can also be signaled by the verb *use,* as in ''John *used the rake* to gather the leaves.'' This sentence type can be prompted by questions, such as ''How did . . .?'' and ''What did John use to . . .?''

Patient/Object
This class may be taught initially using the final position in the sentence as a direct object to transitive verbs. Question prompts such as ''What did Carol throw?'' may be used to elicit this class.
It is somewhat more difficult to teach this class in the subject position, because that position is usually occupied by an agent. If agents are taught in response to a *who* type of question, patients might use *what,* as in ''What grew in the park?''

Dative
The dative class is most frequently and obviously used as an indirect object. This function can be clearly signaled initially by use of the prepositions *to* and *for.* Question prompts can include these cues and the word *whom,* as in ''For whom did Mary buy the flowers?''

Temporal, Locative, and Manner
These classes are relatively easy to teach because each has specific questions that prompt usage. Prepositions, such as *in, on,* and *at,* are used with these functions as are *to, with,* and *by,* which are used to mark other semantic class use.

Accompaniment
The final position in the sentence and the use of the preposition *with* should be used in training to signal this class. *With whom* question prompts can be used to elicit response.

Relational Words
Relational words fulfill many functions in language. Relationships may be based on quantity or quality and may be general or specific. Other relational words are used to mark location and time. Conjunctions are relational words that relate one clause to another. Each type of relational word requires specific considerations.

In general, relational terms can be trained within descriptive tasks, in which the child must differentiate between one entity and another, or in narrative tasks, in which the child must aid the listener to differentiate characters. The speech-language pathologist can help the child initially by keeping the task context-bound and by controlling the number of items or characters. By ''playing dumb'' or acting confused, the facilitator can help the child provide additional or essential information. Narratives are also effective vehicles for the training of conjunctions, especially when the facilitator synthesizes larger, more conceptually-complex sentences based on those of the child.

Quantitative terms.   A child does not need to be able to count to learn quantitative terms. Initial training can begin with the concepts of *one* and *more* *than one.* The second concept can be variously marked by *many, much, some,* and *more.* Such terms as *these* and *those* should be introduced with some caution because of deixis or interpretation from the perspective of the speaker. Deixis is mentioned in the pragmatics portion of this chapter and is covered briefly in the following section.

The distinction between *many* and *much* is complex and should be ignored with children functioning at a preschool level. In general, *many* is used with regular and irregular plural nouns, such as *cats, shoes,* and *women.* In contrast, *much* is used with mass nouns. Mass nouns refer to homogeneous, nonindividual substances, such as *water, sand,* and *sugar.* It is not surprising that children have difficulty with the two terms *much* and *many.*

Before going beyond the quantity words mentioned, the child must learn to count and have a concept of the relative values of different numbers. In other words, the child must know that four is greater than two, not that four merely follows in a sequence.

Later quantifiers can include words such as *few* and *couple.* These can be followed by other quantifiers, such as *nearly, almost as much as,* and *half.* Table 9.4 lists common quantitative words. The ordering of these words in the noun phrase is very important and is discussed in the syntax section of this chapter.

Qualitative terms. Qualitative terms include such words as *bigger* and *tallest,* which use the *-er* and *-est* morphological markers, and such phrases as *as big*

TABLE 9.4
Common quantitative and qualitative terms

Quantitative	Qualitative
One, two, three, four. . .	Big, little, long, short
Many, much, lots of	Large, small, fat, thin
Some, few, couple	Soft, hard, heavy, light
More, another	Same, different, alike
Nearly, almost all	Old, young, pretty, ugly
As much/little as	Blue, green, red,,. . .
Plenty	Hot, cold, warm, chilly
Half, one-fourth, two-fifths	Wide, narrow
10%,75%	Sweet, sour
Units of measure: Inch, foot, mile, cup, pint, quart, gallon, centimeter, meter, kilometer, liter, ounce, pound, gram, kilogram, acre	Nice, mean, funny, sad
	Fast, slow
	Smooth, rough
	Angry, afraid
Clean, dirty	Comparative and superlative
Empty, full	relationships: *-er, -est,*
	as x as, x-er than

as, not as wet as, smaller than, and the like. Table 9.4 also lists common qualitative terms. In general, children learn to use the comparative *-er* before the superlative *-est,* and training should follow that pattern. It is best to begin with the regular use of these two markers before introducing exceptions, such as *better* and *best.* Words can be expanded into phrases, for example, *bigger* to *bigger than.*

Children seem to acquire concepts one semantic feature at a time (Clark, 1973). A corollary to this hypothesis is that broad, nonspecific concepts (e.g., *big*) are learned before more specific concepts (e.g., *long*). In this example, *big* refers to overall size, whereas *long* refers to size only in the horizontal plane. Several studies have confirmed this acquisition order (Richards, 1979).

The speech-language pathologist should introduce terms and relationships in the order in which comparative terms develop. Table 9.5 includes common pairs of comparative terms and the approximate age at which most children can use them correctly.

In general, conceptual word-pairs are acquired asymmetrically, one prior to the other, based on their polarity. Children ages 3 to 7 appear to learn the positive-pole member of conceptual pairs, the one that represents more of the dimension characterized by the conceptual pair, prior to learning the negative member (Bracken, 1988, Greenberg, 1966). For example, *big* and *little* are opposite poles of the dimension *size. Big* represents more size and is, therefore, the positive mem-

TABLE 9.5
Common comparative word-pairs

Positive-Negative (age)	Positive-Negative (age)	Positive-Negative (age)
same-different (36–60 months)	open-close	on-off (24–36 months)
in front of-behind (48–54 months)	inside-outside	up-down (36–60 months)
into-out of	over-under (42–48 months)	high-low (42–60 months)
top-bottom (48–54 months)	front-back (48–52 months)	forward-backward
rising-falling	above-below (66–72 months)	happy-sad
healthy-sick	right-wrong	old-young
big-little (30–48 months)	heavy-light (30–48 months)	large-small (78–84 months)
deep-shallow	tall-short (30–84 months)	long-short (horizontal) (54–60 months)
thick-thin	loud-quiet	hot-cold
hard-soft (30–42 months)	sharp-dull	dark-light
smooth-rough	solid-liquid	tight-loose
more-less (42–72 months)	full-empty (36–48 months)	a lot-little
all-none	with-without (48–54 months)	fast-slow
old-new	arriving-leaving	early-late
before-after (66–72 months)	first-last (60–66 months)	always-never

(The overall order does not reflect the order for teaching conceptual pairs.)

Source: Bracken (1988), Edmonston and Thane (1990); Wiig and Semel (1984).

ber. These data suggest that positive members should be taught first to language-impaired children.

In addition, positive-type comparisons should be taught before negative ones. In other words, *bigger than* should be introduced before *smaller than* and *not as big as.* Positive comparisons seem to be easier for children to process.

Spatial and temporal terms.   Several words are used to mark both space or location and time and, thus, are potentially confusing. Among the most commonly used words in English are prepositions, such as *in, on, at* and *by.* Each of these small, seemingly insignificant words has several definitions. The syntax section of this chapter discusses prepositional training. In addition, other words, such as *first* and *last,* also note place and time.

Spatial concepts are best taught first in relation to the child; then with ''featured'' or fronted objects, such as a television, chair, or person; and finally with nonfeatured objects, such as a wastebasket or a ball (Edmonston & Thane, 1990). The latter is more difficult to learn because it involves deixis. In general, vertical dimensions are learned before horizontal. Horizontal front and back terms, such as *in front of* and *behind,* are learned before horizontal side-to-side terms, such as *beside* and *next to.*

The order of temporal term learning reflects the underlying concepts of order, simultaneity, and duration (Edmonston & Thane, 1990). Terms that denote order, such as *before, after, first,* and *last,* are usually learned before terms for simultaneity, such as *at the same time* and *when.* Duration terms, such as *a long time,* are generally acquired last.

In general, it is better to begin with concrete definitions and progress to more abstract ones. For example, with *first, last, before,* and *after,* training can begin with objects in a line. The facilitator can have the child touch individual objects, then a short sequence of objects, and finally, a reverse sequence. Objects should be used first before terms for events and the concept of time sequencing.

One context is not enough for teaching concepts of space and time. The greater the number of contexts, the more learning and generalization that will occur. Language can be used to help the child organize the environment by marking experiences of space and time. Table 9.6 includes common spatial and temporal terms.

The speech-language pathologist can use direction following and activities to train space and time. It might be best to begin with routines that the child knows, such as those that occur at home or in the classroom, and then move into less familiar activities, such as using a pay telephone or changing a tire, in which the child must rely more on linguistic input.

She can also later use sequenced pictures or storytelling in the training. Pictures may seem very abstract to some children, especially school-aged retarded children, and should be used with caution.

Deixis and the use of deictic terms are very difficult concepts to teach. The facilitator who takes the role of speaker and prompter for the child violates the roles in a conversation. The simple example of *here* and *there* is illustrative.

TABLE 9.6

Common spatial and temporal terms

Spatial	Temporal
Next to	Next
Before	Before
After	After
On, on top	Into
In, into	Soon
In between	Later
Between	Now
Middle	Above
Above	Yesterday
Under	Today
Over	Tomorrow
Below	Calendar dates
Corner	Months
Bottom	Seasons
Inside	Numerals for years
Outside	Morning
Side	Afternoon
End	Evening
In front of	Days
Behind	Weeks
Beside	Hours
Right	Minutes
Left	Through
Through	Away from
High, tall	Toward
Upside down	Sometimes
Together	

The request "Put the ball *here*" is said from the speaker's perspective. To the listener, the speaker's *here* is most likely *there*. If the speaker then shifts to the listener or child's perspective and says "Yes, put it *there*," it may further confuse the child.

When training deictic terms, it is best to sit next to the child so that you can share a perspective. From this shared perspective, some deictic terms, at least those for location, would be similar. Another facilitator, puppet, or prerecorded tape may act as the other conversational partner. The teaching of deixis is also discussed under pronouns in the syntax section of this chapter.

Conjunctions. The facilitator should teach conjunctions in the order in which they develop by noting for the child the relationships expressed in each (Klecan-Aker, 1985). For example, *because* represents cause and effect and may not be fully acquired until about age 12 by both language learning disabled and non-LLD children (Tyack, 1981; Wiig & Semel, 1984). Table 9.7 presents the general order of conjunction acquisition.

TABLE 9.7
Acquisition order for English
conjunctions

And
And then
But, or
Because
So, if, when
Until, before-after
Although, while, as
Unless
Therefore, however

Data from studies are very variable, and this list is
only a rough guide.
Source: Based on Bloom, Lahey, Hood, Lifter, &
Fiess (1980); Clark & Clark (1977); Corrigan (1975);
Hood & Bloom (1979); Kuhn & Phelps (1976); Lee
(1974); Wiig and Semel (1984).

The conjunction *and* can first be taught to combine entities, as in "cats *and* dogs." In a cooking activity, the facilitator might say "Which two types of cookies do you like best?" or "Tell me your two favorite types of cookies." In similar fashion, *but* can be used for like/dislike distinctions ("I like cookies, *but not beets*").

Wiig & Semel (1984) suggest using a "main clause + conjunction + subordinate clause" format initially to help the child acquire the underlying relationship. For example, sentences might be presented as follows:

> We wear a coat *because* it is cold.
> We wear a coat *if* it is cold.
> We wear a coat *when* it is cold.

Once the child understands these relationships, the order of the clauses can be reversed, as in "Because it is cold, we wear a coat."

Next, the speech-language pathologist can present new clauses for the child to complete. She can also use a breakdown and buildup technique in which the child identifies clauses and conjunctions and then reconstructs the sentence (Klecan-Aker, 1985).

Word Retrieval and Categorization

Word-retrieval difficulties can result from two possible sources (Kail, Hale, Leonard, & Nippold, 1984; Kail & Leonard, 1986). The first is lack of elaboration or lack of a well-established, thorough representation of the word within the child's lexicon. The second source of problems is in retrieval. In general, children with this problem are less efficient in retrieving words from storage. Whereas elaboration difficulties may occur alone, retrieval problems usually do not and may be an additional difficulty found in some children with elaborative problems (Kail & Leonard, 1986).

A number of activities have been suggested that facilitate word-finding skills (McGregor & Leonard, 1989; Wiig & Semel, 1984). Children appear to benefit from both elaboration and retrieval activities (McGregor & Leonard, 1989). Word-finding activities can easily be incorporated into a number of everyday activities and conversations about these activities.

In elaboration training, the speech-language pathologist can use nonidentical exemplars and word comparison tasks. She presents nonidentical exemplars, or examples of the word in several different linguistic contexts, to enrich the child's definition and word associations. Nonidentical exemplars for *house* might include *dollhouse, house fly,* and *greenhouse.* In comparative tasks, she expects the child to identify similarities and differences between two words with related meanings, such as *house* and *hotel.*

Children seem naturally to enjoy word games and word play, and these teaching strategies can be incorporated into many different types of activities. As a communication partner, I like to get very "confused" and use words in silly ways. Children laugh and freely correct their somewhat slow-witted communication partner.

Retrieval training may include categorization tasks, such as naming members of a category or identifying the category when given the members. Categories include animals, clothing, grocery items, and the like. Categories may also be formed by the initial sounds of words and by rhyming.

As a group, language-impaired children are less likely than nonimpaired children to discover semantic organization strategies on their own and usually require more examples to determine a basis for organization and to generalize organizational skill. Word-retrieval errors should demonstrate the predominant organizational framework of the child and alert the speech-language pathologist to the patterns that need strengthening.

Categorization tasks, especially such familiar ones as Saturday morning cartoon shows, in which the child names members of the category, facilitate recall by building associational and categorical linkages between words. The child usually recalls a word by first accessing the category to which it belongs.

Categorization tasks can be elaborative in nature when members of more than one category are presented together. For example, the items *chair, bed,* and *table* can be classified as furniture; *chair, swing,* and *bicycle* are things on which you sit; and *bicycle, car,* and *bus* are vehicles. The facilitator could present these items together and ask the child to classify them in as many different ways as possible.

Training might begin with actual objects and children making piles of objects that go together (Cole & Cole, 1981). As a child, I used to sort my comic books by main character and my baseball cards by team. Similar tasks are found in several everyday activities. Children can make collages in school of things that go together. Items might be classified by description (e.g., cold) or by function (e.g., things that you ride on). The facilitator should encourage the child to describe objects using as many different sensory descriptions as possible.

Familiar everyday objects and events should be used. This notion is sometimes difficult for adults to understand, especially if they are attempting to bring interest and variety into the training. I am reminded of a teacher who tried to teach zoo and farm animal categories but found the children very unresponsive. Both categories were outside their realm of experience. When one child suggested the category of animals seen ''squashed'' on the highway, every child became a participant. Although the example is somewhat gruesome, the lesson for teachers is very practical.

The facilitator can help a child note perceptual and functional features and attributes that determine how members are categorized. The child with a language learning disability will have particular difficulty abstracting salient features and, therefore, will have difficulty forming categories based on these features.

It is important that children note a similar attribute on more than one object. Otherwise children may begin to associate certain attributes with specific items. For example, several very different objects may be described as *wet*. This kind of task naturally leads to categorization. Attributes should also appear in many different linguistic forms.

Word-finding difficulties can also be helped by descriptive tasks, associational activities (''Red, white, and _____''), and open-ended fill-ins and completion (''We eat with a _____''). Word-sorting tasks can aid in the development of categorization and recall skills (Bjorkland, Ornstein, & Haig, 1975). Taxonomy charts, especially for newly introduced classroom content, can also help children develop categorization strategies.

Categorical identification seems to be the best aid to recall (Wiig & Semel, 1984). By naming the category, the facilitator can help the child locate the desired word. Partial word cues may also help the child and are less confusing than are synonyms. Sentence completion and nonverbal, gestural cues are also aids.

SYNTAX AND MORPHOLOGY

Although language use improves syntax, the reverse is not true (Lucas, 1980; Mundell & Lucas, 1978). It is important, therefore, that syntactic training be as conversational as possible.

When language forms or constructions are taught outside of a communication context, the forms may be mastered without the knowledge of how to express ideas within and across these forms (Norris & Bruning, 1988). In addition, utterances produced in context strengthen cohesion and relationships across linguistic units. The linguistic techniques discussed in Chapter 8 are particularly applicable to syntactic training.

During training it is important that the facilitator control for vocabulary and/or sentence length, especially when teaching new structures. If the facilitator changes too many variables at one time, it may confuse the child or make the task too complex for successful completion.

The facilitator should also be careful not to require metalinguistic skills beyond the child's abilities. Although recognition and comprehension usually precede production, judgments of correct usage do not. Judging a sentence to be grammatically correct is a metalinguistic skill that develops in the middle elementary school years. Asking children to form sentences with selected words also requires metalinguistic skill. In short, any task that requires the child to manipulate language abstractly takes some degree of metalinguistic skill.

The development of syntactic and morphologic forms is well documented and provides a guide for intervention. The following section discusses hierarchies for intervention with several different forms. The purpose is to offer general guidelines for the ordering of structures to be taught.

Verb Tensing

Verbs are very difficult for language-impaired children, partly because of the many ways they are treated syntactically and morphologically. Although the typical nonimpaired 2-year-old has a notion of action words, the child does not understand the many forms these verbs can take; nor does the child comprehend other verbs that express notions such as state. Verb learning takes several years, with the rules being mastered slowly.

The teaching of verb tensing can be adapted easily to everyday activities in which children discuss what they are doing at present, did previously, or will do in the future. Art projects or building toys are especially useful. Appendix G offers a number of activities for targeting verb tensing.

Training should begin with *protoverbs*, such as *up, in, off, down, no, there, bye-bye,* and *night-night*. These verb-like words are usually used in relation to some familiar action sequence (Barrett, 1983). General purpose verbs, such as *do*, might be targeted next.

More specific action verbs should be introduced in their uninflected or unmarked form. The facilitator can cue by asking what a child is doing or by directing the child "Tell X to verb." To facilitate learning, action word meanings might be taught with specific actions or objects. Children first describe their own actions, not those of others (Barrett, 1983; Huttenlocher, Smiley, & Charney, 1983; Nelson & Lucariello, 1983). While playing, the facilitator can hide her eyes or turn away from the child and ask "What are you doing?" Although the cue requires an *-ing* ending on the verb in the response ("Eating"), this form is not required at this level of training.

Familiar event sequences, such as play or routines, facilitate action verb usage because of the mental representations of these sequences that children possess (Chapman & Terrell, 1988). This enables the child to focus on the communication rather than on the extralinguistic elements of the event (Constable, 1986).

Once the child is able to form simple two- and three-word utterances with an action word, as in "Doggie eat meat," the present progressive verb form can be introduced without the auxiliary verb. The language facilitator can model this form through self-talk and parallel talk. She can cue the child to use this form with "What's doggie doing?" or "What's he doing?" However, pronouns must be used with caution at this level.

At this level of training the child only needs to deal with the immediate context. A sense of time beyond the present, however, is essential for further verb training.

The facilitator can use a few high usage irregular past tense verbs, such as *ate, drank, ran, fell, sat, came,* and *went,* to introduce the past rather quickly and to forestall overgeneralization of the regular past *-ed,* the next target form. With both past tense forms, storytelling, show and tell, and recounting past events are good vehicles for training and use. Initially, the facilitator can ask the child such questions as "What did you eat (or other action verb)?" to teach the child the form. When the child responds with "Cookie" or another entity, the facilitator can reply "What did you do with cookie?" Later, the sequence can begin with the question "What did you do?" The child responds "Ate cookie" or "I ate a cookie." It is important that question cues not violate pragmatic contingency, which requires that questions make sense. Facilitators should not ask questions to which they know the answers. This is easily achieved by asking about unobserved actions.

Before training additional verb forms, the facilitator should introduce singular and plural nouns and subjective pronouns, because the child will need these for the third person singular present tense *-s* marker and for present tense forms of the verb *to be.*

The facilitator can introduce the third person marker with singular and plural nouns. Subjective pronouns can be gradually introduced. She can elicit this form with such cues as "What does he do every day (all of the time)?" or such fill-ins as "Every day, the girls (verb)" or "All of the time, he (verbs)."

She should not target the phonological variations of the *-ed* marker (/d/, /t/, and /Id/) and those of the third person *-s* (/s/, /z/, and /Iz/) in initial training. When the marker is first being emphasized in training, the facilitator should use one form exclusively, such as the /d/ or /s/. As the emphasis on the marker becomes more natural or lessens, its cognate can be introduced.

Facilitators should not expect the child to understand the phonological rules relative to ending sounds and added markers. Usually de-emphasis of the marker's sound will allow the child to produce naturally either two voiced or two unvoiced sounds at the end of each word. The /Id/ and /Iz/ markers should be avoided until much later. Nonimpaired children usually employ the cognates by late preschool. It takes them a few more years to acquire the /Id/ and /Iz/ forms.

Use of pronouns enables the child to begin training on the verb *to be* both as an auxiliary verb and as the copula or main verb. Because the form is noun (or pronoun) + *be* + X, in which the X can be a noun, adjective, adverb, or verb, these two forms can be trained together, thus facilitating carryover. The distinction between auxiliaries and main verbs is too difficult to try to explain here. As a rule, the uncontractible form is taught first, the uncontracted contractible next, and the contracted contractible form last.

The verb *to be* is a regularist's nightmare, with different forms for various persons and tenses. Therefore, different forms should be introduced slowly. Nonimpaired children generally learn the *is* form first.

Other auxiliary verbs, such as *do,* can also be introduced to facilitate the development of more mature negatives and interrogatives. The negative form of *do* can be elicited with "Tell *X* (some person) not to *verb.*" *Do, can,* and *will/would* appear first in the negative form in the language development of nonimpaired children. In other words, *can't, don't,* and *won't* appear before *can, do,* and *will/would.*

Using the present progressive form *be + going,* the child can now begin to form early future tense forms. Facilitators should be willing to accept this form because it marks the concept (Bliss, 1987). The more mature *will* form can be trained later.

Training should begin with *going to noun,* as in "going to the zoo," before *going to verb,* as in "going to eat." The former is more concrete and does not require use of an infinitive phrase, such as *to eat.* The more mature *will* form of the future tense can be introduced later.

Guidelines for training *can, do,* and *will/would* include the following (Bliss, 1987):

1. Allow some delay between mastery of one form and introduction of another in order to avoid confusion.

2. Use self-reference in the form of either first person pronouns or the child's name initially since this is the first referent associated with these forms (Fletcher, 1979).

3. Link these forms with actions because this is the first association of nonimpaired children (Fletcher, 1979).

4. Initially, use short utterances with the word at the end in order to increase saliency ("Can you jump?" "Yes, I *can.*")

5. Provide meaningful situations in which the concepts and forms serve some purpose.

With the addition of the future tense, the child can now discuss the past, present (progressive), and future, somewhat like the preacher whose lengthy sermons "Tell'em what I'm gonna tell'em, tell'em, and tell'em what I told'em." Language activities can include planning, execution, and review.

Finally, the facilitator can introduce modal auxiliaries. These are helping verbs that express mood or feeling, such as *could, would, should, might,* and *may.* The shades of meaning across the various modal auxiliaries are often very subtle, and the facilitator should not expect mature usage for some time.

Procedures should make sense both semantically and pragmatically (Bliss, 1987). Examples include "I bet you can/can't . . .," "Mother, may I?," asking the child to perform various tasks ("Will you please . . .?"), problem solving ("What will happen if . . .?," "What might happen if . . .?"), and role playing ("What should we do if . . .?").

Pronouns

Pronouns are extremely difficult to learn because the user must have syntactic, semantic, and pragmatic knowledge. In general, the facilitator should teach the underlying concept first and should model appropriate use for the child. Use of pronouns requires an understanding of the semantic distinctions of number, person, and case. The noun in the sentence generally determines use, but the conversational context is also a determinant.

Several parent and teacher practices that make language easier for the child to process may, however, confuse pronoun learning and use. Overuse of nouns or of the royal *we* (e.g., "*We* are tired" to mean that the speaker is tired) model inappropriate use.

Children often avoid making an overt pronominal error by overusing nouns. This mistake can be avoided somewhat in training by limiting the number of referents. For example, if the speech-language pathologist uses too many characters in a story format, the child may overuse nouns in an attempt to remember who is being discussed. Using nouns can help children use their memory, which is somewhat more limited than that of adults.

In general, the first person *I* should be trained before the second person *you*, followed by the third person *he/she*. This developmental order reflects increasing complexity with shifting reference and the number of possible referents.

Deictic terms, such as *I* and *you*, are difficult to teach, as noted in the semantics portion of this chapter. A second speech-language pathologist, facilitator, or child can serve as a model to avoid confusing the child's frame of reference.

Development by nonimpaired children would suggest that facilitators target subjective pronouns (*I, you, he, she, it, we, you they*) before objective pronouns (*me, you, him, her, it, us, you, them*). Possessive pronouns would follow (*my, your, his, her, its, our, your, their*), and finally, reflexive pronouns (*myself, yourself, himself, herself, itself, ourselves, yourselves, themselves*). Although there are exceptions to this hierarchy, it approximates normal development (Haas & Owens, 1984).

This hierarchy and the error patterns of young children suggest that reflexives might initially be trained as possessives (*myself*). The exceptions (*himself* and *themselves*) can be introduced later.

One exception to the training hierarchy might be third person singular pronouns. It appears easier for children to learn *her-her-herself* than *him-his-himself*, probably because of the consistency in the feminine gender (Haas & Owens, 1985). The three feminine pronouns might be trained before the masculine.

Conversational training with so many varied forms can be very confusing. Initially, the facilitator must carefully target the desired pronouns and practice cues to elicit these forms.

Plurals

To learn plurals, the child must have the concepts of *one* and *more than one.* Numbers or words such as *many* or *more* may serve as initial aids.

As with the past tense *-ed* and third person *-s* markers, the facilitator should not expect mastery of the phonological rules until later. Again, training should begin with either the /s/ or /z/, gradually introduce the other, and wait some time before introducing /Iz/.

The facilitator may wish to introduce a few common irregular plurals to forestall overgeneralization. As mentioned in the semantics section of this chapter, words such as *water* and *sand* are not irregular plurals and present a special case, especially with the modifiers *any* and *much.*

Articles

Articles are extremely difficult for children to learn because of the two different operations they perform. Articles may mark definite (*the*) and indefinite (*a*) reference and also new (*a*) and old (*the*) information. When in doubt, preschool and early elementary school children tend to overuse *the.*

The facilitator can use objects and pictures and instruct the child to describe what is seen (''A puppy''). Next, she and the child can describe each object or picture, as in the following exchange:

FACILITATOR: Tell me what you see.
CHILD: A duck.
FACILITATOR: A duck? Let's see. I can tell you that *the duck is yellow. What can you tell me?*
CHILD: The duck is swimming.

The *an* should not be introduced until the child is functioning at the early elementary school level.

Once pronouns have been introduced, the facilitator can switch back and forth between pronouns and articles, as in the following:

FACILITATOR: Here's *a* puppy. What can you tell me about *him*?
CHILD: *He* has a cold nose.
FACILITATOR: Who does?
CHILD: *The* puppy.

The possibilities are endless within a conversational paradigm.

Prepositions

Although nine prepositions (*at, by, for, from, in, of, on, to,* and *with*) account for 90% of preposition use, these nine have a combined total of approximately 250 meanings. No wonder some language-impaired children have difficulty with this class of words. Prepositions are discussed briefly in the semantics section under relational terms.

Development of prepositions suggests the following hierarchy of training (Johnston, 1984; Johnston & Slobin, 1979; Washington & Naremore, 1978):

in, on, inside out of

under, next to

between, around, beside, in front of

in back of, behind

Such terms as *in front of* and *behind* should be initially trained using fronted objects, for example, a television. Nonfronted objects can be introduced later.

In general, children will learn more easily when real objects are used in training. Actual manipulation of these objects, however, may interfere with learning (Harris & Folch, 1985). Such experience may be better at the level of conceptual rather than linguistic training. Spatial and directional aspects should be trained with a number of objects and/or examples so the child understands the concept separate from any specific referent. Variety may preclude the child's focusing on the objects and referents in favor of the relationship. Large muscle activities can also be used as children go *in* and *out* of boxes or closets, *on* and *off* tables and chairs, and the like. Thus, the child's body becomes a referent (Messick, 1988). Spatial terms may be taught in a naturalistic context of play with puppets, dolls, action figures, or the child's body. In one lesson, I played the tiger who pursued a preschool child *in* the cage, *out* of the cage, and so on.

Word Order and Sentence Types

Word order and different sentence types are best trained within conversational give-and-take. Devices such as the Fokes Sentence Builder (Fokes, 1976) have been used effectively and efficiently to train sentence structure, but they can become very repetitious. Such devices can be used creatively to allow the child to form his or her own sentences, even nonsensical ones.

Miniature linguistic systems have also been used to teach word combinations (Bunce, Ruder, & Ruder, 1985). In these systems, a matrix is developed with one class of words on the ordinate and another on the abscissa. The child need not learn all possible combinations to acquire the rule. Good generalization to untrained combinations has been reported. Figure 9.1 offers some sample matrices and the teaching models that have been effective.

Noun phrases initially can be expanded in isolation. A question-answer paradigm will enable the facilitator to target specific aspects of the noun phrase. Once placed within a sentence, the noun phrase can be expanded in the object position, followed by the subject position. The order of noun modifiers is discussed in Chapter 5 under analysis of the noun phrase.

Adjectives can be taught in contrastive situations in which the child must

FIGURE 9.1
Miniature linguistic systems

	Cookie	Cake	Pudding	Pie	Bread
Eat	X	X	X	X	X
Bake	X				
Mix	X				
Want	X				
Give	X				

	Pet	Dog	Cat	Horse	Ferret
Feed	X	X			
Bathe		X	X		
Groom			X	X	
Walk				X	X
Brush	X				X

Verbs on one axis are combined with nouns on the other to form short phrases. Each combination taught is marked with an *X*. Rule learning will generalize to the untrained combinations.

distinguish between two objects that differ along one parameter, as in *big ball* and *little ball* (Kamhi & Nelson, 1988). Incorrect or inadequate adjective use in conversation would result in misunderstanding and the misinterpretation of the child's message. In a similar fashion, post-noun modifiers can be used with objects in different locations, as in *the ball in the box* and *the ball on the table*.

Verb phrases and accompanying clause types should be chosen carefully. Specific verbs that clearly illustrate transitive and intransitive clauses might be chosen. Equitive verb phrases and the use of "be" can be trained in elliptical answers to questions, as in *He is* and *We are* responses to questions such as "Who is at the zoo?" The uncontractable form of the verb is very salient in this format. A similar method of teaching transitive and intransitive verbs can also be used to teach auxiliary verbs, as in "Who is eating?" and "Who can jump?" (Kamhi & Nelson, 1988).

Several strategies discussed in Chapter 8 can be used very effectively to strengthen word order. For example, expansion can provide a more mature model than the child's utterance, and buildup/breakdown strategies help the child analyze relationships.

Table 4.7 offers some guidelines on the acquisitional order of certain sentence types. By the time most nonimpaired children begin school, they are using adult-like declaratives, imperatives, and *wh*- and yes/no interrogatives in both the positive and negative forms. Later developing forms include clausal and multiple embedding and conjoining, passive voice, and tag questions.

PHONOLOGY

Not every child with speech sound errors is a candidate for a phonological approach. A child who has limited articulation errors, such as a k/t substitution or a distortion of /s/, would benefit more from traditional articulation training. In general, children use immature phonological processes to make phonology simpler and more manageable. The processes are applied across sound classes and syllable sequences. The child whose errors are not limited to specific sounds, but rather reflect such patterns as producing all error sounds as plosives, is more suited to a phonological approach.

A phonological rather than a phonetically based approach is a more effective and efficient way of remediation because the former focuses on the reduction or elimination of general processes affecting many sounds (Weiner, 1981). Thus, "remediation should focus on phonological patterns to be acquired rather than on isolated phonemes" (Hodson & Paden, 1983, p. 44).

Although consonants may be correct when they occur in stressed syllables, especially in the initial position, the same sounds may be omitted or substituted with a more easily produced sound when they occur at word ends, in consonant clusters, or in unstressed syllables. Naturally, these simplification processes will affect speech intelligibility (Hodson & Paden, 1981).

The best targets for training occur frequently in the child's daily living. Intervention is likely to result in improved overall intelligibility. The more powerful the child's utterance in achieving the child's conversational needs, the better target it is for intervention.

Several other criteria exist for target selection (Edwards, 1984; Louko & Edwards, 1990). For example, the speech pathologist might target position-specific or optional processes because they occur intermittently. She might also target processes that affect stimulable sounds or those that occur early in development. The speech-language pathologist must select the process or processes and the affected sounds to target.

As with other aspects of language training, the speech-language pathologist can train phonological rule use within conversational activities (Low, Newman, & Ravsten, 1989; Hoffman, Norris, & Monjure, 1990). Often she accomplishes this training working with children in a group setting. She uses real-life or role-played situations with natural consequences.

Children with phonological impairments are aware of the effect of their errors on listener comprehension and will make adjustments to enhance vital comprehension (Campbell & Shriberg, 1982; Paul & Shriberg, 1982). These adjustments can be incorporated into training at a conversational level with emphasis on communicative success (Hoffman et al., 1990).

Changes made at the higher levels of communication simultaneously affect lower sound production levels. Compared to children using a minimal pairs strategy, discussed later in this chapter, children using a functional conversational approach make greater improvements in overall expressive language as well as similar changes in improved phonological performance (Hoffman et al., 1990).

A reason for this difference might be found in a metaphonological explanation. Metaphonology is the ability to judge the correctness of phonological productions. It is possible that the child has a model or underlying representation of the message to be sent and that there is a communication breakdown when there is a mismatch between the model and the actual message produced by the child (Mele-McCarthy, 1990). Intervention can target either the underlying representation, as a conversational approach attempts to do, or phonological production.

Training might begin with the child being instructed to tell a narrative. A puppet might serve as the listener while the speech-language pathologist acts as prompter for the child. Following each child turn, the puppet can make requests for clarification, for added information, or for increased sentence complexity using the strategies in Chapter 8. Requests for clarification that require phonological adjustments by the child should be emphasized. For example, the puppet might respond as follows:

> ''You said 'tenny,' that's an old sneaker, and your brother's name is 'Kenny.' Well, I've never been to a party for a sneaker. I don't understand. Did you have a good time?

This strategy can be very effective when used with the minimal pairs strategy discussed later in this chapter.

The clinician can aid the child to clarify or to increase the length and complexity of the narrative. This format emphasizes the importance of communication clarity and offers numerous opportunities for modeling, feedback, and revision.

Many non-conversational language-based intervention approaches incorporate both word meaning and sound contrast aspects of language (Blache, Parsons, & Humphreys, 1981; Ferrier & Davis, 1973; Monahan, 1987; Weiner, 1981; Young, 1983). This method attempts to use the child's semantic and conceptual abilities and to stress the important linguistic function of sounds. Words that differ by one sound, called *minimal word pairs,* are used to teach the sound contrasts necessary to convey meaning (Blache & Parsons, 1980).

Although these approaches are not strictly conversational in nature, they do incorporate different aspects of language into intervention. Sound-meaning contrast training is most appropriate for children with severe phonological impairments, although training should also include conversational approaches similar to those mentioned previously.

One variant of this method, called *perception-production/minimal pairs,* consists of five levels of training: a sound perception level in isolation and in word pairs, and four production levels (Tyler, Edwards, & Saxman, 1987). Perceptual training is accompanied by pictures illustrating each member of the pair, such as *sew/toe.* Production levels include word imitation, independent naming, minimal pairs, and sentences. At the minimal pairs level, the child is required to produce the correct word of the pair in situations in which incorrect production would cause semantic confusion. The CVC type of words are used, and no other error sounds are included.

Each member of the minimal word pair may also be pictured using a *rebus* symbol rather than a printed word or actual picture (Young, 1987). A rebus is a picture or symbol that conveys meaning. For the training of phonological rules, the association is sound referenced. In sound-referenced rebus symbols, the symbol for *their*, *there*, and *they're* would be the same because these words sound alike. The rebus does not relate to the meaning of the word, but merely sounds like part of the word. For example, the rebus *shoe* might be used to facilitate production of ti*ssue*.

Training might also include auditory bombardment at the beginning and end of each session (Hodson, 1980; Hodson & Paden, 1983; Monahan, 1986), during which the speech-language pathologist repeats a list of minimal word pairs emphasizing the process(es) being targeted. Auditory bombardment is designed to heighten the child's awareness of target sounds.

This section discusses the language-based procedure in detail. It can be incorporated into intervention for deletion of final consonants, consonant cluster reduction, and deletion of weak syllables. A modified procedure can also be used with sound substitutions.

Deletion of Final Consonants

Deletion of final consonants is a carryover from the child's early word-making strategy of linking open syllables in a string. Open syllables are formed by a consonant and a vowel, as in *ma*, and are strung to form such words as *mama*. Many early words follow this same syllable form, for example, *baby* and *cookie*.

The facilitator can teach the use of final consonants using two complementary methods—a key word and minimal word pairs approach and a chaining approach. Although the methodology differs, the two apparently do not conflict or confuse children (Johnson & Hood, 1988). In both methods, intervention should begin with sounds already present in the child's repertoire, because the introduction of new sounds might frustrate the child by requiring too much learning.

Key Words and Minimal Pairs

In this method, the speech-language pathologist uses groups of two or three words that contain a key word, differ in meaning on the basis of the final sound, and are easy to illustrate in pictures. For example, the key word *bee* could be used with words that begin with these sounds but differ in their final consonants, such as *bean*, *bead*, *beat*, and *beak*. Other examples include the following (Young, 1983):

four	paired with *fork*, *force*, and *fort*
pea	paired with *peek*, *peel*, and *piece*
bow	paired with *both*, *bone*, and *boat*
see	paired with *seed*, *seat*, and *seal*
tea	paired with *team*, *teach*, and *tease*
die	paired with *dice*, *dime*, *dive*, and *dine*

The key word can be contrasted with the others, all of which are homonyms without the final consonant. Short periods of auditory bombardment may help reinforce the learning of contrasts (Monahan, 1986). Ending markers, such as plural -*s* and past -*ed*, can also be incorporated into this approach. The intervention steps are as follows (Young, 1983):

1. Teach the meaning contrasts between the words, beginning with a single pair, by having the child point to a picture when given a clue or asked a question, for example, "Which one lives in a hive?"

2. Have the child point to pictures when named randomly, as in "Which one is *beat*?"

3. Have the child produce the target words correctly using the following seven substeps. Errors can be managed by returning to contrasting meaning, such as "You said 'bee,' but the picture of the 'bee' is way over here. What do we call a bird's mouth? Yes, a bird's mouth is called a 'beak'." Final consonant substitutions consistent with the child's level of maturity should be accepted. Immature substitution errors can be corrected through traditional articulation therapy. The seven substeps are to (Young, 1983):

    a. Imitate word model correctly.

    b. Name word correctly without model.

    c. Use word correctly in carrier phrase, such as "This is a _____."

    d. Imitate word correctly in a sentence that illustrates the word's meaning, such as "I eat bean soup."

    e. Generate spontaneous sentences with each word.

    f. Use ending consonants consistently in monitored speech in the the therapy setting. Nontrained words should also be monitored.

    g. Use ending consonants outside the therapy setting.

The criterion at each step is 90% correct performance.

Chaining

Chaining can be used along with minimal pairs training (Johnson & Hood, 1988). Emphasizing transitions between sounds, this method targets the ending position of the first word in a two-word phrase, such as "Jum*p* up" or "Pu*sh* in". Training occurs within daily play activities. Other combinations include the following:

jump/take/push/pitch/make—up/out/in/it

A number of consonant sounds from the child's repertoire are used for the target sound at the end of the first word. A variety of consonant sounds are used because this method teaches chaining as a coarticulation rule (Johnson & Hood, 1988).

Initially, correct production of this sound and of the ending or arresting consonant of the second word is not required. Any consonant used in the target position is accepted. Phrases are taught in the CV form that the child already uses. Thus, "Make it" is taught as "May kit" [CV CV(c)] to facilitate production of the final /k/ on *make*.

Production criterion and syllable boundaries are gradually tightened. Despite a lack of research data, it is reported that most children learn to generalize their new learning to closed syllables.

Cluster Reduction

Cluster reduction is one of the most common and longest lasting phonological processes (Haelsig & Madison, 1986; Ingram, 1976). Children use it to simplify complex articulatory demands, and the types of simplification used are often predictable across children. In English, consonant clusters tend to be associated with word beginnings.

An intervention approach that uses a shift in stress and a visual cue in the form of a rebus symbol can be effective with consonant cluster reduction and deletion of unstressed syllables (Young, 1983, 1987; Young & Sacks, 1982). Backward chaining can help to simplify consonant cluster production. The procedure for cluster reduction follows (Young, 1987):

1. Each rebus symbol is introduced and named by the speech-language pathologist and child. The speech-language pathologist slowly produces the target word for the child, demonstrating that the initial sound of that word and the rebus symbol will sound close to the production of the word. For example, the child is introduced to the rebus symbol for *tool* and repeats the word with the symbol. Then, the child is introduced to *stool* and shown that *s* + rebus = target word. The child repeats the target word slowly as two distinct segments (sound + rebus).

2. Using the visual rebus symbol as a cue, the child repeats the facilitator's production of the word with no separation of sound and rebus.

3. The child repeats the speech-language pathologist's production with the rebus obscured.

4. The child produces the target word without a model.

5. The child uses the word in phrases, sentences, and conversation.

The correction procedure at each step is to return to the previous step.

Cluster reductions with the /s/ phoneme are the most predictable and are common among children. The minimal word pair technique using words that differ on the basis of deletion or nondeletion of the /s/ can be applied. Examples include the following (Young, 1983):

/sk/ cool/school, care/scare, cold/scold, key/ski, core/score
/sp/ pool/spool, pin/spin, pie/spy, pot/spot, pill/spill
/st/ team/steam, top/stop, tool/stool

Unstressed Syllables

In English multisyllabic words, the initial syllable is usually emphasized. Children more easily perceive and more consistently produce these primary or maximum stress syllables (Ervin-Tripp, 1966; Martin, 1972). They may delete, reduce, or replace unstressed syllables by a substituted sound or syllable in a simplification purpose similar to deletion of final consonants and cluster reduction (Ingram, 1976; Klein, 1981). Substitutions may be related to reduplication, in which a stressed syllable is repeated; to assimilation, in which the unstressed syllable is modified toward the sounds in the stressed syllable; or to replacement by an overused speech sound.

Disyllabic words can be used in intervention by changing them in two ways: (a) stressing the weak syllable so that both syllables have the same stress, and (b) associating meaning with the unstressed syllable by means of a visual rebus symbol (Young, 1987). These cues focus attention on the difficult portion of the word, the weak syllable.

To emphasize the unstressed syllable, the speech-language pathologist can use a backward chaining technique in which she teaches the final portion of the word and then incorporates it into the word. For unstressed sounds that approximate words but are omitted or substituted, the unstressed syllable can be pictured in a rebus. For example, the second syllable in *cookie, monkey, turkey,* and *donkey* sounds like *key*. The association is sound based not meaning based. The picture of *donkey* and a rebus of *key* can be paired to reinforce the association. Training should begin with sounds that the child uses in the initial position in words but omits in unstressed syllables. Otherwise, *key* can be taught first and then incorporated into *monkey* (Young, 1983, 1987).

The training procedure for weak syllable reduction consists of the following steps (Young, 1987):

1. The speech-language pathologist presents and names the rebus symbol for the child. The child repeats the correct production of the symbol name. The speech-language pathologist then slowly produces the target words with *equal stress on both syllables and use of the rebus symbol* with production of the unstressed syllable. For example, if the target words are *apple, people, purple,* and *chapel* and the key word is *pull,* the child can hear *a-pull* while noting the *apple* picture followed by the rebus *pull.* The child repeats each facilitator production. Both syllables should receive equal stress.

2. The facilitator again presents the disyllabic words and pictures with the rebus symbol, but this time using the natural stress pattern. The child repeats each word.

3. The facilitator presents the rebus symbol, but obscures the card in some manner. The child imitates her production with natural stress.

4. The child correctly produces each word without use of a verbal model or rebus cue.

5. The child uses the words in phrases, sentences, and conversation.

Incorrect production results in the child's receiving the extra cues of the preceding training step.

Other possible word pairs include (Young, 1983):

pea	paired with *happy, sleepy, puppy, snoopy*
bull	paired with *table, label, marble*
knee	paired with *tiny, funny, honey, pony*
sir	paired with *mixer, answer, dancer, boxer*
kit	paired with *rocket, jacket, locket, pocket*

The present progressive can be taught with pictures depicting *sing, ring,* and *king* to be used as follows:

sing	paired with *dancing, chasing, kissing, bouncing*
ring	paired with *cheering, pouring, tearing*
king	paired with *knocking, picking, licking*

Assimilation

Key words and facilitating contexts can be used together to modify assimilation processes (Weiner, 1979). The intervention approach is very similar to the paired stimuli methodology. A word like *dog,* which might be pronounced "[g⊃g]," is paired with a word in which assimilation does not occur with this child, such as *dime.* Through repeated exposure, the child recognizes that both words begin with the same sound. Do not choose a word like *dead* for the paired word because the child might then modify [g⊃g] to [d⊃d] to better approximate *dead.* Conversely, when the child initially produces [d⊃d], the word might be paired with *frog* or *hog* to help the child recognize the final [g] sound.

A facilitative context is one in which the nearby sound fosters production of the correct consonant. For example, [*i*] facilitates [*l*] because both are high front sounds. Consonants placed together, as in *mad dog,* also facilitate production of targeted sounds.

Sound Substitutions

To simplify production, the child can follow production rules relative to unknown sounds. For example, unknown sounds may be produced in the front of the mouth or as plosives, two processes called *fronting* and *stopping,* respectively. To promote generalization and prevent overgeneralization, it is best to work on more than one process at a time (Edwards, 1984).

These processes may be addressed by an approach that incorporates (a) auditory bombardment with several sounds within the pattern, (b) conceptualization training using perceptual sorting tasks and lexical production, and (c) phonemic contrast that enables the child to perceive semantic differences in minimal word pairs (Elbert, Rockman, & Saltzman, 1980; Monahan, 1986; Montgomery & Bonderman, 1989). The training procedure for sound substitutions has the following steps:

1. Auditory bombardment can occur with and without amplification. Two groups of children can work independently, one concentrating on and receiving target words amplified through headphones, and the other completing some project with the words being heard in the background. Rather than concentrating on individual sounds, auditory bombardment can concentrate on enough phonemes within a sound pattern to affect pattern generalization to the child's repertoire (Hodson & Paden, 1983).

2. During the perceptual portion of conceptualization training, individual phonological targets are highlighted. The child is trained to perceive the phoneme contrasts and semantic differences in minimal word pairs or words that differ only in the correct and substituted sounds, as in *toad-code.*

   The contrasting sounds differ only along a single feature or dimension. Using lexically unique words, the child learns that different sounds signal different meanings.

   While presenting a picture that illustrates the word, the speech-language pathologist says each word in the pair, emphasizing the contrasting sounds (*debt-get*), and follows each production with an explanation ("That had a *front* sound—That had a *back* sound"). She then asks the child to sort the pictures into two stacks of front and back sounds. Rebus symbols can be used to emphasize the contrast between the presence or absence of the sounds and the difference in the target words.

3. In the production portion of conceptualization training, the child participates in practice using the pictures and a facilitator's verbal model. The facilitator reinforces the child for each response that does not contain the error process. For example, when producing a word with a back sound, she reinforces the child for producing *any back sound, not just the correct target sound.* This procedure more closely reflects natural phonological process acquisition (Weiner, 1981). In other words, correct production occurs through a gradual process of modification. The following activities can be used (Monahan, 1986):

   (a) Find a card. A specific card is sought from a display of several cards arranged face down. The name of the card is repeated fre quently by both participants in sentences, such as "Find the _____" and "I found the _____." The players take turns being the finder.

(b) Playing teacher. The child as teacher holds up each card and says "This is _____." The actual teacher supplies the missing word. The child as teacher corrects or confirms the teacher's production (often purposely incorrect).

(c) Silly sentences. The facilitator and child take turns making sentences containing both words in the contrast pair. ("I *get* in *debt* if I shop too much.")

The facilitator can also use art activities, music, drama, and circle games with conversation centering on the activity carefully chosen to elicit the specific phonological targets in question (Montgomery & Bonderman, 1989).

4. Using a picture cue, the child repeats the facilitator's productions. Only correct productions are reinforced.

5. The child repeats the productions correctly with the picture obscured.

6. The child produces the word correctly without any model.

7. The child uses the word in phrases, sentences, and conversation.

The minimal-contrast approach is not the only effective methodology. The modified cycles procedure, unlike the minimal pairs method, targets several processes within a short period of time (Tyler et al., 1987). Auditory bombardment is used heavily. Although the program focuses on correct production of a target sound and its sound substitution, it automatically shifts to another process every 3 weeks unless correct production falls below 20%. In this manner, several processes can be targeted nearly simultaneously.

A third approach, maximal opposition, contrasts sounds that differ along several parameters (Elbert & Gierut, 1986; Gierut, 1989). Presumably, children are free to choose and attend to those specific features of the sounds that they identify as relevant. This approach is based on the initial maximal perceptual distinctions of children in which they concentrate on the wide extremes of sound contrasts. In addition, maximal opposition treats children as active participants who form their own hypotheses from examples of language and then generalize these hypotheses to actual use. The overall procedures are similar to those for minimal pairs.

Summary

Although the speech-language pathologist cannot always use all elements of the functional model simultaneously, she usually can use several elements within any given teaching situation. Her target selection certainly should reflect the child's overall communication needs. Facilitators within the environment, everyday activities, and conversational give-and-take can usually be adapted to the individual child and language target(s). Some training, such as phonological intervention, may necessitate the initial use of structured approaches. Generalization to conversational use, however, will require incorporating these settings into the training. Appendix G contains activities that are adaptable for intervention and the multiple training targets within each. The speech-language pathologist can select several targets for a single child or can work on different individual targets with several children within the same activity.

BIDIALECTAL CHILDREN

All speakers of a language use some *dialect* of the idealized standard language. A dialect is a rule-governed form of the standard used by an identifiable geographic, racial, ethnic, or socioeconomic group. Some dialects are closer to the standard than others. Dialects that vary greatly from the standard are called *nonstandard* and offer a special challenge to the speech-language pathologist.

Nonstandard dialects are neither crude approximations of the standard nor haphazard, unpatterned forms. Nor do they reflect disordered language or disorganized thinking on the user's part. These dialects are valid forms of the standard language within themselves, and this validity should be reflected in the intervention planning of public schools. Notions of dialectal superiority reflect prejudicial thinking and have led to educational approaches aimed at eradicating nonstandard dialects. The American Speech-Language-Hearing Association (Position paper, 1983) has labeled this approach inappropriate. Targeting dialectal differences for eradication questions the minority groups that speak these dialects.

Bidialectal education should be fostered instead. This approach recognizes the validity of dialects and also the educational and employment needs of the individual. Smitherman (1985) found that only those speakers of Black English (BE) who master code switching, the successful use of both BE and a second dialect closer to the standard, achieve educational success.

As discussed previously, the speech-language pathologist must not regard dialectal differences as language disorders. Language is impaired when the child demonstrates inappropriate, incorrect, or immature use within his or her dialectal community. This position suggests, therefore, that intervention should teach both nonstandard and standard equivalents for disordered structures (Adler, 1988). For example, if the language-impaired child speaks Black English, use of the verb *to be* should be taught in both BE and the standard. Only this approach truly serves the child who must function within both a dialectal community and the larger society.

CONCLUSION

We have discussed only a few of the intervention techniques for specific disorders. Limited space necessitates a rather cursory examination of the procedures. Speech-language pathologists should seek further information in source materials or in published clinical materials. They should also conceive their own creative and innovative methods for intervening in language impairments. Hopefully, these methods can be adapted to fit the conversational model presented in Chapters 7 and 8.

Not all specific language problems are easily treated with a functional approach, but the entire model does not have to be discarded. Caregivers, for example, are a valuable resource and can be used in various ways, whatever the specific language problem being targeted. Chapters 10, 11, and 12 explore the adaptation of functional intervention to the classroom and with presymbolic and minimally symbolic children.

FOUR
Application to
Special Locations and Populations

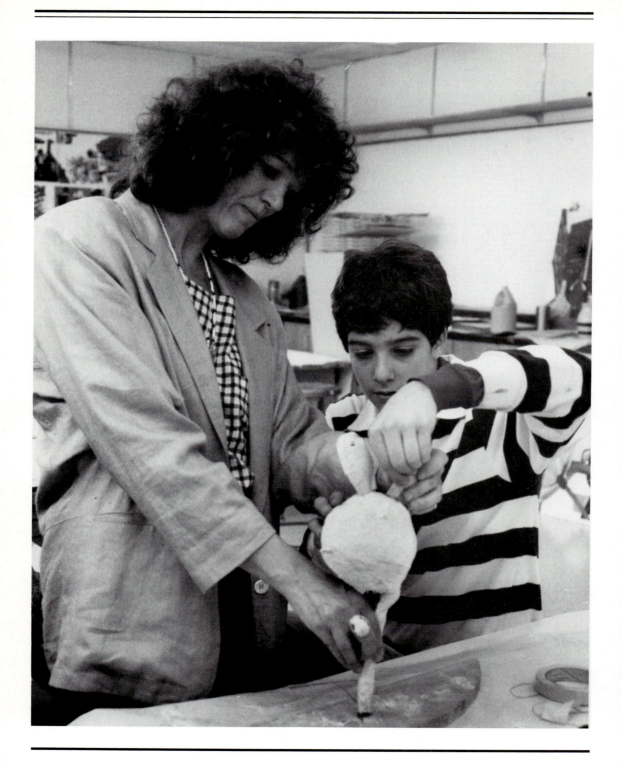

10
Classroom
Functional Intervention

anguage and communication play many vital roles in school success and in the development of reading (Nelson, 1988a; Silliman, 1984; Simner, 1983; Wallach & Liebergott, 1984, Wallach & Miller, 1988; Westby, 1984). Five effective warning signs of potential school failure are (a) in-class attention span, distractability, or memory span; (b) in-class verbal fluency or the use of precise words to convey or describe; (c) in-class interest and participation; (d) ability to recognize numbers and letters; and (e) the number and type of printing errors made when copying (Simner, 1983). Language-impaired school-aged children experience difficulties not only with language but also with academic performance (Catts & Kamhi, 1986; Cooper & Flowers, 1987; Hasentab & Laughton, 1982; Simon, 1985; Wallach & Butler, 1984; Westby, 1985; Wiig & Semel, 1984). The language-impaired child cannot interpret or express ideas at an adequate level to achieve academic success.

In school, children encounter the language of instruction, which presents discourse experiences that are very different from the child's previous conversational interactions (Cook-Gumperz, 1977; Nelson, 1984, 1985; Ripich & Spinelli, 1985). Language is treated in the abstract as children learn to talk about it and to manipulate it to learn about other things. Metalinguistic skills are very important. The child with inadequate language skills or inadequate strategies for making sense of different situations is apt to become lost (Nelson, 1989).

More than communicating with other people, ''in school, language must also be used to regulate thinking, to plan, reflect, evaluate, and to acquire knowledge about things that are not directly experienced'' (Norris, 1989). On an oral-to-literate continuum (Westby, 1985), school tasks are at the extreme literate end, requiring the child to understand and express information displaced from his or her own experiential base. Language itself creates the context in which information is conveyed to other people so that they can comprehend it and understand an event without having shared in the experience (Jorm, 1983; Spekman, 1983).

Language training within the school classroom offers a special challenge for the speech-language pathologist and classroom teacher. School systems throughout the United States and Canada are adopting and modifying many models of classroom intervention to provide more appropriate and effective intervention.

The *pull-out* or *isolated therapy model* of intervention now prevails in public education (Marvin, 1987). In this model, the child is removed from the classroom for speech-language services.

The pull-out model tends to fragment the child's intervention, especially if the child needs more than one pull-out service. Such patchwork schedules are extremely difficult for children with few strategies for making sense of the world. Increased need results in increased fragmentation until there is little continuity, and the child's progress suffers as a result (Bashir, 1987).

Usually, there is little generalization with the pull-out model, and the content of such intervention may be irrelevant to the child's classroom needs (Anderson & Nelson, 1988). Children may resist leaving class because poorer performance results from the classroom absence.

As mentioned in Chapter 1, language intervention should more closely reflect what we know about language development and use (Nelson, 1986a & 1988a; Wallach & Butler, 1984; Wallach & Miller, 1988). Functional intervention theories describe language as it occurs throughout the child's many experiences. Assessment and intervention theories that flow from this model stress language processing within a variety of relevant contexts, such as the classroom (Miller, 1989). Thus, the model is process, not product oriented (Moses & Maffei, 1989).

A functional approach to intervention shifts the focus from the child as the source and solution of the language problem to a holistic view that includes the child and the child's language uses and learning strategies, the contextual demands, the expectations and beliefs of other people within that context, and the child's interaction, the context, and the child's communication partners (Miller, 1989). Thus, the focuses of intervention become the contexts that surround the language-impaired child and the manipulation of these contexts.

The classroom's cognitive activities are an excellent context for stimulating language growth (Moses & Maffei, 1989). Within the classroom's constructive activities, children create, change, relate, and compare entities, set goals, encounter and try to overcome problems, make errors, reflect on success or failure, and note problem-solving procedures.

The negative effects of pull-out are not found in classroom intervention. The ongoing classroom activities can serve as the basis for intervention, with content coming from the child's assignments and projects and the interactions of the classroom (Wallach & Miller, 1988). Thus, intervention is relevant for the environment in which it is being used. In addition, the child can benefit from the social dynamics of the classroom (Nelson, 1988b).

The variety of formats for classroom intervention include the following (Blank & Marquis, 1987; Catts & Kamhi, 1987; DeSpain & Simon, 1987; Dudley-Marling, 1987; Miller, 1989; Simon, 1985):

1. Speech-language pathologist teaches a self-contained classroom, usually at the elementary level, for students needing a focus on language and language processing (Buttrill, Niizawa, Biemer, Takahashi, & Hearn, 1989).

2. Speech-language pathologist team-teaches with the regular classroom teacher and other specialists, usually the resource room teacher (Norris, 1989). This teaching may include both specialists teaching small groups simultaneously, or one specialist, such as the teacher, working with the larger class, while the other, such as the speech-language pathologist, works with a smaller group. Goals and objectives, individualized educational plans (IEPs), and the monitoring and reviewing of individual programs are the team's joint responsibilities.

3. Speech-language pathologist provides one-on-one classroom-based intervention with selected students in the classroom using course materials (Nelson, 1989). The intervention usually centers on language strategies for classroom use.

4. Speech-language pathologist acts as a consultant for the classroom teacher and other specialists. As such, she advises (not supervises) personnel, assisting primary caregivers with intervention strategies. Consultative models of intervention usually involve joint goals and objectives that the classroom teacher implements.

   This collaborative consultation model is the one most frequently suggested in the professional literature (Marvin, 1987). This model is very flexible and may include elements of several other formats. Because this model has obvious advantages for generalization (Damico, 1987), it is the basis for discussion in this chapter.

5. Speech-language pathologist provides staff training and curriculum development to the school or district.

The model for discussion incorporates some elements of each of these formats, although primary emphasis is on the consultative format.

The most promising model to evolve proposes the speech-language pathologist as a direct intervention agent and also as a consultant, identifying targets and training methods and training the classroom teacher and/or aide(s) in these methods (Lyngaas et al., 1983). In partnership, the speech-language pathologist and classroom teacher combine their efforts to serve language-impaired children. Parents are also used, when possible.

This evolving model includes but is not limited to the following elements:

1. The classroom teacher helps to identify potential language-impaired children through observation of classroom behavior. The speech-language pathologist evaluates the speech and language skills of these children and others who fail speech and language screenings. Such evaluations are an ongoing and integral part of the intervention process.

2. The speech-language pathologist continues to provide individual or small group therapy outside the classroom to children in need. In addition, the speech-language pathologist, classroom teacher, and aide provide small and large group intervention services within the classroom.

3. The classroom teacher, aide, and parents interact daily with the children in ways that facilitate the development of language skills.

To use the context of the natural environment, the speech-language pathologist should be in that environment and use communication situations occurring in that context (Spinelli & Terrell, 1984). Thus, the speech-language pathologist increasingly provides individual and group intervention within the classroom and conducts small group activities in which newly acquired language skills are used.

ROLE OF THE SPEECH-LANGUAGE PATHOLOGIST

Any classroom intervention model raises questions about the speech-language pathologist's role and about others' expectations of the intervention team. These questions include the following:

☐ What is my new role? Who am I?
☐ Are there special language needs within the routines of the classroom situation?
☐ How do I address individual needs within a classroom?
☐ How do I justify my new role to an administration that gauges my work in individual contact hours?
☐ What is the relationship of language arts and language remediation?
☐ How do I educate teachers?

The classroom model is still evolving, and there are no quick answers. Our discussion of the elements of the classroom model addresses some of these questions.

The speech-language pathologist is a problem solver who, with the guidance of a few principles, applies and adapts a variety of methods in seeking solutions. In the final analysis, the model that evolves is a blend of the child's needs and the desires of the school, the individual teacher, and the speech-language pathologist.

The speech-language pathologist is the school's language expert. As such, she advises administrators, teachers, and committees on the handicapped about children and language impairment. She is also responsible for speech and language assessment, for the planning and implementation of all speech and language programming, for record keeping, and for training personnel who will work with the language-impaired children.

Relationship with Classroom Teachers

The speech-language pathologist helps the teacher identify children with language impairments and suggests techniques to facilitate development. This is an ongoing process, accomplished through in-service training and individual consultation and training, as well as co-teaching within the classroom.

The speech-language pathologist and the classroom teacher have unique skills that they can use to help each other and the language-impaired child. The speech-language pathologist understands language development and the remediation of speech and language impairments. The classroom teacher knows each child and understands the use of large and small group interactions for teaching.

Difficulties usually arise over turf or territory. The classroom teacher may feel threatened by the presence of another ''teacher'' in the classroom and may resent being shown how to talk to students to maximize each child's language learning. The speech-language pathologist may feel like a classroom aide, undervalued for her expertise. These differences and potential problems should be discussed openly prior to beginning intervention. Each professional's roles should be delineated and clearly understood.

The speech-language pathologist and the classroom teacher should exchange clear and valuable information. This ongoing exchange is especially important at the beginning of intervention.

The speech-language pathologist and classroom teacher are part of the intervention team and should contribute in that fashion. Each has special expertise to impart. Neither one is there to spy on the other, and their personal opinions of each other have no place in the teachers' room.

Relationship with Parents

Not all parents can or wish to participate in their children's speech-language intervention. Parents tend to fall into three identifiable groups, the largest being those who desire participation. Next are those who desire no participation, and the smallest group is composed of parents who want more information (Andrews, Andrews, & Shearer, 1989). The first group of parents can be involved in planning and implementation of intervention, and parents who want information can be served through parent meetings and in-service training.

Relationship with School Administrators

The speech-language pathologist's new role may require some education of the administration. Traditional patterns of instruction change slowly, and administrators may not understand generalization and the need to provide language remediation within the classroom. Caseload dictates and contact hour requirements may have to be modified to accommodate the classroom model.

Administrators will need to be impressed with the increased efficiency gained through the co-teaching of the speech-language pathologist and classroom teacher. Discussion should center on how best to serve the children and how to use professional time commitments most efficiently.

Finally, the speech-language pathologist's new role should be viewed within the perspective of a comprehensive school or districtwide program that includes early childhood intervention, bilingual and bidialectal services, and the training of English as a second language (Koenig & Biel, 1989). Public law is dictating an extension of speech-language and educational services to these children.

Language Intervention and Language Arts

Classroom teachers and administrators are sometimes confused about the difference between language arts and language remediation. Unless this distinction is clear, the speech-language pathologist's role also may be misunderstood, especially as it relates to classroom intervention. Language arts accomplishes several things:

1. Provides children with labels for the language units that they have been using in their speech.
2. Requires children to stretch their language abilities into new areas, such as fictional and expository writing.
3. Enables children to have language growth experiences, such as performances.
4. Helps children to reason and problem solve using linguistic units.

All of these valuable accomplishments presuppose that each child has a well-formed language system.

Language remediation cannot make this supposition. In language remediation, the child is taught language units or behaviors that are not present or are in error in the primary mode of communication, that is, in language transmitted via speech. Through training, teachers and administrators become aware of this distinction and of the valuable contribution of each to the child's education.

The classroom model raises other questions that are addressed in the explanation of the overall model.

ELEMENTS OF THE MODEL

The model consists of identification (assessment), intervention, and facilitation. In each phase, the classroom teacher and the speech-language pathologist, although a team, have individual inputs that affect the delivery of quality services for the child.

Identification of At-Risk Children

Teachers play a vital role in identifying children with speech and language impairments. Most teachers are not trained in language development or impairment, and the speech-language pathologist must alert them to the behaviors that signal a possible impairment.

Teacher training can be accomplished in in-service sessions. Teachers can also be given aids to use in identifying a potential speech and language problem. Table 10.1 lists some behaviors that the speech-language pathologist might point out to the classroom teacher for identification of children having language problems. Appendix H contains an analysis format for classroom interactions that can guide teachers in determining the locus of breakdown in communication interactions in the classroom (Vetter, 1982).

In addition, the speech-language pathologist and the classroom teacher can identify the individual classroom or grade level's special communication requirements as a gauge against which each child can be measured to assess achievement. Called *curriculum-based assessment,* this method uses the child's progress within the school curriculum as a measure of his or her educational success (Tucker, 1985). Children are assessed against the curriculum within which they are expected to perform. Thus, intervention focuses on changes in the child's behavior that are relevant to the educational setting.

From preschool through high school, the curriculum not only becomes more difficult but also changes in the types of demands made on the student. Wiig and Semel (1984) outline these changes as follows:

> Preschool: Learning focuses on sensorimotor, language, and socio-emotional growth with materials that are manipulative, three dimensional, and concrete.

TABLE 10.1
Identifying children with language problems in the classroom

The following behaviors may indicate that a child in your classroom has a language impairment that is in need of clinical intervention. Please check the appropriate items.

_____ Child mispronounces sounds and words.

_____ Child omits word endings, such as plural *-s* and past tense *-ed.*

_____ Child omits small unemphasized words, such as auxiliary verbs or prepositions.

_____ Child uses an immature vocabulary, overuses empty words, such as *one* and *thing,* or seems to have difficulty recalling or finding the right word.

_____ Child has difficulty comprehending new words and concepts.

_____ Child's sentence structure seems immature or overreliant on forms, such as subject-verb-object. It's unoriginal, dull.

_____ Child's question and/or negative sentence style is immature.

_____ Child has difficulty with one of the following:

_____ Verb tensing	_____ Articles	_____ Auxiliary verbs
_____ Pronouns	_____ Irreg. verbs	_____ Prepositions
_____ Word order	_____ Irreg. plurals	

_____ Child has difficulty relating sequential events.

_____ Child has difficulty following directions.

_____ Child's questions often inaccurate or vague.

_____ Child's questions often poorly formed.

_____ Child has difficulty answering questions.

_____ Child's comments often off topic or inappropriate for the conversation.

_____ There are long pauses between a remark and the child's reply or between successive remarks by the child. It's as if the child is searching for a response or is confused.

_____ Child appears to be attending to communication but remembers little of what is said.

_____ Child has difficulty using language socially for the following purposes:

_____ Request needs	_____ Pretend/imagine	_____ Protest
_____ Greet	_____ Request information	_____ Gain attention
_____ Respond/reply	_____ Share ideas, feelings	_____ Clarify
_____ Relate events	_____ Entertain	_____ Reason

_____ Child has difficulty interpreting the following:

_____ Figurative language	_____ Humor	_____ Gestures
	_____ Emotions	_____ Body language

_____ Child does not alter production for different audiences and locations.

_____ Child does not seem to consider the effect of language on the listener.

_____ Child often has verbal misunderstandings with others.

_____ Child has difficulty with reading and writing.

_____ Child's language skills seem to be much lower than other areas, such as mechanical, artistic, or social skills.

Early grades (K–2): Learning focuses on perceptual-cognitive strategies with materials that are one dimensional, abstract, and symbolic.

Middle grades (3–4): Learning places higher demands on linguistic and symbolic skills with less direct instruction. The child is expected to make inferences, analyze data, and synthesize information.

Upper grades (5–6): Learning focuses on content areas with the child expected to recall past learning and display fluency with basic academic skills.

Middle and high school: Learning emphasizes lectures in content areas with students expected to reorganize material as they listen and to gain the main or important points. Anywhere from 75–90% of the day may be spent receiving information.

By identifying the overall requirements for the class, the teacher has provided a list of potential skills with which the language-impaired child may experience difficulty. Some school districts have identified skills children need to succeed in each grade. Table 10.2 presents some of the skills needed in the first three grades.

In addition to the school's official curriculum, which is an outline of the material to be learned in each grade, children encounter several other curricula (Nelson, 1989). These include the *de facto curriculum* that is actually taught and the cultural and school curricula needed to succeed within each context. The expectations of the latter are often very confusing for the child with language-processing problems. The implicit expectations of individual teachers and other children form a fourth curriculum.

The speech-language pathologist must first become familiar with the curricula that affect the individual language-impaired child. She can assess the child through a combination of interview and observation of the child's ability to meet the language demands of the curricula. The interview phase can provide information on the curricular expectations, and observation can focus on the specific linguistic demands made of the child.

An analysis of the linguistic demands must consider all aspects of language and the many reception and production modes. Such an analysis should also note metalinguistic skills demanded in these various aspects and modes (Nelson, 1989).

The speech-language pathologist may gain additional information by informally sampling the child's performance. For example, Larson and McKinley (1987) recommend a procedure for comparing a secondary school child's notes with those of a good student in the same class. Audiotapes of classroom instructions can be analyzed to determine the level of complexity that each child must be able to process. The speech-language pathologist might collect samples of the child's oral reading or help the child complete assignments, noting the child's language-related work skills.

Teachers should also be trained to observe and describe classroom behaviors as precisely as possible. The speech-language pathologist's complaint that teachers refer children who have rather nonspecific vocabulary problems or are

TABLE 10.2
Some possible language skills needed in the first three grades

First Grade. The student will be able to:

Recognize correct word order auditorily.

Identify singular and plural common nouns and proper nouns.

Identify regular and irregular, past and present verbs.

Identify descriptive and comparative adjectives.

Use nouns and pronouns, adjectives, and verbs correctly in sentences, including verb-noun agreement.

Give and write full sentences.

Categorize words by opposites, by sequence, by category, and as real/nonreal.

Retell a story.

Identify the main idea in a paragraph.

Classify narrative and descriptive writing.

Rhyme words and identify words that begin with the same sound.

Identify declarative and interrogative sentences and use correct ending punctuation for each.

Capitalize the first word in a sentence, days, months, peoples' names, and the pronoun *I*.

Alphabetize.

Give directions and explanations and follow two-step directions.

Read aloud.

Listen attentively and courteously to others.

Second Grade. In addition to the skills needed for first grade, the child will be able to:

Use correct word order.

Identify incomplete sentences.

Recognize singular and compound subjects of a sentence.

Identify possessive and plural nouns, contracted verbs, and superlative adjectives and use correctly.

Capitalize holidays, titles of people, books, stories, and places.

Identify correct comma use.

Use an apostrophe in contractions.

Identify the topic sentence and sentences that do not relate in a paragraph.

Write an explanation or set of directions.

Address an envelope.

Write rhyming words to complete a poem.

Identify figurative language and synonyms.

Recognize characters, plot, setting, and the major divisions in a story or play, and the difference between fiction and nonfiction.

TABLE 10.2 *(continued)*

Tell and write a clear, original story.

Use the title page and table of contents in a book.

Use the dictionary for spelling and meaning.

Read critically for sequence, main idea, and supporting details.

Use tables and graphs as sources of information.

Recognize types of poetry.

Listen discriminately for rhyming, sequences, and details.

Third Grade. In addition to the skills needed for first and second grade, the child will be able to:

Identify imperative and exclamatory sentences, simple and compound sentences, and run-on sentences.

Recognize compound predicates in a sentence.

Recognize articles and conjunctions in sentences.

Use an exclamation point.

Use an apostrophe in possessive nouns.

Define a paragraph and identify the main idea and supporting sentences.

Write a paragraph, a book report, and a letter with correct capitalization and punctuation.

Write a clear, original story with title, beginning, middle, and end.

Recognize the difference between biography and autobiography.

Use a dictionary for pronunciation.

Use an encyclopedia, telephone book, newspapers, and magazines as references.

Identify compound words, homophones, and homographs.

Use prefixes and suffixes.

Read critically for sequence, main idea, and supporting details.

Organize information by category and sequence.

Recognize real and make-believe, relevant and irrelevant, and factual and opinionated statements.

Identify characteristics of different types of narratives.

---

inattentive reflects poorly on the speech-language pathologist's training of teachers in language impairment and its manifestations. Teachers are a valuable source of raw data on classroom performance when they know what to observe and measure.

The speech-language pathologist must follow up these reports and collect her own data within the classroom setting. These data can be corroborated by further testing and sampling.

Teachers should be informed about the results of such testing and sampling and advised on the best methods of intervention. Teachers can be periodically apprised of the child's progress and intimately involved in the intervention process.

Individual Intervention within the Classroom

Within the classroom, the speech-language pathologist can work with small groups of children. Group projects can provide the context for intervention using the techniques discussed in Chapter 8. Other children can serve as models. The teacher can work with the rest of the class at this time. If they are working on similar projects, the teacher can observe the speech-language pathologist and use some of her techniques.

An axiom of the classroom is "Busy little hands are productive ones" (Pearson, 1988). Group activities may center on art or construction projects using modeling clay or Play-Doh®, pegboards, beads, puzzles, construction paper and glue, and the like.

Children's individual needs can be addressed if the speech-language pathologist or teacher carefully interacts with each child in ways that foster the targeted aspects of language. Signs posted conspicuously will remind the teacher or aide how to interact with each child. With planning, this training can be individually accomplished even in groups of children.

The goals of classroom intervention are for the child to learn new ways of communicating and to have ample opportunity to practice newly acquired skills (McCormick, 1986). The environment should be responsive so that the child learns that language can have some effect on that environment. "Communication intervention should focus on increasing the frequency of communicative behaviors, shaping production of increasingly more sophisticated language functions, and encouraging expression of familiar functions with more advanced language forms" (McCormick, 1986, p. 125). The language of effective classroom communicators is characterized by fluency of word-finding skill, coherence or content organization, and effectiveness and control (National Council of Teachers of English Report, 1976).

The child's learning within the classroom is a function of individual learning style and the environment (Samuels, 1983; Schumaker & Deshler, 1984). Both must be considered when assessing or attempting to intervene with learning. The language of the child's classroom and materials can provide the context and content for intervention. A number of sources provide intervention materials for use within the classroom curriculum (Cosaro, 1989; Hoskins, 1987; Larson & McKinley, 1987; Nelson, 1988a; Pidek, 1987; Simon, 1985; Wallach & Miller, 1988).

With advancing grades, the emphasis shifts increasingly to independent work and to listening and note-taking abilities. Each of these tasks is extremely complex. Intervention helps students learn strategies for analyzing various tasks and determining the steps to take to accomplish them. The speech-language pathologist might teach language-impaired students time management skills, study skills, critical thinking, and language use (Buttrill et al., 1989). She might develop a book of listening activities for teacher use within the classroom (Cosaro, 1989).

Study skills training might include text analysis, study strategies, note taking, test-taking strategies, and reference skills. Through text analysis the child can be helped to understand the organization of texts and their more efficient use.

Study strategies might include active processes for reading (Greene & Jones-Bamman, 1985), such as identifying the main ideas and reviewing periodically to organize the material. Children also can learn associative and other memory strategies.

Critical thinking is the collection, manipulation, and application of information to problem solving (Alley & Deshler, 1979). Language is an integral part of this process (Narrol & Giblon, 1984). Therefore, the language-impaired child may experience difficulties with organizing information and with decision making. Likewise, sophisticated metalinguistic judgments would also be difficult. Critical thinking training might target the three components of general thinking, problem solving, and higher level thinking (Buttrill et al., 1989).

General thinking includes observation and description, development of concepts, comparisons and contrasts, hypotheses, generalization, prediction of outcomes, explanations, and alternatives. Problem-solving skills include analyzing the problem into smaller parts, developing options, predicting outcomes, and critiquing the decision (Alley & Deshler, 1979; Schwartz & McKinley, 1984). Higher level thinking includes deductive and inductive reasoning, solving analogies, and understanding relationships. These tasks are increasingly more abstract and require greater reliance on linguistic input.

With increased emphasis on lectures at the secondary level, listening skills become even more important. In general, good listening skills are highly correlated with good overall language performance (National Council of Teachers of English Report, 1976). Students can be taught to tune in to what they hear and to actively listen (Kail & Marshall, 1978). Subsequent training can focus on recognition and understanding of lecture material. The child's semantic, syntactic, and morphological repertoire can be expanded as a base for comparison with new information from lectures. Such training might include word meanings, relationships and categories, sentence transformations, active and passive voice, embedding and conjoining, and segmentation (Buttrill et al., 1989). Through critical listening training, the child learns to supply missing information, complete stories, find important information, and recognize absurdities in spoken information.

In oral language production, the child can express the language repertoire trained receptively. In addition, the child can sharpen word retrieval and figurative language skills. The speech-language pathologist can teach children to verbalize important critical reasoning skills, such as questioning, comparing, and analyzing, and to discuss a task or topic and give examples.

She can enhance written language training by using computers and topics of interest to the child. Organizational skills gained in critical thinking training can be used in expressive writing training.

Finally, she can enhance conversational skills by role playing and practice (Schwartz & McKinley, 1984). The language-impaired child can be helped to identify different communication contexts and their requirements.

Written information can also be used to train oral language skills. Within a conversational or small group framework, this written information can be used for practice in communicating between speaker and listener (Norris, 1989). Written material can be systematically controlled to ensure that it is well organized and cohesive and that it offers a variety of topics, roles, and situations.

Prewritten textual information allows the speech-language pathologist to teach language holistically, using all aspects of language rather than fragments (Laughton & Hasenstab, 1986). The use of social interactions enables the child to learn language as an integrated social-cognitive-linguistic experience.

The overall intervention model might incorporate elements of two instructional approaches called *strategy-based* and *systems* models. The strategy-based model of intervention assumes that learning problem-solving strategies is more powerful than learning factual content and will generalize more readily (Deshler, Alley, Warner, & Schumaker, 1981; McKinley & Lord-Larson, 1985; Schwartz & McKinley, 1984; Wong & Jones, 1982). Teaching includes strategies for verbal mediation and for the organization and retrieval of linguistic information (Buttrill, Niizawa, Biemer, & Takahashi, & Hearn, 1989; Norris, 1989; Tattershall, 1987; Wallach & Miller, 1988; Wiig & Semel, 1984). This model is highly appealing because of its potential for generalization outside the intervention setting.

In contrast, a systems model assumes that the source of the language impairment lies in the interactions of the child, the primary caregivers, and the content to be learned. Thus, learning is a function of this complex system (Nelson, 1986a). Intervention strategies should reflect the child's varying learning needs across several learning contexts (Nelson, 1989; Wallach & Miller, 1988).

Throughout this text, we discuss the benefits of teaching rules or strategies rather than discrete bits of language. The model presented assumes that this would occur within the interactions of the child and significant others.

Although classroom intervention may suffice for some children with mild language problems, others will also need individual intervention. This can be accomplished in the classroom or through the more traditional pull-out model. The functional conversational model is still very appropriate, as noted in Chapter 7. Children may also work individually within the classroom using computer-aided instruction (Schetz, 1989).

The speech-language pathologist can demonstrate individualized targets and techniques for the teacher with the child or discuss them in meetings with the child's teachers, aides, and parents. Parents who cannot receive instruction in individualized training techniques are better used as facilitators rather than direct trainers.

Language facilitator education can be accomplished in in-service workshops and at parent meetings. The speech-language pathologist should not try to impart all her knowledge to teachers, aides, and parents at these meetings. A general outline of language development and an introduction to principles of instruction will suffice.

Language Facilitation

Language facilitation includes (a) identifying the needs of certain contexts and giving children the opportunity to experience this context successfully and (b) talking to children in ways that facilitate growth and highlight production. The classroom is a special context with its own demands. Facilitative techniques can be used there and in conversational interactions with children.

Classroom Language Requirements

Much of the classroom training should focus on the interactional patterns of the caregiver/facilitator and the language-impaired child. Most teacher-child classroom interaction consists of providing the right information. The child is taught to provide the correct answer and then be quiet. This behavior does not encourage an interactive conversational pattern (Rieke & Lewis, 1984).

Whereas conversations are relatively egalitarian and observe the rules of turn taking, classroom interactions are usually controlled by the teacher, who allocates turns. In contrast, conversational partners evaluate the acceptability of each utterance, but they are not expected to guess the correct utterance the other desires, as children must do in classroom responding. Finally, conversational turns may be expected but only rarely required. In the classroom, the teacher asks questions that require responses. The abstraction level of certain question forms is difficult for some children. Some question forms demand statement of fact whereas others expect the child to reason and explain processes that may require inductive or deductive reasoning.

Often, the type of language used in the classroom is very different from what the child experiences at home. For example, the teacher's language consists of many indirect requests and statements. Questions or statements, such as ''Can you show us where the answer is written'' or ''I can't hear Lori because others are being impolite,'' contain requests or demands.

There is still plenty of room for conversational give and take in nondidactic exchanges, however, and these contexts must also be considered. The children have classroom time to participate in social conversation. Classroom programs and materials can be manipulated to maximize the opportunity for interaction. Language functions found in a typical classroom are enhanced through such manipulation.

Often the work occurs in small groups working on some common project. Children working alone have little opportunity to interact with others. Groups should reflect the classroom's composition, with opportunities for high- and low-functioning children to interact.

The skill of knowing how to get things done in the classroom is not usually taught to children, but rather taken for granted by teachers (Wilkinson & Milosky, 1987). The lack of such knowledge can be problematic for the language-impaired child asked to work with others to accomplish some task. The usual instructions are to help each other.

The child must be able to request and give information, action, and materials and to make judgments on the correct language and communication behaviors in and out of context. Each child is expected to be able to identify the information needed by all involved to complete a task and also to judge the appropriateness of information that is given.

Classroom language functions include (a) relating socially to others while stating personal needs; (b) directing others and self; (c) requesting and giving information; (d) reasoning, judging, and predicting; and (e) imagining and projecting into nonclassroom situations (Tough, 1973, 1979). Relating socially to others while stating one's own needs contains a number of behavior categories, such as referring to psychological or physical needs (''I want to leave now'' or ''I'm hungry''), protecting one's self and self-interest (''That's mine''), agreeing or disagreeing (''You're wrong''), and expressing an opinion (''I hated that dessert'') (Staab, 1983). This function can be elicited through activities organized around a highly desirable object that is not available to all participants, such as one beanbag for a toss game involving three children.

The directing self and others function includes the categories of directing one's own actions, directing the actions of others, collaborating in the actions of others (''You be the mommy and I'll be the daddy''), and requesting direction (''How do you do this?''). This function can be elicited by requiring children to accomplish some task that they cannot do without help (Staab, 1983). There will also be a need to direct others and to follow others' directions.

The giving information function includes labeling (''That's a camel''), referring to events (''Yesterday, we got a kitty''), referring to detail (''That kitty is black and white''), sequencing (''We went to the party, and then we went to the movies''), making comparisons (''Yours is bigger''), and extracting the general point (''We're making Hanukkah presents''). To elicit this function the child shares an experience with someone who did not originally share it, as in show and tell (Staab, 1983).

Often, classroom discussions involve activities in which the entire class has participated, and children do not feel the need for their information to be as precise or detailed. They presuppose that their classmates share much of the information. This presumption cannot be made when classmates do not share the information.

Requests for information vary with the type of information sought. For example, adults and children tend to use more direct requests when there are few, if any, obstacles to receiving the answer, as in checking short answers to problems (Francik & Clark, 1985; Milosky & Wilkinson, 1984). In this situation, the request is very direct: ''What's the answer to number 4?''

As children mature, they learn to identify the type of information needed to help a requester. In general, children become more aware of the importance of information specificity. Children are also more likely with maturity to provide information on the process of solving a certain problem rather than just the answer requested. In responding to the previous question about problem number 4, the child might try to presuppose the difficulties of the requester and respond, ''6 5/8; I converted to 8ths after solving the problem in 16ths.'' School-aged children who provide specific information and process explanations are more likely to be high achievers (Peterson & Swing, 1985).

The reasoning, judging, and predicting function includes explaining a process (''When you get lost, you should find a policeman''), recognizing causal relationships (''The bridge fell because it was weak''), recognizing problems and solutions (''This box is too small; get another one''), drawing conclusions (''We couldn't finish the project because there wasn't enough glue''), and anticipating results (''If we pull this cord, the bell should ring''). In general, problem-solving tasks, such as designing or building an object, will elicit this function (Staab, 1983). Problem solving includes predicting, testing hypotheses, and drawing conclusions.

Finally, the imagining and projecting function includes projecting feeling onto others (''I think he's afraid of the ghost'') and imagining events in real life or fantasy (''I'm captain of the spaceship *Izits*. All aboard''). This function can be elicited by fantasy play (Staab, 1983).

Many activities can be projected into imaginings by asking children to imagine that they are some character in a story or imagine what they would do in a particular situation. With older children, different situations can be role played.

To be successful, children must be able to use all of these language functions with some facility. As noted, activities can be designed to aid this growth.

Talking with Children

As mentioned, language input is important for later output, and adult interactions with children must facilitate language growth and learning. In a nonthreatening way, whenever possible, the speech-language pathologist should observe and comment on the use of language by teachers and parents. Teachers are often unaware of the effect their language has on the processing of children with language impairments. For example, teachers' oral directions may contain a large proportion of figurative expressions and indirect requests (Lazar, Warr-Leeper, Nicholson, & Johnson, 1989).

Teachers' responsiveness to delayed children's initiations is below an optimal level (Pecyna Rhyner, Lehr, & Pudlas, 1990). In general, teachers respond infrequently and, often, in such a manner as to terminate the interaction. The teacher's frequent use of directives may also limit child-teacher interactions.

The speech-language pathologist can efficiently introduce teachers, aides, and parents to facilitative conversational techniques at in-service training sessions or parent meetings. She should help teachers, aides, and parents understand the importance of adult modeling and responding to communicative behaviors. She should attempt to decrease the directive style of some parents and teachers in favor of a more conversational approach.

The speech pathologist can provide teachers, aides, and parents with examples of good interactive styles. A handout, such as that in Table 10.3, is often helpful. She should stress the importance of different facilitator behaviors and the need to tailor techniques to the child's individual style and language level.

Whenever possible, she should review these techniques and use them in demonstration with the individual child. Teachers, aides, and parents can then attempt certain facilitative behaviors while the speech-language pathologist observes.

INSTITUTING A CLASSROOM MODEL

The most difficult aspect of the classroom model is its initial institution. The transition from pull-out service to classroom-based service takes careful planning. Central to success is the resolution of the following issues:

TABLE 10.3
Guide for parents' and teachers' interactive style

Talk about things that interest the child at least once a day.

Follow the child's lead. Reply to the child's initiations and comments. Get excited with the child.

Don't ask too many questions. If you must, use such questions as *how did/do, why,* and *what happened* that result in longer explanatory answers.

Encourage the child to ask questions. Respond openly and honestly. If you don't want to answer a question, say so and explain why ("I don't think I want to answer that question; it's very personal").

Use a pleasant tone of voice. You need not be a comedian, but you can be light and humorous. Children love it when adults are a little silly.

Don't be judgmental or make fun of the child's language. If you are overly critical of the child's language or try to "shotgun" all errors, the child will stop talking to you.

Allow enough time for the child to respond.

Treat the child with courtesy by not interrupting when the child is talking.

Include the child in family discussions. Encourage participation and listen to the child's ideas.

Be accepting of the child and the child's language. Hugs and acceptance go a long way.

Provide opportunities for the child to use language and to have that language help the child accomplish some goal.

☐ Training of the speech-language pathologist.

☐ Training of other professionals.

☐ Establishment of a clear source of authority for intervention.

☐ Administrative support in the form of adequate space, scheduled time slots, and financial commitment (Miller, 1989).

☐ Identification criteria for students to receive services based not on standardized test scores but on classroom language processing and use (Miller, 1989).

☐ Responsibility for IEPs (Miller, 1989).

The task of changing an entire model of intervention seems overwhelming. It is essential, therefore, to begin slowly and to prepare parents and other professionals for the change.

First, the individual speech-language pathologist must train herself. This training includes education in the use of a functional conversational approach. This text provides one step in that education. Workshops, convention presentations, and further professional reading are also essential. In addition, the speech-language pathologist should role play the use of various techniques because they differ considerably from the more traditional behavioral patterns.

Classroom teachers can help the speech-language pathologist become familiar with small and large group instruction. Possibly, the speech-language pathologist could spend an hour per week in some group activity within a classroom.

Second, the speech-language pathologist must train other people. The initial purpose of this training is to educate teachers and administrators about the need for classroom intervention. This is best accomplished with in-service training stressing (a) the importance of the environment for nonimpaired language learning, (b) questions of generalization, (c) the verbal nature of the classroom, (d) the practicality and efficiency of classroom intervention strategies, and (e) the need for and desirability of team approaches.

Once convinced of the need for such a model of intervention, the teachers can begin to learn specific intervention techniques. These techniques may be introduced in in-service training with individual instruction to follow. Videotaped lessons with language-impaired children are excellent training vehicles to demonstrate the use of various techniques.

Third, clear lines of authority for language intervention must be established. It is vital to the success of this model that roles and responsibilities as well as authority be clearly established. This step requires administrative support and a definite statement of policy.

Fourth, administrative support in the form of space, scheduled time, and necessary financial outlays must be established. It is too easy for administrators to declare a change in procedures without giving adequate support to ensure success.

The biggest single impediment to implementation is the lack of time. The speech-language pathologist and the classroom teacher must allow time each week to discuss each child's success and to review targets and techniques. Unfortunately, administrators are often unwilling to grant time for these conferences. My experience is that these meetings often occur over lunch or during breaks in the schedule. Although this arrangement is less than optimum, it does allow these essential interactions to occur.

Administrators also have difficulty seeing the need to lessen dependence on standardized measures of language. Language test scores offer a quantifiable measure of behavior that can be used for determinations of student needs and progress. Yet, similar measurement can be made against the curriculum and from conversational samples. The implementation of this step requires the joint educational effort of the speech-language pathologist and the classroom teacher.

Finally, IEPs will need to be written or modified to reflect the change in service delivery. Other members of the intervention team, including parents, will need to be educated on the rationale for such changes. Parents usually accept the classroom model when shown the increased service that their child will receive if the classroom teacher is also a language trainer. Many parents are also happy with the decreased amount of pull-out time.

The implementation phase should progress slowly and carefully because it is new to both the speech-language pathologist and the classroom teacher. At first, one child in one classroom can be targeted. This can gradually be expanded to include several children in this classroom or one child in each of several classrooms.

Undoubtedly, there will be problems in initiating classroom intervention. The speech-language pathologist is advised to choose the initial child and classroom carefully to ensure some measure of success and to minimize friction with the classroom teacher. Once the speech-language pathologist and the teacher begin to experience success, other teachers will be more willing to adopt the model.

Finally, there will always be administrators, classroom teachers, and/or parents who refuse to accept or cooperate with the implementation of the classroom model. Rather than become discouraged, the speech-language pathologist should work with those individuals who accept the model and continue to try to educate those who do not. Usually, success with a few children is all that is needed to convince the foot-draggers.

CONCLUSION

Functional environmental approaches, as represented by the classroom model, are among the most progressive trends evidenced today (McCormick, 1986). In many school districts throughout Canada and the United States, this model is becoming a reality. Some districts are mandating the change from above, whereas others are experiencing a quiet revolution from below. No change as radical as this one can be accomplished without some difficulties.

The role of the speech-language pathologist is changing. In many cases, speech-language pathologists are being asked to implement intervention models for which they have minimal training. Although this is expected in a professional field that is changing and growing as rapidly as speech-language pathology, it does highlight the need for continuing professional education.

Still, the speech-language pathologist is the language expert responsible for identifying children with language impairments and for implementing intervention. In this new role of consultant, the speech-language pathologist enhances this intervention process through others.

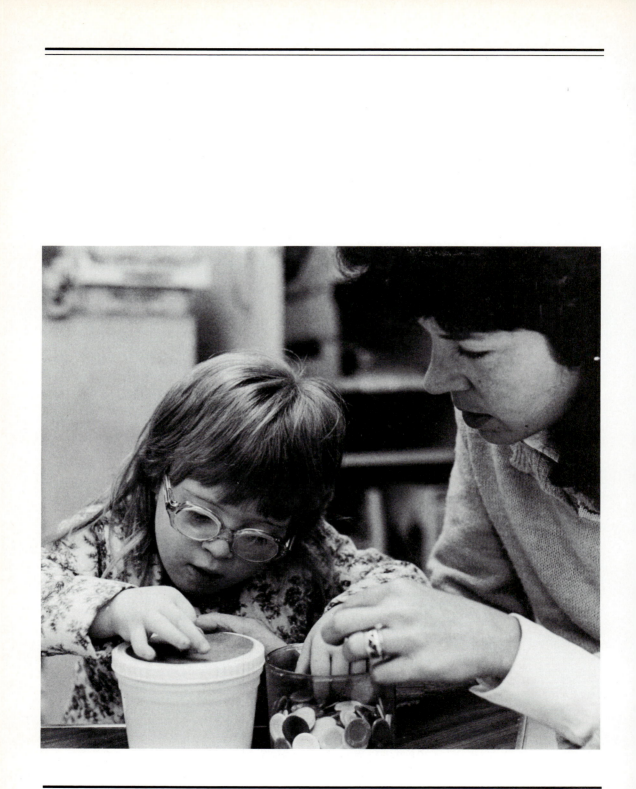

11

Assessment of Presymbolic and Minimally Symbolic Children

Children communicating at a level below 2 years of age have very unique needs. The language and communication skills of these children may be extremely limited. Often, the goal of intervention is the *initiation* of effective communication. Such children may have rudimentary communication skills or use only single-symbol or short multisymbol communication. Because of their special circumstance and their increased need for functional intervention, these children represent a special case of intervention.

Presymbolic children do not use conventional signs, words, or pictures for communication. They may possess no recognizable communication system or may use gestures, such as pointing or touching or moving objects. *Minimally symbolic* children use some visual, verbal, or tactile symbols alone or in combination. These functioning levels may be the result of a handicapping condition, such as mental retardation or deafness, a delay in the onset of language, or a language impairment. This chapter addresses a number of issues relative to the assessment of presymbolic and minimally symbolic children.

Intervention with presymbolic and minimally symbolic children usually focuses on initial communication, presymbolic skills, lexical growth, and/or early symbol combination rules. At this level, it is especially important for training to incorporate functional procedures that will actively induce generalization (Spradlin and Siegel, 1982).

The needs of this population are discussed first. Next, a brief history of intervention with this population is explored to better understand current methodology. Finally, an integrated functional model is introduced, and assessment procedures for presymbolic and minimally symbolic children are discussed. This section also briefly touches on issues relative to assessment for augmentative communication.

NEEDS OF PRESYMBOLIC AND MINIMALLY SYMBOLIC CHILDREN

Any model of assessment and intervention should address the needs of presymbolic or minimally symbolic children, while being cautiously mindful of presymbolic development provided by nonimpaired children. This section explores both the needs of language-impaired children and the development of non-impaired children.

Presymbolic Language-Impaired Children

Presymbolic and minimally symbolic children are a very diverse group representing a variety of etiological and diagnostic labels. Their one common trait is the lack of or minimal ability to use symbols. An early difficulty with communication, such as lack of responsiveness, may result in a less than optimal language-learning environment. These children may also experience cognitive and/or sensory difficulties that impede the development of symbol-referent associations.

As with the nonimpaired, the interactional patterns of language-impaired children and their caregivers are important for the development of communication. Frequently, due to a lack of responding, the interactions of the children with their caregivers are less than optimal (Mirenda & Donnellan, 1986, Rieke & Lewis, 1984). There may be a lack of appropriate verbal interactions. Caregivers may be directive, providing little opportunity for children to engage in verbal or vocal give-and-take (Nakamura & Newhoff, 1982). Such directives typically elicit few verbal responses from the children (Prizant & Rentschler, 1983; Semmel, Peck, Haring, & Theimer, 1984).

It is important to note that the breakdown of communicative interaction is not the fault of any one communicative partner. Parents of impaired children usually respond to them in ways that are age appropriate but reflect the lack of responsiveness on the part of the children. There may be a cycle in which caregivers gradually initiate and respond less as their children do.

For similar reasons, extended institutionalization also results in general deterioration of language abilities (Phillips & Balthazar, 1979; Shane, Lipshultz, & Shane, 1982). The most frequent verbal behaviors of institutional staff are directives. These behaviors result in the fewest client verbalizations. In turn, when clients do verbalize, they are often ignored by staff or receive nonverbal staff responses (Tizard, Cooperman, Joseph, & Tizard, 1973).

In the classroom, multiply handicapped children have few opportunities to initiate communication (Guess & Siegel-Causey, 1985; Houghton, Bronicki, & Guess, 1987). Teachers are usually highly directive.

In home, institutional, or educational settings, there may be little motivation to develop more appropriate communication. Many daily activities are predictable routines. In addition, the caregivers may anticipate the children's needs. Thus, the children have little need to make requests, to ask questions, or to comment (Calculator, 1988b). In this situation, the child may initiate very little communication or exhibit immature or idiosyncratic communication patterns. Idiosyncratic patterns are individualistic and do not generalize beyond such children and their immediate communication environment.

Presymbolic and minimally symbolic language-impaired children residing in a nonresponsive communication environment or one that offers little opportunity to communicate are at risk for failure to develop useful presymbolic communication systems. Useful communication would, in turn, provide the motivation for learning symbols. This situation may be very different from the language-learning environment of nonimpaired children, which can serve as an intervention model.

Nonimpaired Children

Twelve-month-old nonimpaired children's cognitive and social knowledge is evident in the things they talk about and in their use of language. Cognitively, these children have been acquiring the ability to *represent* or re-present reality within their minds. These images stand for concepts, as linguistic symbols will do later.

Children's first words are symbols for what they know (Palermo, 1982). Early meanings relate to objects, actions, locations, and descriptors. Usually, children talk about entities within their own world that they can manipulate and that are immediate. In other words, children *map* their cognitive knowledge onto language (Roberts & Horowitz, 1986).

Children spend the first year learning about the physical constancy and functions of objects and about object permanence, disappearance, and reappearance (Bloom & Lahey, 1978). More important, they learn means-ends or that an object or a person can be used to attain something else (Bates, Bretherton, Shore, & McNew, 1983). A gesture, vocalization, or verbalization can summon aid. Finally, children learn that certain sound sequences are paired consistently with certain entities to represent these entities. It is within the conversational context of children and caregivers that children acquire these words and their cognitive knowledge.

From birth, caregivers interpret children's nonvocal and vocal responses as meaningful. They treat children as conversational partners (Newson, 1979; Tronick, Als, & Adamson, 1979). Gradually, children learn patterns of conversational exchange (Kaye, 1979).

At first, children's behavior is unintentional, although it may convey information about their condition or draw attention to them. By about 8 months, children's nonvocal behaviors have been conventionalized into a recognizable system of gestures (Bates et al., 1983). With these gestures, children demonstrate a definite intention to communicate with their partners by considering these partners in their behavior. First, children secure their partner's attention, then gesture and possibly vocalize (Scoville, 1983). These gestures enable children to request, signal notice, ask questions, and offer objects. First words or symbols develop to fill these communicative functions (Bruner, 1978; Bullowa, 1979). By the time nonimpaired children use their first word, they have a well-established communication system.

TOWARD A MODEL OF ASSESSMENT AND INTERVENTION

A model of assessment and intervention might reflect both the premises of this text and the history of assessment and intervention with the presymbolic and minimallly symbolic population. To comprehend such a model fully, it is necessary to understand past and current models of assessment and intervention.

A Brief History of Therapy Models

Prior to the early 1960s, intervention efforts with presymbolic and minimally symbolic children stressed a language stimulation approach. Direct intervention services were very limited. The stimulation approach was followed in the late 1960s by a behavioral paradigm that was, in turn, replaced by a more cognitive and sociocommunicative design. Early behavioral approaches stressed speech as the means of production with little regard for presymbolic learning. The cognitive and sociocommunicative designs stressed selected presymbolic skills that were assumed necessary prerequisites for symbol use. Displeasure with the results of all of these methods led to a communication-first approach in which initial communication is established at some level and then altered toward a more symbolic communication system.

Although each approach has been able to demonstrate success with some language-impaired children, intervention with increasingly more severely involved clients has questioned the efficacy of each approach. Even with these many approaches, minimally symbolic children "often fail to use language responses spontaneously in appropriate situations" (Wulz, Hall, & Klein, 1983, p. 2).

Currently, communication-training programs for presymbolic and minimally symbolic children reflect two general intervention strategies—presymbolic training and communication training. In the first, children are taught presymbolic skills prior to the introduction of symbolic communication (Bricker & Bricker, 1974; MacDonald, Blott, Gordan, Spiegal, & Hartmann, 1974). Presymbolic training usually includes cognitive, perceptual, social, and/or communicative targets identified as significant in nonimpaired children's acquisition of symbol use. The presymbolic approach has been used most frequently and most successfully with young children who exhibit mild/moderate retardation.

Cognitive presymbolic training might include motor imitation, object permanence, symbolic play, and means-end. These skills represent important presymbolic cognitive abilities that the Swiss educator Jean Piaget and his followers recognized. It is reasoned that object permanence, or recognition that an object exists even when no longer visible, is a necessary step in the development of symbol use. First, the child learns to hold visual images in the mind, then more abstract symbols. Unfortunately, the complex nature of the cognition-language relationship makes the value statements about such training tentative at best (Rice, 1983). The relationship of language and the specific cognitive areas mentioned is correlational, and skill attainment may initially be evidenced in either language or cognition (Kelly & Dale, 1989). Perceptual targets are usually awareness and recognition of sound and symbol production and symbol discrimination. Social and communicative targets could consist of nonvocal and vocal turn taking, eye contact, and gestures.

The specific behaviors selected for training vary in number, kind, and scope with the various commercially available training procedures (Horstmeier and MacDonald, 1978a; Manolson, 1983; McLean & Snyder-McLean, 1978; Owens, 1982c). This diversity reflects differing opinions on the relative worth of certain presymbolic behaviors. In general, a greater number of training targets reflects an attempt to include more presymbolic skills, while also increasing the number of small or incremented training steps as an aid for more severely language-impaired children.

In recent years, a communication-first approach has evolved in which initial emphasis is on the establishment of a communication system that can later be expanded toward symbol use (Keogh & Reichle, 1985; Reichle, Piche-Cragoe, Sigafoos, & Doss, 1988; Sternberg, McNerney, & Pegnatore, 1985; Sternberg, Pegnatore, & Hill, 1983; Stillman & Battle, 1984; Stremel-Campbell, Johnson-Dorn, Guida, & Udell, 1984; Yoder, 1985). Proponents of this approach reason that communication training, especially with young children, should occur during the first 6 years of life, when the brain is experiencing its greatest physiological growth, rather than waiting until presymbolic skills have been learned (Wilbur, 1987).

The communication-first approach attempts to establish an early *signal* system, such as touch, to enhance the child's opportunities for interaction. One of the most promising methods of initiating this system is through *behavior chain interruption* strategies, in which a pleasurable activity, such as rocking or listening to music, is stopped and the child must signal to have it begin again (Goetz, Gee, & Sailor, 1985).

Followers of the communication-first approach usually consider the presymbolic approach to be a *wait-until-the-client-is-ready* approach. The communication-first approach reflects (a) the frustration of many speech-language pathologists with the slow rate of client progress in acquiring presymbolic skills, (b) the realization that many clients communicate prior to acquiring language and prior to professional intervention, and (c) an acceptance that some clients may never communicate symbolically.

It is reasoned that there are insufficient data to exclude children from communication intervention while presymbolic training occurs. As noted, the relationship between cognition and language is correlational at best, not causal (Kelly & Dale, 1989).

Even though presymbolic language-impaired individuals pass through the same Piagetian sensorimotor stages as nonimpaired children, there is less congruence within each stage (Kangas & Lloyd, 1988). Children with language impairments may exhibit behaviors from more than one stage. In addition, there is a disparity in some language-impaired children between sociocognitive level and language performance (Cardoso-Martins, Mervis, & Mervis, 1985; Cunningham, Glenn, Wilkinson, & Sloper, 1985; Smith & vonTelzchner, 1986; Thal & Bates, 1988). For example, late talkers begin combining gestures prior to combining words; nonimpaired children combine both at about the same time.

Piagetian measures must be applied cautiously because they rely heavily on experience that may be altered significantly for children with language impairments. The relationship of cognition to language must be questioned even more when applied to presymbolic adolescents and adults (Calculator, 1988a; Snyder-McLean, Etter-Schroeder, & Rogers, 1986). Speech-language pathologists must be cautious not to overextend normative data.

In recent years, there has been a recognition that fewer presymbolic behaviors than originally believed are necessary for symbol use and that some augmentative communication systems can be successfully implemented with little or no presymbolic training (Carr & Durand, 1985; Horner & Budd, 1985; Keogh & Reichle, 1985; Reichle & Yoder, 1985; Rice, 1983). *Augmentative communication* systems (e.g., signs, gestures, communication boards, or computer-assisted devices) support, enhance, or augment the communication of nonspeaking children (Beukelman, Yorkston, & Dowden, 1985). In general, speech-language pathologists use these systems with clients for whom the vocal-verbal mode of communication is dysfunctional, the symbol-referent relationship is difficult to establish, or the need to communicate is seemingly nonexistent.

The presymbolic skills and communication-first approaches are not mutually exclusive, however, and aspects of each may be incorporated into an integrated model. It is important to focus on the goal of symbol use to communicate. The purpose of this chapter is to bring the many intervention approaches together into a unified whole that reflects a functional approach based on the children's actual needs.

An Integrated Functional Model

As noted in Chapter 1, traditional speech-language clinical services rely primarily on isolated therapy within a segregated climate (Sternat, Nietupski, Messina, Lyon, & Brown, 1977). More appropriate for presymbolic and minimally symbolic children than such "episodic intervention" (Brown, Nietupski, & Hamre-Nietupski, 1976) is a 24-hour per day, sustained service delivery model (Falvey, Bishop, Grenot-Sheyer, & Coots, 1988; Graham, 1976; Halle, 1987; Kopchick & Lloyd, 1976). The remainder of this chapter describes assessment and intervention techniques that support this goal.

A functional model of intervention targets each child's present communication system and presymbolic and symbolic behaviors within many natural communication environments throughout the day. This approach also targets the communication behaviors of each child's primary caregivers who serve as natural interactional partners. The goal is to establish communicative environments that target the child's specific needs.

The speech-language pathologist's roles, as one of many communication partners, are to interact clinically with the child and to train other language facilitators within the classroom, unit, home, or community residence. Thus, the speech-language pathologist becomes both direct service provider and consultant. As such, she designs the individual communication intervention plan with input from others, modifies that plan as necessary, provides in-service training for the professional and paraprofessional staff, trains each child-caregiver dyad, and maintains records.

The trainers or language facilitators are crucial to this integrated functional approach, and several commercially available language-training programs for presymbolic and minimally symbolic children use caregiver-trainers, such as parents (Horstmeier & McDonald, 1978; Manolson, 1983; Owens, 1982c). Child-caregiver conversational interactions are natural environments for language acquisition, and as many primary caregivers as possible should be enlisted as change agents.

As language facilitators, these caregivers are also clients of the speech-language pathologist, and their behavior should be monitored closely. Caregiver behaviors can be modified through training, modeling, role playing, and feedback (McNaughton & Light, 1989; Owens et al., 1987).

Training for the presymbolic child might use the dual approach mentioned previously, consisting of a primary thrust to establish an initial communication system and a secondary program of prerequisite skills training. Figure 11.1 diagrams this approach. An initial signal communication system is instituted and continually modified for each child, while training the prerequisite skills necessary for modification of that communication system to more conventional symbols, such as spoken words, signs, or pictured symbols. Social and cognitive skills are trained while the child's communication skills continue to improve, although not every child will progress to symbol use.

Content should reflect the child's environment and the entities the child knows and/or may desire. For example, presymbolic individuals learn symbols taught within the context of requests more rapidly than those taught as labels (Litt & Schreibman, 1982; Reichle et al., 1984; Saunders & Sailor, 1979; Stafford, Sundberg & Braam, 1978). The resultant communication becomes more pur-

FIGURE 11.1

Dual intervention approach
with presymbolic children

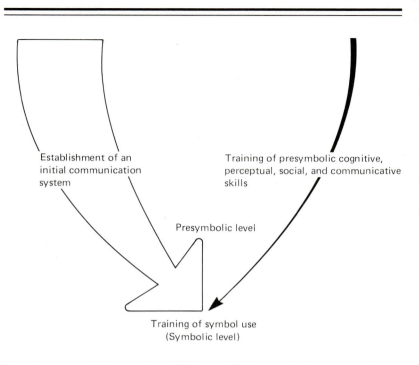

The primary presymbolic approach establishes an initial communication system, whereas
the secondary approach teaches skills believed essential to symbol use. These two approaches join at the symbolic level in which the child is taught to use symbols within the
context of the previously established communication system.

poseful and is reinforced by natural contingencies rather than by learned reinforcers.

In summary, an integrated functional intervention approach offers instruction within natural conversational contexts in everyday activities, emphasizing
introduction of a communication system and acquisition of presymbolic skills.
Caregivers fulfill the role of language facilitators under the guidance of the
speech-language pathologist. The vehicle for change is the child-caregiver interaction.

Evaluation: Getting the Whole Picture

The evaluation process is part science and part art. Although systematic procedures are used to gather data, it is the speech-language pathologist's creative or
artistic skill that synthesizes this information into a useful whole and designs the
appropriate intervention procedures. A variety of methods, including direct observation, caregiver interviews and questionnaires, behavior scaling and rating,

and direct testing, are used to attain an accurate description of each child's unique competencies within each communication context.

Communication intervention requires both training of the child and adaptation by the child's environment (Cirrin & Rowland, 1985; Donnellan, Miranda, Mesaros, & Fassbender, 1984; Vicker, 1985). If children change their behavior but environmental expectations do not change accordingly, then the children may have little or no opportunity to use these new behaviors. For example, if people in the environment do not expect a child to use a communication board, there will be little chance for the child's behavior to generalize. Therefore, the speech-language pathologist is interested in evaluating the child's abilities and needs and also the communication expectations and demands of the communication environment and the interaction of the child and the environment.

The child's abilities and needs. The speech-language pathologist is primarily interested in the child's current communication system, including the mode of communication, and in the level of presymbolic and/or symbolic functioning. A holistic description of the child's communication abilities and needs requires a variety of data collection methods. Of interest are the manner and content of both social and nonsocial communication.

With presymbolic and minimally symbolic children, it is essential that a variety of collection methods be used to obtain an adequately diverse sample of each child's communication system. For example, observation may provide examples of the commenting or declaring intention but fail to elicit negative requests or protests (Coggins, Olswang, & Guthrie, 1987). In contrast, elicitation tasks may yield protesting but little commenting.

The child may have a rich and varied, albeit idiosyncratic, communication system. Some forms may be situationally controlled. Only by using various methods to collect data from a number of sources can the speech-language pathologist hope to gain a complete description.

The child's presymbolic and/or symbolic functioning should also be fully described. Table 11.1 lists presymbolic behaviors that a number of intervention specialists and programs consider important for assessment and training. Not all professionals agree on which presymbolic behaviors to target (Miller & Chapman, 1984). Each speech-language pathologist should add or delete presymbolic behaviors based on the literature and her experience with the presymbolic population.

The assessment of presymbolic abilities is important even if children are possible candidates for augmentative communication systems. A number of tools offer effective guidelines for selecting the most appropriate augmentative system for a particular child based on the child's abilities (Calculator, 1988c; Chapman & Miller, 1980; House & Rogerson, 1984; Musselwhite & St. Louis, 1982; Owens & House, 1984; Shane & Bashir, 1980).

Symbolic assessment should include more than a list of the symbols the child uses. The range of functions these symbols represents is important, regard-

TABLE 11.1
Possible presymbolic skills for assessment and training

Presymbolic Skills	Rational

Sensory skills: Any and all modalities
  Startle and notice
  Search for stimuli
  Localization to stimuli
  Following moving stimuli
	To locate and train use of various sensory modalities for communication input and output.

Motor imitation
  Gross motor imitation
  Fine motor including facial and vocal imitation
  Imitation with objects
  Deferred imitation
	Piagetian early cognitive skill. Later used as mode of training for other skills. Facial and vocal imitation to be used for speech.

Object permanence	Piagetian cognitive skill
Turn taking with motor and vocal imitation	Early communication skill
Functional use of objects	Establish early meanings
Means-ends	Learn to control environment, communicate
Communicative gestures	
Receptive language and symbol recognition	Recognize symbol value

Sound imitation
  Vocal shaping
  Vocal sequencing
	Prerequisites to speech

Sources: Compiled from Bricker and Bricker, 1974; Hanna, Lippert, and Harris, 1982; Horstmeier and Mac-Donald, 1978b; Manolson, 1983; Owens, 1982c.

less of the means or manner of communication. Various researchers suggest different combinations of illocutionary functions, such as requesting information or making comments (Page, 1982; Wexler, Blau, Dore, & Leslie, 1982); semantic functions, such as agent + action and negative + X (MacDonald, 1978a); or a combination of both (Owens, 1982b). Symbols are initially acquired to fulfill illocutionary functions already in children's repertoires. Children also treat symbols as representing various semantic functions that form building blocks for early multisymbol utterances. Table 11.2 lists some common semantic and illocutionary functions found in initial symbolic communication. Definitions are listed in Appendix I.

Questionnaire and interview. The speech-language pathologist can initially ascertain the manner and content of the child's communication and some indication of functioning level by questionnaire and/or interview and by observation. Responses can enhance the validity of later testing. Of interest are the child's actual skills rather than an age equivalency, which is of minimal value in making intervention decisions.

TABLE 11.2
Semantic and illocutionary functions of early symbolic communication

Semantic Functions	Illocutionary Functions
Nomination	Answer
This/that + Nomination	Question or requesting
Location	information
Location + *X*	Reply
Negation	Elicitation
Negation + *X*	Continuant
Modification (Types:	Declaration
Attribution, possession, and recurrence)	Practice or repeat
Modifier + *X*	Name or label
Notice	Command, demand, request,
Notice + *X*	protest
Action (signaled by agent, action, or object)	
Agent + action	
Action + object	

Sources: Compiled from Dore, 1975; MacDonald, 1978a; Owens, 1982c.

Questionnaires or scales often comprise a portion of published language intervention programs (Hanna, Lippert, & Harris, 1982; MacDonald, 1978b; Owens, 1982a) and can be modified to conform to the speech-language pathologist's model of initial language training. Table 11.3 lists the questions of primary interest collected from a number of different sources.

Because presymbolic or minimally symbolic children can provide little information on questionnaires, caregivers are encouraged to participate in the intervention process. Questionnaire administration also provides an opportunity to acquaint caregivers with presymbolic skills that are of interest although not readily obvious. The Oliver (MacDonald, 1978b), a caregiver inventory, actually instructs caregivers to engage in some test exercises with the child, thus providing valuable data for later testing.

Some scales attempt to establish a developmental age (Bzoch & League, 1971; Sacks & Young, 1982) by asking questions relative to skills acquired at various age levels. Generally, these tools do not weight scores in terms of the importance of these behaviors for later training. Thus, all behaviors appear equally important, which, of course, they are not. Nevertheless, such developmental scales can be helpful when normative age equivalencies are required.

Observation.   Through structured observation, the speech-language pathologist attempts to describe the communicative environment of the child. Descriptive factors include the amount of time the child spends in certain environments;

TABLE 11.3
Questionnaire or interview content for presymbolic or minimally symbolic children

---

How does the child communicate primarily?
  Does the child use vocalizations, gestures, postures, eye contact, or other means of
  communication?
  Who understands the child's communication efforts?
Does the child play alone or with others?
Does the child demonstrate any turn-taking behaviors?
Does the child enjoy making sounds? How often does the child make sounds?
Does the child ever initiate communication? How? In which situations?
Which situations seem to be high communication contexts?
Which caregivers seem to engage in the most interaction with the child?
Does the child
  Make wants known?
  Request help?
  Point to objects or actions, name, or both?
  Request information?
  Seek attention?
  Demonstrate emotion?
  Protest?

Sources: Compiled from Calculator, 1988a; MacDonald, 1978b; Owens and Rogerson, 1988.

the frequency of communication in these environments; and the partners, activities, and objects present (Carlson, 1981).

One important aspect of evaluation is determining the communicative intention of the child's behaviors, whether appropriate, inappropriate, or anywhere in between. It is not the behavior itself, but its relationship to the context, that indicates communication.

Communication behaviors are consistent, identifiable responses associated with environmental events or with the child's state. Children with sensory, mental, and/or physiological impairments often do not use clearly recognizable communication (Clark & Seifer, 1982; Odom, 1983). The child who turns away from another person or becomes self-abusive or increases self-stimulation when someone approaches is communicating a desire not to communicate. Some communication may be unrecognizable as such and may be misinterpreted (Houghton et al., 1987).

Communication behaviors may be message-specific, each communicating a single message, or may communicate a variety of messages (Iwata, Dorsey, Slifer, Bauman, & Richman, 1982; Schuler & Goetz, 1981). For example, loud vocalizations may signal attention getting or several functions, such as attention getting, desire for an object, and/or need for assistance. Communication may also be intentional or unintentional based on whether the listener is considered.

Requesting is an important skill that enables children to regulate other people by asking for entities or for information. A wide variety of methods are acceptable for requesting objects and actions, for example, gestures, vocalizations, and verbalizations. In general, the more specific the child's request, the more effective the child is in eliciting a response. In assessing the pragmatically impaired child who exhibits little or no requesting, the speech-language pathologist should ask the following questions (Olswang, Kriegsmann, & Mastergeorge, 1982):

1. How does the child code requests?
2. Does the child attempt to regulate the behavior of other people or appear to have the desire to do so?
3. Does the child's behavior indicate a recognition that other people can act as agents?
4. Are opportunities for requesting available?
5. How do caregivers encourage and respond to requests?

Requesting will be severely limited if the child sees no need to engage in the behavior or if there is little opportunity to do so.

The two aspects of the environment for the speech-language pathologist to monitor are the child's elicited and spontaneous requests along with the activities in which they occur and the caregiver antecedents used in eliciting requests. She can code children's requesting behaviors and caregiver's eliciting behaviors as in Table 11.4.

Intentional or social communication is typically addressed to and modified for the receiver. This may be signaled by establishing eye contact, awaiting a turn, responding, interrupting, and/or moving to a conspicuous position or toward the receiver. Even self-injurious behavior may signal a message, such as a desire to escape or a feeling like "Leave me alone; I don't want to do this" (Carr, Newson, and Binkhoff, 1980).

In contrast, unintentional or nonsocial communication, such as speaking when no one is present, does not consider the receiver. Situational responses, such as an eye blink following a loud noise, are also considered unintentional communication unless the child interacts in some way with the receiver.

Finally, random or stereotypic behaviors, such as incessant rocking, that do not seem to be related to environmental events or to the child's state, appear to be noncommunicative (although this is not always the case). Some professionals contend that all behaviors have some functional message value (Schuler & Goetz, 1981; Watzlawick, Beavin, & Jackson, 1967).

In the past, intervention has begun with the elimination of inappropriate or aberrant behavior, ignoring the communication potential of these behaviors and their role in the limited communication repertoires of some children. Through systematic observation, the speech-language pathologist can form initial tentative hypotheses regarding intentions. In turn, she can confirm these hypotheses

TABLE 11.4
Observation of requesting behaviors

Child Request Behaviors
Types
Spontaneous request—Child initiated, not preceded by verbal or nonverbal adult behavior.
Elicited request—Child produces request following adult verbal or nonverbal elicitation.
Intention
Request for objects/people—Names or points to object/person, directing listener to provide.
Requests for action—Child directs listener to perform in a certain manner.
Requests for information—Uses rising intonation or *wh-* word to direct listener to provide information.

Adult Elicitation Behaviors
Direct model—Adult directs child to produce model provided ("Tell me, 'open door' ").
Direct question—Adult asks question that elicits request ("What do you want?").
Obstacle presentation—Adult gives command or direct verbal instruction, but some obstacle, such as a missing piece or broken object, is provided ("Get some candy" [jar sealed tightly]).
General statement—Adult gives a verbal comment that refers in a general way to some object or activity that the child might want to request ("I have some funny books over here").

Source: Adapted from Olswang, L., Kriegsmann, E., and Mastergeorge, A. (1982). Facilitating functional requesting in pragmatically impaired children. *Language, Speech, and Hearing Services in Schools, 13,* 202–222.

by systematic and meticulous manipulation of antecedent and/or consequent events during testing.

She can record hypotheses regarding the child's intentions on a simple form similar to Figure 11.2 (Donnellan et al., 1984). Although designed for aberrant behavior, the form can be adapted, and other child behaviors listed across the top. The communicative functions or intentions on the left are derived from a number of taxonomies of the intentions of nonhandicapped children. Facilitator hypotheses of intent are marked in the space corresponding to the behavior and to the possible intention. In the examples shown, tantruming is believed to signal an intention to attract attention, and touching an object may signal a desire for some item.

Direct testing.   The final step in evaluation is direct testing to determine the optimum input and output modes for communication, the desirability of an augmentative system of communication and the selection of type, and the presymbolic or symbolic functioning level of the child. This process is ongoing and may tax the creativity of even the best speech-language pathologist because of the difficulty in testing some children.

FIGURE 11.2
Functions of children's behavior

Behaviors (columns, left to right):
AGGRESSION · BIZARRE VERBALIZATIONS · INAPP. ORAL / ANAL BEHAVIOR · PERSEVERATIVE RITUALS · SELF-INJURIOUS BEHAVIOR · SELF-STIMULATION · TANTRUM · FACIAL EXPRESSION · GAZE AVERSION · GAZING / STARING · GESTURING / POINTING · HUGGING / KISSING · MASTURBATION · OBJECT MANIPULATION · PROXIMITY POSITIONING · PUSHING / PULLING · REACHING / GRABBING · RUNNING · TOUCHING · DELAYED ECHOLALIA · IMMEDIATE ECHOLALIA · LAUGHING / GIGGLING · SCREAM / YELL · SWEARING · VERBAL · WHINING / CRYING · COMPLEX / PHYSICAL THREATS · COMPLEX SIGN / APPROX. · ONE-WORD SPEECH / APPROX. · ONE-WORD SIGN / APPROX. · PICTURE / WRITTEN WORD

FUNCTIONS

I. Interactive

A. Requests for
Attention — X (under SELF-INJURIOUS BEHAVIOR)
Social interaction
Play interactions
Affection
Permission to engage in an activity
Action by Receiver
Assistance
Information / clarification
Objects — X (under REACHING / GRABBING)
Food

B. Negations
Protest
Refusal
Cessation

C. Declarations / comments
About events / actions
About objects / persons
About errors / mistakes
Affirmation
Greeting
Humor

D. Declarations about feelings
Anticipation
Boredom
Confusion
Fear
Frustration
Hurt feelings
Pain
Pleasure

II. Non-interactive

A. Self-regulation
B. Rehearsal
C. Habitual
D. Relaxation / Tension release

This form can be adapted to list the individual child's behaviors across the top. Hypotheses regarding the illocutionary functions of these behaviors can be recorded in the appropriate space.

Source: Donnellan, A., Mirenda, P., Mesaros, R., & Fassbender, L. (1984). Analyzing the communicative functions of aberrant behavior. *Journal of the Association for Persons with Severe Handicaps, 9*, 210–222. Reprinted with permission.

If the child already has some type of rudimentary communication system, the speech-language pathologist attempts to describe this system as accurately as possible. Of particular interest are input and output means. The three primary expressive and receptive modes of communication are manual/visual, vocal/verbal/auditory, and tactile. Manual/visual means include gestures, signs, body movement, and/or visual contact or pointing. Vocal/verbal/auditory means include intonation, speech sounds, phonetically consistent forms, and/or spoken words. Tactile means include touch, signing in the hand, and physical manipulation, such as moving a partner's hand to a desired object. A skillful communicator uses a combination of methods depending on context. Some language-impaired children rely on one mode primarily or on different input and output modes. For example, a child may understand and comply with single words or short phrases received auditorily, but rely on a gestural form of expressive communication.

For very low functioning presymbolic children, the speech-language pathologist assesses each of the three means for consistent responding and for focused or directed behavior. The speech-language pathologist should also assess the oral mechanism for motor development and control (Morris, 1982; Morris & Klein, 1987; Sleight & Niman, 1984). Part of the evaluation may include a probe to determine the difficulty in establishing an initial communication system.

As mentioned earlier in this chapter, communication can be established by a behavior chain interruption method in which some pleasurable behavior, such as listening to music, is interrupted. (Goetz et al., 1985). During the evaluation, the speech-language pathologist can attempt to determine activities pleasurable to the child that she can use in this training. These activities may include rocking, listening to music, eating or drinking, or playing with some toy. Physical rocking, in which the child is cradled, has been used very successfully to establish initial communication (Sternberg et al., 1983; Sternberg et al., 1985). Through this pleasurable activity, the child can build a consistent responding behavior to signal for the rocking to continue.

During testing, the speech-language pathologist can confirm hypotheses about illocutionary function formed during observation. The speech-language pathologist can manipulate events that precede and follow the behaviors in question and note the effect of these changes on the behavior's frequency and intensity. Changes in the behavior should indicate some relationship between the behavior and the environment. For example, if the speech-language pathologist suspects that rocking signals requesting of objects, she might give objects in the immediate context to the child when rocking occurs and observe the result.

Formal direct testing of age-related communication can be accomplished by using any number of infant communication or development measures (Bayley, 1969; Boyd, Stauber & Bluma, 1977; Griffith & Sanford, 1975; Rogers, D'Eugenio, Brown, Donovan & Lynch, 1978; Song et al., 1980). Many items are not appropriate for older children and may have little application to their experiences. Such instruments may also be difficult to use with multiply handicapped children. For example, the child with cerebral palsy may be unable to exhibit many of the motor behaviors listed. Necessary modifications in testing procedures may preclude the outright use of a test's age norms. At best, these instruments provide only a gross estimate of the child's overall communication abilities.

Functional or behavioral level data from questionnaires, interviews, and observations provide initial data for evaluating actual presymbolic or symbolic skills through direct testing. Certain commercially available instruments assess varying numbers of presymbolic and symbolic behaviors (Hanna et al., 1982; MacDonald, 1982b; Horstmeier & MacDonald, 1978b; Owens, 1982b; Rescorla, 1989). Most of these tools were created by modifying developmental scales to reflect more accurately the population being tested and the skills specifically needed for symbolic communication. Because the speech-language pathologist is interested in not only the skill level of the child but also the ease of teaching presymbolic skills, a necessary portion of the assessment should include teaching.

One widely used tool is the Ordinal Scales of Psychological Development (Uzgiris and Hunt, 1975). Based on a Piagetian model of early cognitive development, the Ordinal Scales and their adaptation by Dunst (1980) comprise a stage-oriented, assessment tool. Behaviors tested help to place the child in one of the sensorimotor stages of cognitive development. Because the scales were not originally designed for special needs children, each evaluated behavior must be adapted for the child's specific physical limitations. Other similar tools, such as the Callier-Azusa Scale (Stillman, 1978), are designed for multiply handicapped populations (e.g., children who are deaf-blind). Because these tools are based on a hierarchical model of development, the results describe general cognitive functioning and suggest goals for further training. The speech-language pathologist can choose subtests most directly related to presymbolic development, such as those that relate to gestures, means-ends, and imitation (McLean & Snyder-McLean, 1988).

No specific skills, such as the imitative behavior of clapping hands, will aid in the development of symbols. Hand clapping is one example of a larger behavioral class of imitation. The speech-language pathologist is more interested in the presence or absence of these general classes of behavior, and she probes overall conceptual development of these classes.

Such assessments may tax the best creative methods. However, stereotypic or perseverative behavior can be used if the speech-language pathologist can elicit this behavior within a few seconds of her model. The speech-language pathologist who knows she can elicit this behavior is able to control the behavior for training purposes, such as modifying it.

She should encourage caregivers to attend the evaluation and to assist by providing suggestions and actual test items from the child's environment, such as toys or grooming items. The presence of both the caregiver and familiar objects enhances the validity of the testing procedure. Often, presymbolic and minimally symbolic children have very concrete meanings for symbols or demonstrate very ritualized behavior. A cup may not be *cup* for the child unless it is the one used every day. This information would be unavailable without the caregiver's presence, and the speech-language pathologist might assume that the child does not know the symbol *cup*.

Certain minimal presymbolic skills even seem necessary for use of some augmentative communication systems. The level of functioning necessary depends on the system selected. In short, the more symbolic the system, the higher cognitive skill involved. For example, some forms of gestural signaling may be accomplished at a relatively young developmental age when compared to speaking or signing.

Cognitive abilities are especially important for the size and quality of the augmentative repertoire that the child will develop (Silverman, 1989). Although late Piagetian sensorimotor stages IV and early V are correlated with true symbol use, this correlation should not preclude augmentative instruction at a less than symbolic level that is useful to the child (Calculator, 1988c).

The speech-language pathologist frequently assesses social skills, such as turn taking, eye contact, joint attending, and gesturing, when considering a child for an augmentative communication system. She may classify gestures as coverbal or paraverbal, signaling emotional state, attitude, or station; referential, referring to an object or event; or iconic, replicating some entity with hand shapes or movements (Yorkston & Dowden, 1984).

Assessments for augmentative communication should also include a physical evaluation of manual dexterity, range and accuracy of movement, physical placement, oral-peripheral structure and functioning, and visual acuity. Various systems should be tried to determine those best suited to the child. It is not unusual to find children communicating via a number of augmentative modes simultaneously.

Although the decision process involved in selecting or designing an augmentative system for a child is a first step, the assessment does not need to be (Reichle & Karlan, 1985). An assess-teach model, in which the child attempts to learn various systems while being assessed, seems promising (Reichle et al., 1988).

Sampling.   At a symbolic level, whether verbal or through some augmentative means, the speech-language pathologist is interested in the number of symbols in the child's lexicon and in the variety of semantic and illocutionary functions the child displays. The relative merits of sampling and more formalized testing are discussed in Chapter 3.

The speech pathologist collects a conversational sample and rates each utterance for the semantic and illocutionary functions found in early child language (MacDonald, 1978a; Owens, 1982b). Although such categories may be inappropriate for older retarded children, they do suggest a standard set of functions with which to begin (Leonard, Steckol & Panther, 1983). Normative distributions are not available for these functions, which are usually situationally related. Of greater interest is the range of functions the child uses.

The speech-language pathologist collects samples by observing everyday activities or routines with the child's primary caregivers, such as teachers, parents, and classroom aides. Children engaged in familiar meaningful activities with age-appropriate materials are likely to interact more and to produce more language than do children in other situations.

Analysis can be accomplished at the utterance level. For speaking children, an utterance consists of one or more symbols separated from other symbols by a pause, a drop in the voice, or an inhalation. Children using augmentative communication may look at their partner or pause between utterances. Whatever the mode of transmission, the speech-language pathologist records and rates each utterance for both semantic and illocutionary function and for the number of symbols used. Appendix I provides definitions of the most common functions listed in Table 11.2. A form such as Figure 11.3 may be helpful for recording and analyzing the data. The speech-language pathologist records the number of symbols per utterance under the appropriate functions demonstrated by the utterance.

Repetitive utterances, such as ''baby baby,'' may function as single-symbol utterances. If this is suspected, the speech-language pathologist should credit the child with only one symbol for that utterance. Likewise, certain combinations may also function as single-symbol utterances. The child may repeatedly produce ''dog here'' yet not use either symbol independently or in combination with other symbols. If this is suspected, it can be confirmed by the caregivers or through observation, and the utterance rated accordingly.

The speech-language pathologist then uses the total number of symbols and the total number of utterances within each function to compute the mean length of utterance (MLU) of each function. She can use the results as follows to select training objectives (Owens, 1982c):

- ☐ Teach relevant functions that do not occur.
- ☐ Provide opportunities for low frequency functions to occur.
- ☐ Teach longer forms for functions with low MLUs.
- ☐ Reduce or modify stereotypic, perseverative, or echolalic utterances that seem nonfunctional.

Such detailed collection and analysis procedures are very time-consuming, but they are necessary for presymbolic and early symbolic children who may exhibit a low incidence of communicative behavior and use inappropriate and unconventional signal systems.

The speech-language pathologist may also collect semantic functions within a structured format using conversational and/or imitative cues to elicit function-specific two-, three-, and four-word utterances (MacDonald, 1978a). Although less naturalistic than sampling, these techniques can elicit a broader range of

FIGURE 11.3

Functional analysis of a language sample of a minimally symbolic child

Utterances	SEMANTIC FUNTIONS Nom.	L.	Neg.	P.	Att.	R.	Not.	O.	Act.	Ag+	+Ob	ILLOCUTIONARY FUNCTIONS A.	Q.	R.	D.	P.	N.	S.	O.	Semantic-Illocutionary Functions
1. BALL	1																1			
2. WANT BALL									2		2							2		
3. THROW BALL									2		2							2		
4. THROW ME		2																2		
5. WANT THAT?	2											2								
6. NO THAT			2															2		
7. MORE THROW						2			2									2		
8. BALL?	1											1								
9. THROW BALL ME		3							3		3							3		
44.																				
45.																				
46.																				
47.																				
48.																				
50.																				
OVERALL TOTAL (Words)	4	5	2	0	0	2	0	0	9	0	7	3	0	0	0	0	1	13	0	
TOTAL NO. OF UTT.	3	2	1	0	0	1	0	0	4	0	3	2	0	0	0	0	1	6	0	
MLU by functions (Divide total words by total utterances)	1.3	2.5	2	0	0	2	0	0	2.3	0	2.3	1.5	0	0	0	1	2.2	0		

Nom. = Nomination
L. = Location
Neg. = Negation
P. = Possession
Att. = Attribution

R. = Recurrence
Not. = Notice
O. = Other
Act. = Action
Ag+ = Agent + Action

+ Ob = Action + Object
A. = Answer
Q. = Question
R. = Reply
D. = Declaration

P. = Practice
N. = Name
S. = Suggestion, Command, Demand, Request
O. = Other

In the first utterance, the child pointed at the object and said one symbol ("Ball") clearly a semantic Nominative and an illocutionary Name. Utterances 4 ("Throw me"), 6 ("No that") and 7 ("More throw") are two-symbol examples of the semantic rules X + Locative, Negative + X and Recurrent + X, respectively. At the two-symbol level, these semantic functions are expanded by adding another symbol. This format applies to the first seven semantic functions. In contrast, utterance 3 ("Throw ball") is an example of a different type. The Agent, Action, and Object categories are expanded by combining categories. Thus, utterance 3 is an example of a two-symbol Action and a two-symbol Object. Utterance 2 is similar. Utterance 9 represents a combination of X + Locative and Action + Object to form Action + Object + Locative, a three-category combination scored under each appropriate category.

Source: Owens, R. (1982). From the manual for the *Program for the Acquisition of Language with the Severely Impaired (PALS)*. Copyright © 1982 by The Psychological Corporation. Reproduced by permission. All rights reserved.

functions than may be possible within interactional samples. She can then compare these data with the spontaneous sample.

The Communication Environment. The speech-language pathologist is interested in more than just the functioning level of the child. Given the effect of context—both linguistic and nonlinguistic—on communication, the speech-language pathologist must also evaluate the communication potential of the child's natural environment. Again, she gathers initial information through interviews with caregivers and by observation. Of interest are the situations, activities, and locations that are high-communication contexts and the child's communication behavior in each. The speech-language pathologist is also interested in identifying caregivers who evoke the most communication from the child and in describing their behaviors, especially the communication demands they place on the child.

The speech-language pathologist may wish to conduct a four-step survey of the child's communication needs and uses (Brown, Branston, Hamre-Nietupski, Pumpian, Certo, and Gruenewald, 1979; Yoder, 1985). First, she describes the functionally most relevant and least restrictive communication environments, at present and in the foreseeable future. These might include the classroom or the home. In step two, she divides these environments into subenvironments by the most relevant and functional activities in each, such as snack time or bathing. Next, she determines the skills needed to participate in each activity. Finally, the speech-language pathologist describes how each activity and/or environment may be adapted to allow or enhance the child's participation. This process provides the data needed to design intervention programs to teach interactional skills and environmental adaptation.

The Interaction of Child and Environment. Although the child and environment are important in themselves, the data gathered from each are most meaningful when we consider how each affects the other. Communication is an interaction between the child and caregivers, and learning can only be measured by the effect that the child's newly trained behaviors have on the environment of which these caregivers are a part. For maximum generalization the child's caregivers must become language facilitators.

In determining the language facilitator potential of each caregiver, the speech-language pathologist must first determine the quality of the interaction between the child and caregiver. The speech-language pathologist can then, when appropriate, suggest modifications in the caregiver's behavior that may, in turn, change the child's communicative behavior. For example, the caregiver who demonstrates a relatively directive style, such as anticipating the child's needs or talking incessantly, might be instructed to wait for the child's request for assistance and to pause for verbal and nonverbal turns by the child.

Qualitative judgments of child-caregiver interaction might be based on the presence or absence of certain behaviors by both individuals. Behaviors to observe might include the caregivers' uses of natural reinforcement, physical proximity, imitation of the child's behaviors, expansion, reply/extension, and content appropriate to the child's experience and functioning level. The child might be rated for attending to the interaction, referencing or signaling notice, physical proximity, and vocal/verbal responding. The presence of these 10 characteristics has been associated with subjective judgments of quality interaction (Russo & Owens, 1982). Although useful, such prepackaged scales might overlook information valuable for any specific child and caregiver dyad. A more descriptive scale that delineates child strategies for engagement, termination, and re-engagement and the primary modes of signaling might be more useful (Wilcox & Campbell, 1983).

In general, prelanguage children engage in a greater frequency and higher level of communication when they initiate interactions. Norris and Hoffman (1990) propose a six-stage rating scale of nonverbal interactions, based on Piaget, that compares the child's level of responding in both adult-initiated and child-initiated interactions. Using descriptors of vocalizations, limb movements, and facial and body postures, the speech-language pathologist classifies the child's behaviors into levels of response.

MacDonald and Gillette (1982) propose the use of four scales, called *ECO-maps*, covering interaction/conversation, mode, content, and use within the interaction. Each scale is further divided into child performance, significant other performance, significant other teaching strategies, and potential problems. In the first two classes of child and significant other performance, the scales rate behavior as an approximate percentage of the time that each interactant engages in the specific behaviors listed. Results allow for an estimate of communication match for that behavior; severe inequities signal a potential mismatch. If the caregiver is rated 9 on "initiates contact," and the child receives only 1, the inequity in this area requires intervention. A progressive match in which the caregiver is monitoring the child's performance and modeling slightly above that level is more desirable. The Teaching Strategies ECOmap rates the caregiver's use of events and strategies the child needs to communicate at a higher level. Finally, the Problems ECOmap identifies specific potential interactional problems.

CONCLUSION

Prior to initiating therapy and throughout the intervention process, the speech-language pathologist must conduct a thorough evaluation of the child's communication system and environment. A variety of data collection procedures are needed to attain an adequate description. Of interest is the child's present communication system and potential for modification and the child's presymbolic or early symbolic level of functioning. The speech-language pathologist will also want to identify the communication characteristics of the child's environment and of the child-caregiver interaction and describe the communication behaviors of all primary caregivers. She would continue to monitor these variables through-out intervention to ensure the child's performance at the optimum communication level.

The goal of a truly functional communication training program necessitates a thorough understanding of the dynamics of the child-caregiver interaction. From initial contact with the child, it is critical that the speech-language pathologist consider the contextual variables that affect communication and are, in turn, affected by it.

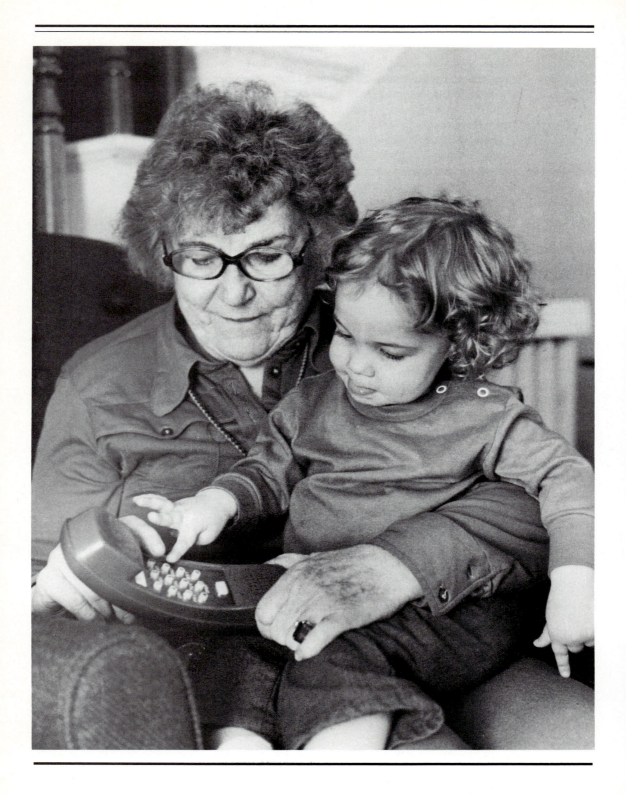

12
Intervention with Presymbolic and Minimally Symbolic Children

The child's intervention plan should be based on and should address the needs of all three major areas assessed—child-related variables, environmental variables, and interactional variables—within an overall integrated functional approach. This section discusses strategies and techniques applicable to each area.

AN INTEGRATED FUNCTIONAL INTERVENTION MODEL

Ideally, the speech-language pathologist sees the child daily for individual or group therapy within a classroom or unit setting with the caregiver. If this is not possible, the caregiver should attend at least once a week. When this attendance is not possible, the speech-language pathologist can inform the caregiver about the training through detailed reports and instructions, and she can train the caregiver periodically in evening group sessions. The speech-language pathologist can observe the teachers and aides in the natural classroom environment and make suggestions for improving the quality of the child-caregiver interaction. With instructional staff, training can occur at in-service sessions or in direct instruction following the brief observation and data review sessions in the classroom environment. Each caregiver should maintain a record of all formal training for review along with the speech-language pathologist's records when making decisions about the intervention plan. Staff should also participate in assessments and in setting intervention goals (McNaughton & Light, 1989).

Activities within each child's various interactional environments form the bases for communication and training. Communication and language training occur at natural junctures within each child's ongoing activities (Rowland & Schweigert, 1989). Three intervention techniques are beneficial: incidental teaching, stimulation, and formal training (Owens, 1982c).

Incidental teaching is a strategy that arises naturally within the child's and caregiver's daily activities or in unstructured situations. In this child-directed strategy, the child controls the focus of the interaction by signaling interest. While enhancing these naturally occurring communication interactions, the caregiver trains or strengthens presymbolic or early symbolic behaviors. In other words, the behavior is trained within the child's daily activities in which it would naturally appear. For example, the child learning about object permanence could encounter natural teaching situations while bathing with nonfloating soap or while searching for misplaced toys. *Incidental teaching is not formal training disguised as fun.* Hidden training, such as preschool action songs, may be just as irrelevant to the context and to the child as formal training, although action songs in another context can aid in valuable concept development.

The caregiver's tasks are to be aware of the learning potential within each situation and to structure events to enhance learning. In unstructured activities, such as free play, the child's expressed interest is the key. Caregivers can learn to follow the child's lead and to incorporate training into these interests. Table 12.1 lists examples of incidental teaching.

A number of studies have reported success, albeit limited, in the use of incidental techniques. For example, institutionalized adolescents increased their verbal initiations for food at meals following a delaying procedure in which the trainer awaited client signals (Halle et al., 1979). In addition, teacher use of the procedures spread to other settings. Similar results have been reported with the use of sign (Oliver & Halle, 1982). Autistic adolescents have been taught object labels within a lunch preparation activity in a kitchen area (McGee et al., 1983).

TABLE 12.1
Examples of incidental teaching

Type of Training	Example
Establishing eye contact	During feeding, the child looks at the facilitator in order to receive a spoonful of food.
Object permanence	While bathing, the facilitator "loses" nonfloating soap in the bath water and states, "Oh, I lost the soap; can you find it?"
Imitation with objects	During daily living skills training, the child imitates the facilitator's use of a comb.
Requesting gesture	At snack time, the child requests a special snack from those on the table.
Symbol recognition	The child picks out clothes named during dressing.

Unfortunately, this incidental aspect of training is most difficult for caregivers to comprehend. Although it is relatively easy to train caregivers to engage in formal training with children, and relatively easy for these caregivers to adapt the training to other environments, it is not as easy for them to adapt the training to less structured, informal, everyday activities unless directly taught these behaviors (Alpert & Rogers-Warren, 1984; Salzberg & Villani, 1983).

The speech-language pathologist can assist caregivers in using incidental techniques by following these suggestions:

1. Keep the training procedures simple.
2. Role play potential situations with the caregiver.
3. Target a few frequently occurring everyday situations rather than try to cover every possible situation.
4. Do not require record keeping of incidental teaching.
5. Demonstrate in the actual environment or within real situations.

Caregivers are easily overwhelmed by the plethora of training advice to be used in numerous different potential teaching situations.

Following a review of incidental teaching research, Warren and Kaiser (1986b) concluded that "incidental teaching (a) teaches target skills effectively in the natural environment; (b) typically results in generalization of those skills across settings, time, and persons; and (c) results in gains in the formal and functional aspects of language" (p. 296). Incidental teaching is useful for generalization and for relevancy of training. Without such techniques, the 24-hour-a-day approach is impossible.

Many caregivers express reservations about their ability to implement formal training and to make the assumed time commitment. Thus, incidental teaching is a practical response to the need for more child instruction and more useful child-caregiver interaction.

Warren and Kaiser (1986b) further concluded that "because research with mentally retarded children is limited . . . the extent to which incidental teaching can remediate serious communication deficits . . . is less clear" (p. 296). This concern is addressed by using the two additional teaching strategies of stimulation and formal training in conjunction with incidental teaching.

Stimulation, the way caregivers interact with the child, should be just slightly more complex than the child's functioning to serve as a model. The child will learn best, according to the minimal discrepancy principle, when the model is far enough above his or her competency level to maintain interest but not so far as to frustrate (Hunt, 1961). Our best guide is the communication behavior of mothers of nonimpaired infants.

These mothers treat their children as conversational partners who exhibit meaningful communication. After addressing their children, these mothers usually wait for a response and treat any following behavior as meaningful. The mothers use a variety of techniques, such as exaggerated movements, to gain and maintain their children's interest.

First and foremost, caregivers must expect and be alert for the child's communication and must structure situations to encourage it. Once communication occurs, caregivers provide appropriate models and feedback and allow the child to make choices that can affect change (Owens, 1982c; Page, 1982; Tapajna & Finn-Scardine, 1981). Even nonimpaired peers can serve as excellent language stimulation models (Cole, Vandercook, & Rynders, 1987). Table 12.2 lists some suggested stimulation techniques.

Because research has not identified which behaviors are the most effective, caregivers should use as many as are practical. It is best for caregivers to change their own behavior slowly, possibly incorporating one or two techniques and waiting until these feel comfortable before using more. It will not be necessary to use all of the stimulation techniques with every child. Small changes in the current method of interacting, such as increasing the number of verbalizations addressed to the child, may have dramatic effects (Owens et al., 1987). Augmentative symbols, such as signs, can be learned singly, possibly in a ''signs of the week'' program (Spragle & Micucci, 1990).

Formal training, the third strategy, occurs a few brief times daily. The speech-language pathologist monitors this training closely for content, procedures, and the child's progress. She analyzes each skill to be taught for antecedent and consequent events and constructs a hierarchy that includes the steps needed for successful completion. With presymbolic children, especially those

TABLE 12.2
Stimulation techniques for presymbolic and minimally symbolic children

---

Presymbolic Children
  Speak in short sentences of three to five words containing one to two syllables each.
  Speak about entities in the immediate context.
  Speak slowly with pauses and emphasize content words.
  Use self-talk and parallel talk to describe your own and the child's actions, respectively.
  Gesture or use simple signs when it may aid comprehension.
  Allow time for the child to respond even though he or she may not.
  Establish a communication position vis-a-vis the child's face that is comfortable for the child and that demonstrates a genuine interest in the child's communication efforts.
  Maintain the child's attention by varying the intensity and pitch of your verbalizations.

Minimally Symbolic Children
In addition to the techniques above:
  Attend to all symbolic initiations.
  Gently correct with feedback.
  Expand the child's communication into a more mature form.
  Reply to the child's communication with a relevant and appropriate comment.
  Do not ask too many adult-like questions. They are difficult to process.

Source: Adapted from Owens, R. (1982). From the *Program for the Acquisition of Language with the Severely Impaired (PALS)*. Copyright © 1982 by The Psychological Corporation. Reproduced by permission. All rights reserved.

above preschool age, it is essential that training hierarchies consist of small increments of change. This necessitates a task analysis approach that reflects the child's individual style and sequence of learning, the individual cues necessary, reinforcers, success criteria, and content.

Generalization will be affected by the content selected and by the manner and sequence of formal training. As mentioned in this section, content or training items should come from the child's natural environment. It does little good to train requesting of cookies if the child is unable to have refined sugar or, on a larger scale, to train requesting if the child has little opportunity to use this behavior. The speech-language pathologist must analyze the child's communication environment to determine if there are natural opportunities for the behavior to occur.

The reinforcement should also reflect the child's environment in order to aid generalization. Parents should be trained to respond as naturally as possible. Conversational replies may be best. Consequences, such as "Good talking," occur infrequently in the child's daily interactions and provide little conversational input beyond their reinforcing quality. Conversational responding, such as "Um-hm, that is a horsie, big horsie," is more appropriate and aids generalization to conversation because of its inherent conversational nature.

Child development studies have demonstrated the reinforcing power and teaching potential of expansion, extension, and imitation. Expansion is a more adult model of the child's utterance that maintains the child's word order. If the child says "That bes horsie," the facilitator might respond by expanding to "Um-hm, that is a horsie." In contrast, an extension is a reply to the content or topic of the child's utterance. In the previous example, the facilitator might extend to "Um-hm, Uncle Ed has a horse." Finally, imitation is a whole or partial repetition of the child's utterance. In response to "That bes horsie," the facilitator might repeat "That bes horsie" or simply say "Horsie." All three provide feedback on acceptability of the child's utterance within a conversational context.

CHILD TRAINING

As in assessment, training should focus on both the child's communication system and presymbolic or early symbolic skills. The communication system is expanded and moved ever closer to symbolic communication while the child is learning presymbolic cognitive, social, and communicative skills.

Establishing and Expanding the Communication System

Many training programs begin with the punishment of self-injurious and self-stimulatory behaviors. As noted previously, facilitators should be careful to note the signal value to the child of these excess behaviors before beginning intervention. Self-injurious, tantruming, and aggressive behavior may signal either frustration and a desire to escape or a call for attention (Carr & Durand, 1985). Although excess behavior cannot be allowed to continue to the child's detriment, punishment should be paired with reinforcement of less destructive, more socially acceptable communication behaviors. To the degree that such behavior signals escape or attention getting, the frequency should decrease with the learning of more socially acceptable methods of signaling this information (Carr, 1979; Carr & Durand, 1985; Carr & Lovaas, 1982; Donnellan et al., 1984; Durand, 1982; Durand & Kishi, 1986; Horner & Budd, 1983, 1985; Meyer & Evans, 1986).

Self-stimulatory behaviors can be treated differently and used as reinforcers for behaviors that are less likely to occur. The child is allowed to engage in self-stimulatory behavior when the speech-language pathologist elicits a social or communication behavior. This training is an application of the *Premack Principle,* in which a behavior that is highly likely to occur acts as a reinforcer for one less likely to occur.

The child's limited repertoire of behaviors may be expanded through gradual modification or the introduction of more appropriate alternative behaviors to signal intentions. The speech-language pathologist must decide whether to maintain the child's present method of signaling intentions, modify it, or train new signals. In general, such signals may be maintained if they are not part of a perseverative pattern, if their intention is easily discernible, and if they do not call undue attention to the child (Reichle et al., 1988). The speech-language pathologist must find ways to prompt or cue the acceptable communicative behavior prior to the inception of excess behavior in order to decrease and control the excess behavior. It must be stressed that not all excess behavior is socially motivated and, therefore, amenable to reduction with the introduction of functional communication.

Establishment of a communication system might begin with behavior chain interruption strategies, such as the resonance training mentioned in Chapter 11. In resonance training, the facilitator cradles the child and rocks slowly while speaking about the action. This training should not be attempted without consultation with the physical therapist to ensure that handling and positioning are optimal. A large mirror in front of the pair provides feedback on the child's reaction.

Initially, the facilitator is interested primarily in child responses that signal the child's realization that someone has intruded on his or her space. The child may try to help the facilitator to rock by pushing in the direction of the rocking. Although such behavior signals compliance and acceptance, this movement should not serve as a signal when the rocking stops, because it is part of the movement itself (Sternberg, 1984). The pushing is, however, an indication that the child is motivated to signal, and the facilitator physically prompts a signal, such as touching the facilitator's foot or tapping the floor. The prompted signal is followed by continuation of the rocking and the facilitator's talking about the activity. The prompt is faded gradually.

After several sessions in which the child has signaled for the activity to continue, the facilitator changes the criterion and will not begin rocking initially until the child signals. The facilitator and child assume the rocking posture but do nothing until the child signals. At first, this signal will probably need to be prompted. More important than the signal is the lesson that through communication the child can affect the environment. As the facilitator moves from a cradling position to a side-by-side or facing one, she is in a better position to attempt such training as physical imitation, an important presymbolic skill.

The facilitator can attempt similar training with any behavior pleasurable to the child, such as listening to music. The behavior is interrupted and a signal prompted for it to resume. Once the signal is used consistently, training moves to initiation, as mentioned previously.

Close physical proximity, touching, and a gentle, pleasant manner and voice may also help establish an initial communication system. The child may respond with any of the means already mentioned. With one child, a primitive communication system using eye contact with a spoon to signal ''Feed me'' was established in a few hours. If the child does not respond well to touching or to close proximity, initial assessment and training may have to focus on toleration and desensitization, which are usually accomplished by pairing touching with a pleasurable or reinforcing stimulus.

The speech-language pathologist can also expand the communication system to include environmental *signs*, or signals and gestures, such as having the child reach for, touch, or look at common objects prior to beginning everyday activities in which they will be used. For example, she might require the child to look at or touch a toothbrush before brushing. The toothbrush becomes a sign for brushing and can later signal that activity. Initially, to avoid confusion, the toothbrush used to signal may be the one actually used for brushing, but later brushes should be separate to preserve the signal quality of the nonused one. The object becomes a sign for the event.

Sternberg (1984) recommends the use of *anticipation shelves* in which each daily activity is represented by related objects arranged sequentially in boxes on a shelf. At the beginning of each activity, the child removes the sign from its box. When the activity is completed, the child places the object sign into a ''done'' box. Gradually, the sign and the event become associated. At the next level of training, the child uses the sign to initiate the event. Even at the environmental sign level, success requires at least sensorimotor stage III functioning by the child (Sternberg, 1984). The child is using a primitive augmentative system based on these environmental signs.

The speech-language pathologist must be careful at this point in training to ensure that the child engages in communication interaction with the environmental signs, not just in associational tasks. The objects should also be used to request, protest, and signal notice (Rowland & Schweigert, 1989b).

Natural settings contain naturally arising stimuli, such as materials, partners, and physical surroundings, that influence communication (Halle, 1987). Generalization is best when these stimuli are included in the training.

The speech-language pathologist may also use contrived instructional settings effectively, especially if there is concurrent instruction in the natural environment (Glennen & Calculator, 1985; Nietupski, Hamre-Nietupski, Clancy, & Veerhusen, 1986). For best generalization, the simulated environment should be varied to reflect the natural environment, and instruction in the simulated and natural environments should occur as close as possible in time (Nietupski et al., 1986).

Consistent routines and expected daily schedules within the natural environment enhance communication by providing redundancy that cues interactions (vanDijk, 1985). Behaviors associated with each activity become signals for that activity and natural environmental cues for communication (Snell & Zirpoli, 1987).

As noted elsewhere in this chapter, this environment must be an interactive one. This interaction may involve encouraging turn taking, recognizing and responding to the child's communication, and creating opportunities for the child to communicate (Cirrin & Rowland, 1985; Vicker, 1985). For many presymbolic children, the need to communicate has been eliminated (MacDonald, 1985). Children need to have choices that influence their environment in order to increase their communication skills and independence (Glennen & Calculator, 1985; Guess, Benson, & Siegel-Causey, 1985; Klein et al., 1981; Shevin & Klein, 1984).

Role of augmentative communication. Augmentative communication systems can serve as initial methods of communication, in addition to augmenting speech or becoming the primary mode of symbolic communication. The use of augmentative systems can improve speech intelligibility, increase communication initiations, and improve overall communication skills (Calculator & D'Altilio-Luchko, 1983; Glennen & Calculator, 1985; Hurlbut, Iwata, & Green, 1982; Kouri, 1989; Kraat, 1985; Pecyna, 1984, 1988; Reichle & Karlan, 1985; Romski, Sevcik, & Joyner, 1984; Romski, White, Millen, & Rumbaugh, 1984).

The ease in learning augmentative communication systems depends on the child's overall developmental and communication level, the system chosen, and the training method (Mirenda & Locke, 1989; Mizuko, 1987; Pecyna, 1984). Although the exact level of development necessary for a truly functional communication system is unknown, this factor should not be ignored even for low level gestural systems.

Symbol transparency or "guessability" is one consideration in system selection and training. In general, there is a positive correlation between the resemblance of representations or symbols to the real object and transparency (Clark, 1981; Ecklund & Reichle, 1987; Hurlbut, Iwata, & Green, 1982; Mirenda & Locke, 1989; Mizuko, 1987; Sevcik & Romski, 1986; Vanderheiden & Lloyd, 1986). Pictures or manual signs that resemble their referents are more transparent and easier to learn. Figure 12.1 lists the order of visual augmentative systems by transparency. Readers should note the location of miniature objects in this figure. Presymbolic children may not see miniatures as representing real objects (Vanderheiden & Lloyd, 1986). In addition, it should be noted that judgments of transparency by nonimpaired children do not necessarily reflect the perceptions of presymbolic language-impaired children (Dunham, 1989).

Other determiners of the ease of manual sign learning are symmetry, inclusion of a portion of the body, and concreteness. In general, signs are easier to

FIGURE 12.1
Transparency of visual augmentative communication systems

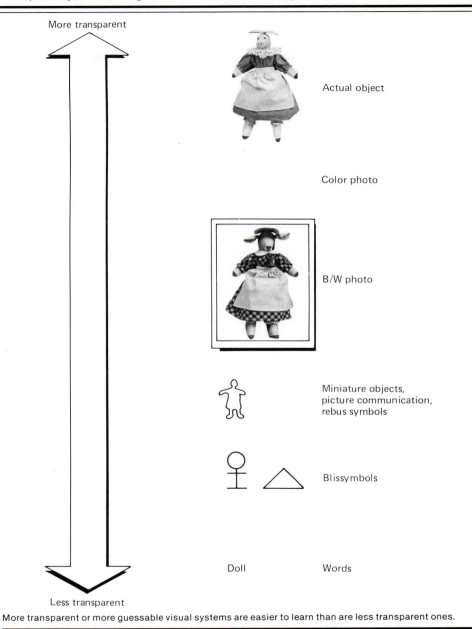

More transparent

Actual object

Color photo

B/W photo

Miniature objects,
picture communication,
rebus symbols

Blissymbols

Doll   Words

Less transparent

More transparent or more guessable visual systems are easier to learn than are less transparent ones.

Source: Adapted from Mirenda, P., and Locke, P. (1989). A comparison of symbol transparency in nonspeaking persons with intellectual disabilities. *Journal of Speech and Hearing Disorders, 54*, 131–140.

learn if both hands move symmetrically and the body is touched in some way, and if the signs are concrete rather than abstract (Kohl, 1981).

Often, the concept that symbols have a function is the most difficult aspect of training for presymbolic children (Romski, Sevcik, & Pate, 1988). Children must learn that they can effect change through symbol use. The speech-language pathologist can encourage the child to select from among desired items to gain some control of his or her world. Initially the child selects the one item presented. Foils, such as an uninteresting item or a blank picture, are then introduced. Two-item choices are trained next. The facilitator can use a modified vending machine device using light, sound, and symbol cues to train children to choose from among several desired items (Romski et al., 1988). In similar fashion, a child might use eye contact with a television or stereo to signal a request for TV or music, respectively.

Once communication is established with other people, the maintenance of that interaction can be attributed to the reciprocity inherent in communication (Kohler & Fowler, 1985). In other words, the reciprocal nature of communication is reinforcing for both partners.

Individuals with more severe or multiple disabilities may have difficulty moving from gestural communication to abstract symbols. These children have difficulty with the one-to-one relational concept of symbol-to-referent. This learning is made more difficult by the simultaneous shift from context-bound gestural systems to more context-free symbols. "Tangible symbols" (Rowland & Schweigert, 1989a), or representations in the form of objects or pictures with a clear perceptual relationship to the referent, can form a link between gestural and symbolic systems of communication. Actual objects or identifiable packaging might be used. Between the actual object and color photo levels of transparency on Figure 12.1, the following three levels of representation might exist (Rowland & Schweigert, 1989a):

1. Associated objects, such as a shoelace to represent a shoe.
2. Shared feature objects, such as a cookie refrigerator magnet to represent a real cookie.
3. Artificial associations in which an object appears on the communication board and is also attached to the referent, such as a wooden apple on the cafeteria door to represent meals.

As with other aspects of communication training, there is often a lack of generalization of augmentative system use. This problem may result from (a) facilitator-centered or -controlled training, (b) unintelligibility of the child's system as used, (c) the precedence within training of the system over the communication process, (d) nonuse of natural settings, and (e) nonusers' lack of response in the natural environment (Calculator, 1988b).

As in verbal symbolic training, the means of transmission and/or the code is often taught separately from the communication function of the symbols. The goal of training becomes learning the system rather than optimizing communication. This is obvious when a nonspeaking child is required to rely on an augmentative response, such as signing *no* when a head shake would suffice. Instead, intervention should focus on encouraging flexible use of various modes of communication (Downing & Siegel-Causey, 1988).

Targets should be functional, such as requesting aid or objects from other people, rejecting or protesting, and commenting (Brown et al., 1984; Reichle, 1990; Reichle, Rogers, & Barrett, 1984). Thus, the child learns to control acquisition and refusal of specific entities within the environment. In general, requesting is easier to train than are the other functions (Reichle et al., 1988). The child might touch desired items to signal a request (Klein et al., 1981). Both preferred and nonpreferred items should be offered so that the child must make an active choice. Otherwise, the signal becomes a general request rather than a discriminating one (Reichle, 1990). Once a choice is made, the facilitator can probe the child's choice by offering two items, the requested one and another. The speech-language pathologist can expand requesting behaviors with the use of a generalized request signal, such as *want* or *more*. She can place the printed symbol for *want* or *more* before the child as he or she reaches for desired items. The child touches the signal in the process of reaching for the item.

The child might signal protest or rejection by pushing away unwanted objects (Stremel-Campbell et al., 1984). An instructional prompt to touch a rejection or protest signal can be delivered prior to offering items that are predictably refused (Reichle, 1990). The child might also be taught to use a general rejection signal (*no*) in several different situations (Keogh & Reichle, 1985). The comment function can be taught using object names or labels (Koegh & Reichle, 1985). Initially, commenting serves a notice function that directs the attention of others and may be signaled by a generalized ''look'' or ''notice me'' signal. For ease of learning, separate lexical items should be used for different functions.

Targets should enhance the child's functioning in multiple environments frequently throughout the day, be age appropriate, and be valued by both the child and the caregivers (Brown et al., 1988). General signals for *want* or *more* have broad application and will occur frequently (Stremel-Campbell et al., 1984; Reichle, 1990). These facts enhance generalization to the transfer environment. More explicit symbols, such as ''hamburger,'' place less burden for interpretation on the listener but have narrower application than do general signals. At a symbolic level, these general illocutionary signals can be paired with object and event names to form longer utterances.

Because generalization from simulated environments to the transfer or natural environment is difficult for many presymbolic clients, augmentative communication systems should be trained within a wide variety of functional activities as these naturally occur in the transfer environment (Calculator, 1988b; Falvey et al., 1988; Guess & Helmstetter, 1986; Kangas & Lloyd, 1988; Light, Collier, & Parnes, 1985; Orelove & Sobsey, 1987, Siegel-Causey & Downing, 1987). Training, even with augmentative systems, too often consists of unnatural, out-of-context, mass-trial formats (Helmstetter & Guess, 1987).

The spontaneous use of augmentative systems can be a problem for both the user and the communication partner or nonuser. Compared to speakers, augmentative users have fewer conversational partners and engage in shorter exchanges (Kraat, 1985). Although augmentative systems can improve the quality of the communication, at present there is still considerable delay with most users as they produce their responses. Production time can be decreased by the placement of items on a communication board, by the vocabulary selected, by careful analysis of the child-device interface, and by multimodality responding.

In general, the nonuser partner assumes a disproportionate responsibility for the conversation (Buzolich & Wiemann, 1988; Farrier, Yorkston, Marriner, & Beukelman, 1985). With little expectation that the user will participate, nonusers may talk around the user, fall into a yes-no probing strategy, answer their own questions or comment before the user can answer, use less mature language, and anticipate a response and preempt (Calculator & Dollaghen, 1982; Goosens & Kraat, 1985; Shane et al., 1982). These modifications cause the user to lose control of the conversation. In turn, children may underfunction or behave as if they are much more limited.

This underfunctioning is reported frequently for augmentative communication users (Calculator, 1985; Houghton et al., 1987). It is the result of insufficient motivation to communicate, which may be caused by lack of opportunity or reason to communicate or by a lack of responsiveness by nonusers.

Nonuser partners can change their behavior, but this requires that the speech-language pathologist instruct them in the use of the augmentative system also (Calculator & D'Altilio-Luchko, 1983). Instruction is especially important if the expectations and demands of the environment are dissimilar from those used in teaching the user. The speech-language pathologist can teach even preschool nonuser peers to become good partners and to initiate, turn take, and respond (Goldstein & Ferrell, 1987). She also can effectively and efficiently train and integrate caregivers into the training process through a combination of in-service and direct training and by including them in the assessment and goal-setting process (McNaughton & Light, 1989).

The facilitator should encourage use of the child's augmentative communication system whenever possible throughout the day, using incidental and stimulation techniques. She reinforces both the child and caregivers for augmentative system usage. In general, the more the child and caregivers use the system, the more it will generalize.

Presymbolic Training

Obviously, not every behavior of the nonimpaired child is an appropriate training target. Nor should the speech-language pathologist assume that infant development scales identify the skills that language-impaired children need. These scales often include a variety of activities, many unrelated to symbol use. The speech-language pathologist should select presymbolic targets judiciously. A long list of prerequisites may actually prevent presymbolic children from learning to communicate (Wulz et al., 1983).

Although some presymbolic children may attain initial language skills when trained first on prerequisite cognitive behaviors, such as means-ends and object permanence, rather than on language alone (Kahn, 1982), the precise presymbolic skills to teach have not been identified. Therefore, each speech-language pathologist must consider ''which developmental behaviors and what sequences of mastery'' (Switzy, Rotatori, Miller, & Freagon, 1979, p. 169) by determining her own theoretical position.

McLean and Snyder-McLean (1988) suggest, as Table 12.3 demonstrates, that presymbolic targets be determined by beginning with skills important for nonimpaired children's language development, such as means-ends, turn taking, and gestures, and modifying these targets based on some training rationale. Each possible presymbolic target should be evaluated on the basis of how it will facilitate the development of symbol use for a specific child.

A general hierarchy of presymbolic skill training was presented in Chapter 11. Even within presymbolic training, such communication skills as turn taking and gestures are targeted. Several commercially available programs also provide extensive information (Bricker & Bricker, 1974; Hanna et al., 1982; Horstmeier &

TABLE 12.3
Determining presymbolic training targets

Presymbolic Cognitive and Social Skills	+	Client Communication Needs	=	Training Targets
Object permanence		Semantic knowledge of objects		Functional use of objects. Appearance, disappearance, and reappearance of objects.
Means-ends		Semantic knowledge of objects		Repeat action with pleasurable outcome. Object manipulation. Indirect means, such as pulling string or winding toy. Tool use.
Gestures		Influence others		Generic (basic, constant) behaviors used to signal. Hierarchy from contact to distal signals. Range of signals.
Turn taking		Interact with others		Joint action routines— Ritualized pattern with a specific theme, following a logical sequence in which each participant plays a specific role, with specific response expectations essential to successful completion.

Source: Adapted from McLean, J. and Snyder-McLean, L. (1988, September). Assessment and treatment of communicative competencies among clients with severe/profound developmental disabilities. Workshop presented for Craig Developmental Disabilities Service Office and State University of New York, Geneseo.

MacDonald, 1978b; Manolson, 1983; Owens, 1982c). Although programs differ on particulars, it is generally accepted that the child should be functioning at Piagetian sensorimotor stage late IV or early V when symbols are introduced (Calculator, 1988c; Owens & Rogerson, 1988).

All training is considered in relation to the three strategies of incidental teaching, stimulation, and formal training. The speech-language pathologist and the other language trainers must keep accurate records of the child's performance and continually adjust the training to meet the child's changing abilities and needs.

Training procedures and sequences mentioned are equally applicable whether the child's ultimate form of communication is speech, an augmentative system, or a combination. Recognition and receptive training with augmentative systems can begin at a relatively low level of presymbolic functioning. Presymbolic training is not ignored, however, because augmentative symbol systems require a level of cognitive functioning at least as high as that for verbal symbols.

Symbolic Training
Symbolic training is superimposed on a gestural, gestural-vocal, or augmentative base trained previously. At the symbolic level, the dual nature of training in communication and prerequisite skills becomes one as the child's communication system becomes more symbolic in nature.

Symbols should be taught for referents that are clearly established in the client's meaning system. Attempts to teach referential concepts and symbols simultaneously may confuse the child (Romski & Sevcik, 1989). The child may associate the symbol with the teaching context rather than with the referent.

It is important that symbolic training remain functional and fulfill a broad range of communication intentions. All too often training deteriorates to the child's responding to such cues as ''What's this?'' in the hope that the response will be used spontaneously on some future occasion.

Initially, each lexical item should correspond to a specific pragmatic function. General symbols, such as *want* and *no*, might be used. Specific symbols, such as *juice* or *hot*, may also be trained, but they should be function-specific also. Minimally symbolic children have difficulty generalizing the use of a symbol across several illocutionary functions (Calculator & Delaney, 1986; LaMarre & Holland, 1985).

Whether the child is using an augmentative or a verbal communication mode, the speech-language pathologist should select vocabulary that is ''individualized, functional, and dynamic'' (Yorkston, Honsinger, Dowden, & Marriner, 1989, p. 102). Standardized vocabulary lists do not provide a sufficiently thorough lexicon for the individual child. Such lists, if adopted, are inefficient because they contain many words that are rarely used (Yorkston, Smith, & Beukelman, 1990).

Even lists of the most frequently used words of nondisabled peers may be of little value in vocabulary selection because they include such words as *to, a, it, am,* and *and* (Beukelman, Jones, & Rowan, 1989) that are abstract and difficult to teach, especially at the single-symbol level of communication. Lexicons based on frequency of occurrence by the individual child within different natural communication contexts may yield a small but highly useful list of symbols.

Careful selection of individual symbols requires a study of the child's environment that is sensitive to the child's needs. Symbols such as *please, thank you,* and *toilet* reflect caregiver desires and may have little relevance for the child. Symbols learned but not used by the child are of little value. The lexicon should be "open-ended," capable of modification as the needs of the child change (Carlson, 1981; Blau, 1983).

The speech-language pathologist can use a combination of the gestural intentions already present and verbal and nonverbal cues to vary the child's behavior. For example, symbols are first trained in imitation to cues, such as "Say _____" ("Sign _____," "Point to _____," etc.), when the child demonstrates an interest in or desire for an entity. This verbal cue is accompanied by a nod that signals the child to respond. The trainer may also prompt by beginning the response for the child.

The verbal cue "Say" ("Sign," "Point to") can be gradually faded and the response shifted to the visual nodding cue. The child will now respond with the name after the trainer names the object and nods. Gradually, the verbal model is also faded. Because the child will name in response to a nod, he or she can be cued in other ways to get a range of illocutionary and semantic functions. It is possible to train a variety of functions for each symbol, thus increasing the child's repertoire.

Initially, the speech-language pathologist should require both gestures and verbalizations of the child because there is often a lack of correspondence between the two with young learners (Baer, Williams, Osnes, & Stokes, 1984; Guevremont, Osnes, & Stokes, 1986a, 1986b). Unless the child chains the verbal and nonverbal behaviors, correspondence between the two may not occur. Through training that uses two items, one desirable and one not, the child can learn to make specific requests for the desirable one (Piche-Cragoe, Reichle, & Sigafoos, 1986).

The trainer modifies intonation and gestures that accompany a single symbol to model a variety of functions. For example, "cup" said while pushing it away might indicate a semantic function of negation and an illocutionary function of protest or command. Such a behavior might be termed a *negative command.* The trainer might cue questioning by saying "Guess what's behind my back" and prompting questions. Responses would fulfill a *nominative question* function.

Speech-language pathologists should also target a variety of semantic functions. Routinely they train agent and object symbols while giving less attention to other categories, such as action (Chapman & Terrell, 1988). Initially, children use action-related symbols called *protoverbs.* These verb-like symbols, which accompany specific actions the children perform, include *up, down, no, on-here, inside, there, get-down, bye-bye, night-night,* and *out* (Barrett, 1983; Benedict, 1979; Clark, 1979). Gradually, each symbol acquires broader meaning and becomes decontextualized.

COMMUNICATION ENVIRONMENT MANIPULATION

The speech-language pathologist can modify the child's communication environment in several ways to enhance communication and training. After a thorough analysis of the communication demands placed on the child, she identifies high and low communication contexts by location, activities, and communication partners.

High communication contexts are encouraged and increased. Modifications would change the interactional quality between the child and the environment. For example, the child's daily routine might be changed to provide more opportunity to interact with a certain classroom aide with whom the child vocalizes frequently. These high communication contexts often offer ideal opportunities for incidental teaching. For example, the aide mentioned might be trained to elicit a variety of vocalizations from the child within their daily routine. Because the child is communicating at a high level, presumably because the context is reinforcing, the speech-language pathologist can change the manner of that communication and modify the context to enhance communication training while leaving the interaction intact.

The facilitator modifies or eliminates low communication contexts. For example, the child's communication behavior may elicit no response from the school bus aide. The facilitator might instruct this person in a few simple methods of conversational responding to increase the communication learning potential of this situation. If the child spends long periods each day in solitary play, these times might be eliminated or changed to parallel or group play.

INTERACTIONAL CHANGES

As noted in the previous section, caregivers can become effective agents of change for presymbolic and minimally symbolic individuals if trained and monitored appropriately (Baker, 1976; Heifetz, 1980; Owens et al., 1987; Salzberg & Villani, 1983). Even minimum instruction is beneficial and enables some caregivers to adopt suitable teaching strategies spontaneously (Cheseldine & McConkey, 1979). Feedback from the speech-language pathologist regarding the application of newly acquired teaching skills, however, is the critical element (Polk, Schilmoeller, Emboy, Holman, & Baer, 1976; Salzberg & Villani, 1983). Caregivers cannot be expected to function in a vacuum with little input from the speech-language pathologist.

The speech-language pathologist can train caregivers to perform formal training, elicit trained responses, and provide appropriate language input for the child. Training caregivers to provide structured formal training has been very successful (MacDonald et al., 1974; Salzberg & Villani, 1983).

The caregiver can also elicit trained responses within the home or classroom through environmental manipulation (McNaughton & Light, 1989; Wulz et al., 1983). After the child is taught to respond to *need to communicate* situations, the caregiver restructures needs-meeting situations within daily routines so that the child's needs are not anticipated but are dependent on the communication behavior. Child-caregiver interactions may also be formally restructured to encourage and to require communication (Horstmeier & MacDonald, 1978a). The caregivers can structure elicitation situations, such as turn-taking games, choice-making, enticement with desirable items, and assistance requesting (McNaughton & Light, 1989). Once a skill is learned, the child is required to use that skill to attain desired entities or privileges for which it was not formerly required. Previously accepted behaviors are no longer sufficient.

A strategy of waiting or time delay has also been used effectively to enhance spontaneous use of trained communication behaviors (Charhop, Schreibman, & Thebodeau, 1985; Gobbi, Cipani, Hudson, & Lapenta-Neudeck, 1986). This procedure is most effective when the child desires some item or has to communicate to complete a task. The presence of a language trainer may also act as a nonlinguistic cue to stimulate production (Carr & Kologinsky, 1983).

Children may omit the initial step of obtaining their partner's attention when necessary. The two-step procedure of attention getting and message transmission is difficult to teach (Sobsey & Reichle, 1986). Children assume that other people will always attend when they communicate if this is the training situation. It may be difficult for the child to discriminate between situations that require attention getting and those that do not.

Other effective strategies for child initiation are introduction of novel elements, oversight, and sabotage (McLean & Snyder-McLean, 1988). Novel items usually spark a notice or referential response. Oversight is simply forgetting to complete some task or add a crucial step, such as intentionally leaving the peanut butter out of a peanut butter sandwich. Finally, sabotage is the introduction of challenging actions or events that prevent some activity, such as tying shoes together prior to giving them to the child to put on. The goal is for the child to request assistance.

Finally, the stimulation behaviors discussed previously can be a helpful guide for caregiver interactional behaviors. The following are additional conversational suggestions (MacDonald and Gillette, 1986):

- ☐ Structure the activity for give and take.
- ☐ Follow the child's lead.
- ☐ Imitate the child.
- ☐ WAIT for the child to take a turn.
- ☐ SIGNAL the child to take a turn.
- ☐ Chain responses by using turnabouts, in which a turn includes both a response to the child's turn as well as a cue for the child to take another turn.

MacDonald and Gillette's ECOmaps offer further guidance.

Summary

Communication training should be ongoing for presymbolic and minimally symbolic children. Caregivers should administer training under the speech-language pathologist's direction. Within each child's natural communication environment, caregivers use simultaneously the three intervention techniques of incidental teaching, stimulation, and formal training. An effective program must target the child's behavior, environmental factors, and the child-caregiver interaction.

CONCLUSION

Presymbolic and minimally symbolic children have special needs that often relate to the very purposes for communication. If these children are going to communicate, there must be a reason for doing so. In addition, the environment must provide models and respond to the child appropriately. Initial communication training cannot be an isolated affair; by its nature, communication is central to all human interactions. Communication will not generalize to the use environment unless that environment becomes a facilitative one for such behavior. Only an integrated functional intervention that targets both the child and the environment can hope to change effectively the child's current behavior.

Appendixes

A
Language Test Content

TABLE A.1

Tests	Possessives	Plural (reg.)	Plural (irreg.)	Derivational Suffix	Present	Present Participle	Present Progressive	Past (reg.)	Past (irreg.)	Future	Present Perfect	Past Perfect	Past Progressive	Present Perfect Prog.	Passive	Modals	Copula	Auxiliary Verbs	Third Per. Sing. (reg.)	Third Per. Sing. (irreg.)	Infinitives/Gerunds	Subject Pronouns	Object Pronouns	Possessive: Nom./Deter.	Indefinite Pronouns	Reflexive Pronouns	Adjectives	Demonstratives	Articles	Comparatives	Superlatives	Adverbs	Prepositions	Wh-Questions	Yes/No Questions	Embedding	Coordinated/Conjunction	Negatives	"Do" Insertions	Response to Commands	Quantity	Body Parts	Common Nouns	Color	Categorization	Miscellaneous
ACLC		X				X																					X						X										X			
Bankson		X	X		X	X	X			X	X								X	X		X	X	X			X			X	X		X					X		X	X	X	X	X	X	X
Berko	X	X		X			X	X	X										X								X			X	X															X
CELI	X	X	X	X	X		X	X	X	X	X	X		X	X	X	X	X	X	X	X	X	X	X	X	X	X	X	X	X	X	X	X		X	X	X	X	X				X	X		
ITPA	X	X	X				X	X	X						X											X	X			X			X										X			
Miller-Yoder	X		X		X		X	X			X				X			X	X			X	X				X	X					X											X		
NSST	X	X			X		X	X		X					X		X	X	X			X	X	X		X							X	X	X			X					X			
OLSIDI	X				X		X	X	X	X						X	X	X	X	X	X	X	X	X		X			X				X	X	X	X	X	X	X							
OLSIST	X				X		X	X	X	X						X	X	X	X	X	X	X	X	X		X			X				X	X	X	X	X	X	X							
PLST					X																																									
SICD		X	X	X	X	X	X	X	X	X	X						X	X	X			X	X	X			X			X	X	X	X	X	X	X	X	X		X	X			X		X
TACL		X		X	X	X	X	X	X	X	X			X	X	X	X	X	X	X	X	X	X	X			X	X		X	X	X	X	X	X	X			X	X	X	X		X		
TSA				X						X							X	X	X			X	X	X		X	X		X					X	X	X	X			X		X	X		
TSA-Screening															X				X			X				X			X					X		X	X	X								
Sampling Tools: Assign. Struc. Stage	X	X			X		X	X	X	X	X	X	X			X	X	X	X			X		X		*	X	X	X				X	X	X	*	*	X	X							*
DSS					X	X	X	X	X	X	X	X	X	X	X	X	X	X	X		X	X	X	X	X	X	X	X						X	X	X	X	X	X							
DST	X	X			X	X	X															X	X				X	X	X			X	X				X	X	X		X		X			
LSAT	X	X			X			X				X	X			X	X	X	X		X	X					X	X	X			X	X	X	X	X	X	X					X			

*Miller's Complex Sentence Development rating format.

Source: Language Test Content: A Comparative Study by R. Owens, M. Haney, V. Giesow, L. Dooley, and R. Kelly, 1983, *Language, Speech and Hearing Services in Schools*, 14, 7–21. Reprinted with permission.

B
Dialectal and Bilingual Considerations

Most regional and ethnic dialects differ only slightly from the standard or are used by a limited number of individuals. Three ethnic dialects, however, represent rather large segments of the U.S. population and have some very important differences with Standard American English. These dialects are Black English, Hispanic English, and Asian English. Black English is used primarily by working class Blacks in the northern U.S. and rural Blacks in the south. Not every African-American uses Black English and not everyone who uses it is an African-American.

Hispanic English and Asian English are probably misnomers. Hispanic English, as used here, is a composite of the English used by many bilingual speakers who learned English as a second language. Individual variations represent the age of learning and level of mastery, the Spanish dialect used, socioeconomic status, and where the person lives in the United States. Asian English is also a composite, but of bilingual Asian speakers who learned English as a second language. As such, Asian English probably does not exist except to simplify our discussion. Asians speak many different languages, and each has a different effect on the learning of English. In addition to the original language learned, other individual differences may reflect factors the same as those of Hispanic English.

Each dialect is discussed in some detail. Where possible, information has been reduced to tables to aid presentation. Each dialect is compared with Standard American English, an idealized norm uninfluenced by the dialectal differences each person possesses.

Black English

Black English reflects the complex racial and economic history of the United States and the migration of African-Americans from the rural south to the urban north after World War II. Regional differences exist to some degree. The major variations between Standard American English and Black English in phonology, syntax, and morphology and in pragmatics and nonlinguistic features are presented in Tables B.1, B.2, and B.3.

TABLE B.1
Phonemic contrasts between Black English and Standard American English

SAE Phonemes	Position in Word		
	Initial	Medial	Final*
/p/		Unaspirated /p/	Unaspirated /p/
/n/			Reliance on preceding nasalized vowel
/w/	Omitted in specific words (*I 'as, too!*)		
/b/		Unreleased /b/	Unreleased /b/
/g/		Unreleased /g/	Unreleased /g/
/k/		Unaspirated /k/	Unaspirated /k/
/d/	Omitted in specific words (*I 'on't know*)	Unreleased /d/	Unreleased /d/
/ŋ/		/n/	/n/
/t/		Unaspirated /t/	Unaspirated /t/
/l/		Omitted before labial consonants (*help–hep*)	"uh" following a vowel (*Bill–Biuh*)
/r/		Omitted or /ə/	Omitted or prolonged vowel or glide
/θ/	Unaspirated /t/ or /f/	Unaspirated /t/ or /f/ between vowels	Unaspirated /t/ or /f/ (*bath–baf*)
/v/	Sometimes /b/	/b/ before /m/ and /n/	Sometimes /b/
/ð/	/d/	/d/ or /v/ between vowels	/d/, /v/, /f/
/z/		Omitted or replaced by /d/ before nasal sound (*wasn't–wud'n*)	

Blends
/str/ becomes /skr/
/ʃr/ becomes /str/
/θr/ becomes /θ/
/pr/ becomes /p/
/br/ becomes /b/
/kr/ becomes /k/
/gr/ becomes /g/

Final Consonant Clusters (second consonant omitted when these clusters occur at the end of a word)

/sk/	/nd/	/sp/
/ft/	/ld/	/dʒ d/
/st/	/sd/	/nt/

* Note weakening of final consonants.
Sources: Data drawn from Fasold and Wolfram (1970); Labov (1972); F. Weiner and Lewnau (1979); R. Williams and Wolfram (1977).

TABLE B.2
Grammatical contrasts between Black English and Standard American English

Black English Grammatical Structure	SAE Grammatical Structure
Possessive -'s	
Nonobligatory where word position expresses possession.	Obligatory regardless of position.
Get *mother* coat.	Get mother*'s* coat.
It be mother*'s.*	It's mother*'s.*
Plural -s	
Nonobligatory with numerical quantifier.	Obligatory regardless of numerical quantifier.
He got ten *dollar.*	He has ten dollar*s.*
Look at the cat*s.*	Look at the cat*s.*
Regular past -ed	
Nonobligatory; reduced as consonant cluster.	Obligatory.
Yesterday, I *walk* to school.	Yesterday, I walk*ed* to school.
Irregular past	
Case by case, some verbs inflected, others not.	All irregular verbs inflected.
I *see* him last week.	I *saw* him last week.
Regular present tense third person singular -s	
Nonobligatory.	Obligatory.
She *eat* too much.	She eat*s* too much.
Irregular present tense third person singular -s	
Nonobligatory.	Obligatory.
He *do* my job.	He *does* my job.
Indefinite an	
Use of indefinite *a.*	Use of *an* before nouns beginning with a vowel.
He ride in *a* airplane.	He rode in *an* airplane.
Pronouns	
Pronominal apposition: pronoun immediately follows noun.	Pronoun used elsewhere in sentence or in other sentence; not in apposition.
Momma *she* mad. She . . .	Momma is mad. *She* . . .

(continued)

TABLE B.2 *(continued)*

Black English Grammatical Structure	SAE Grammatical Structure
Future tense	
More frequent use of *be going to* (gonna).	More frequent use of *will*.
I *be going to* dance tonight.	I *will* dance tonight.
I *gonna* dance tonight.	I *am going to* dance tonight.
Omit *will* preceding *be*.	Obligatory use of *will*.
I *be* home later.	I *will* (I'll) *be* home later.
Negation	
Triple negative.	Absence of triple negative.
Nobody don't never like me.	*No* one ever likes me.
Use of *ain't*.	*Ain't* is unacceptable form.
I *ain't* going.	I*'m not* going.
Modals	
Double modals for such forms as might, *could,* and *should.*	Single modal use.
I *might could* go.	I *might be able to* go.
Questions	
Same form for direct and indirect.	Different forms for direct and indirect.
What *it is*?	What *is it*?
Do you know what *it is*?	Do you know what *it is*?
Relative pronouns	
Nonobligatory in most cases.	Nonobligatory with *that* only.
He the one stole it.	He's the one *who* stole it.
It the one you like.	It's the one (that) you like.
Conditional *if*	
Use of *do* for conditional *if*.	Use of *if*.
I ask *did* she go.	I asked *if* she went.
Perfect construction	
Been used for action in the distant past.	*Been* not used.
He *been* gone.	He left a long time ago.
Copula	
Nonobligatory when contractible.	Obligatory in contractible and uncontractible forms.
He sick.	He's sick.
Habitual or general state	
Marked with uninflected *be*.	Nonuse of *be*; verb inflected.
She *be* workin'.	She*'s working* now.

Sources: Data drawn from Baratz (1969), Fasold and Wolfram (1970), Williams and Wolfram (1977).

TABLE B.3

Pragmatic and nonlinguistic contrasts between Black English
and Standard American English

Black English	Standard American English
Touching of one's hair by another person is often considered offensive.	Touching of one's hair by another person is a sign of affection.
Preference for indirect eye contact during listening, direct eye contact during speaking as signs of attentiveness and respect.	Preference for direct eye contact during listening and indirect eye contact during speaking as signs of attention and respect.
Public behavior may be emotionally intense, dynamic, and demonstrative.	Public behavior is expected to be modest and emotionally restrained. Emotional displays are seen as irresponsible or in bad taste.
Clear distinction between ''argument'' and ''fight.'' Verbal abuse is not necessarily a precursor to violence.	Heated arguments are viewed as suggesting that violence is imminent.
Asking ''personal questions'' of someone one has met for the first time is seen as improper and intrusive.	Inquiring about jobs, family, and so forth of someone one has met for the first time is seen as friendly.
Use of direct questions is sometimes seen as harassment, e.g., asking when something will be finished is seen as rushing that person to finish.	Use of direct questions for personal information is permissible.
Interruption during conversation is usually tolerated. Access to the floor is granted to the person who is most assertive.	Rules of turn-taking in conversation dictate that one person has the floor at a time until all his points are made.
Conversations are regarded as private between the recognized participants. ''Butting in'' is seen as eavesdropping and is not tolerated.	Adding points of information or insights to a conversation in which one is not engaged is seen as being helpful.
Use of expression ''you people'' is seen as pejorative and racist.	Use of expression ''you people'' tolerated.
Accusations or allegations are general rather than categorical, and are not intended to be all-inclusive. Refutation is the responsibility of the accused.	Stereotypical accusations or allegations are all-inclusive. Refutation or making exception is the responsibility of the person making the accusation.
Silence denotes refutation of accusation. To state that you feel accused is regarded as an admission of guilt.	Silence denotes acceptance of an accusation. Guilt is verbally denied.

Source: Taylor, O. (in press). Clinical practice as a social occasion. In L. Cole & V. Deal (Eds.), *Communication disorders in multicultural populations.* Rockville, MD: American Speech-Language-Hearing Association. Reprinted with permission.

English

...eakers may move back and forth between both languages in a process called ...g. The amount of code switching depends on the speaker's mastery of the two ...nd on the audience being addressed. Naturally, a large amount of code switch-...he speaker's English incomprehensible to the monolingual American English

TABLE B.4
Phonemic contrasts between Hispanic English and Standard American English

SAE Phonemes	Position in Word		
	Initial	Medial	Final*
/p/	Unaspirated /p/		Omitted or weakened
/m/			Omitted
/w/	/hu/		Omitted
/b/			Omitted, distorted, or /p/
/g/			Omitted, distorted, or /k/
/k/	Unaspirated or /g/		Omitted, distorted, or /g/
/f/			Omitted
/d/		Dentalized	Omitted, distorted, or /t/
/ŋ/	/n/	/d/	/n/ (*sing–sin*)
/j/	/dʒ/		
/t/			Omitted
/ʃ/	/tʃ/	/s/, /tʃ/	/tʃ/ (*wish–which*)
/tʃ/	/ʃ/ (*chair–share*)	/ʃ/	/ʃ/ (*watch–wash*)
/r/	Distorted	Distorted	Distorted
/dʒ/	/d/	/j/	/ʃ/
/θ/	/t/, /s/ (*thin–tin, sin*)	Omitted	/ʃ/, /t/, /s/
/v/	/b/ (*vat–bat*)	/b/	Distorted
/z/	/s/ (*zip–sip*)	/s/ (*razor–racer*)	/s/
/ð/	/d/ (*then–den*)	/d/, /θ/, /v/ (*lather–ladder*)	/d/

Blends
/skw/ becomes /eskw/*
/sl/ becomes /esl/*
/st/ becomes /est/*

Vowels
/I/ becomes /i/ (*bit–beet*)

* Separates cluster into two syllables.
Sources: Data drawn from Sawyer (1973); F. Weiner and Lewnau (1979); F. Williams, Cairns, and Cairns (1971).

TABLE B.5
Grammatical contrasts between Hispanic English and Standard American English

Hispanic English Grammatical Structure	SAE Grammatical Structure
Possessive -'s	
Use postnoun modifier.	Postnoun modifier used only rarely.
This is the homework *of my brother*.	This is my brother*'s* homework.
Article used with body parts.	Possessive pronoun used with body parts.
I cut *the* finger.	I cut *my* finger.
Plural -s	
Nonobligatory.	Obligatory, excluding exceptions.
The *girl* are playing.	The *girls* are playing.
The *sheep* are playing.	The *sheep* are playing.
Regular past -ed	
Nonobligatory, especially when understood.	Obligatory.
I *talk* to her yesterday.	I *talked* to her yesterday.
Regular third person singular present tense -s	
Nonobligatory.	Obligatory.
She *eat* too much.	She *eats* too much.
Articles	
Often omitted.	Usually obligatory.
I am going to store.	I am going to *the* store.
I am going to school.	I am going to school.
Subject pronouns	
Omitted when subject has been identified in the previous sentence.	Obligatory.
Father is happy. Bought a new car.	Father is happy. *He* bought a new car.
Future tense	
Use *go + to.*	Use *be + going to.*
I *go to* dance.	I *am going to* the dance.
Negation	
Use *no* before the verb.	Use *not* (preceded by auxiliary verb where appropriate).
She *no* eat candy.	She does *not* eat candy.
Question	
Intonation; no noun-verb inversion.	Noun-verb inversion usually.
Maria is going?	*Is Maria* going?
Copula	
Occasional use of *have.*	Use of *be.*
I *have* ten years.	I *am* ten years old.
Negative imperatives	
No used for *don't.*	*Don't* used.
No throw stones.	*Don't* throw stones.
***Do* insertion**	
Nonobligatory in questions.	Obligatory when no auxiliary verb.
You like ice cream?	*Do* you like ice cream?
Comparatives	
More frequent use of longer form (more).	More frequent use of shorter *-er.*
He is *more* tall.	He is tall*er*.

Sources: Data drawn from Davis (1972), Taylor (1986).

TABLE B.6
Pragmatic and nonlinguistic contrasts between Hispanic English
and Standard American English

Hispanic English	Standard American English
• Hissing to gain attention is acceptable.	• Hissing is considered impolite and indicates contempt.
• Touching is often observed between two people in conversation.	• Touching is usually unacceptable and usually carries sexual overtone.
• Avoidance of direct eye contact is sometimes a sign of attentiveness and respect; sustained direct eye contact may be interpreted as a challenge to authority.	• Direct eye contact is a sign of attentiveness and respect.
• Relative distance between two speakers in conversation is close.	• Relative distance between two speakers in conversation is farther apart.
• Official or business conversations are preceded by lengthy greetings, pleasantries, and other talk unrelated to the point of business.	• Getting to the point quickly is valued.

Source: Taylor, O. (in press). Clinical practice as a social occasion. In L. Cole & V. Deal (Eds.), *Communication disorders in multicultural populations.* Rockville, MD: American Speech-Language-Hearing Association. Reprinted with permission.

Most characteristics of Hispanic English reflect interference points or points where the two languages differ, thus making learning somewhat more difficult. For example, the Hispanic English speaker may continue to use the Spanish possessive form in which the owner is preceded by the entity owned, as in "the dress of Mary." The major variations between Standard American English and Hispanic English in phonology, syntax, and morphology and in pragmatics and nonlinguistic features are presented in Tables B.4, B.5, and B.6.

Asian English

Chinese culture and language have for centuries influenced all other Asian cultures and languages. Other cultures, such as that of the Indian subcontinents, have influenced nearby Asian neighbors. Colonial occupation, especially by the French in Indochina, has also influenced the culture and language of the affected region.

The most widely used languages, Chinese, Filipino, Japanese, Khmer, Korean, Laotian, and Vietnamese, represent only a portion of the languages of the area. Each language contains many dialects and has distinct linguistic features. It is, therefore, impossible to speak of an Asian English dialect. Instead, we shall attempt to describe the major overall differences between Asian English and Standard American English. These major differences in phonology, syntax, and morphology and pragmatics and nonlinguistic features are listed in Tables B.7, B.8, and B.9

TABLE B.7
Phonemic contrasts between Asian English and Standard American English

	Position in Word		
SAE Phonemes	Initial	Medial	Final
/p/	/b/****	/b/****	Omission
/s/	Distortion*	Distortion*	Omission
/z/	/s/**	/s/**	Omission
/t/	Distortion*	Distortion*	Omission
/tʃ/	/ʃ/****	/ʃ/****	Omission
/ʃ/	/s/**	/s/**	Omission
/r/, /l/	Confusion***	Confusion***	Omission
/θ/	/s/	/s/	Omission
/dz/	/d/ Or /z/****	/d/ or /z/****	Omission
/v/	/f/***	/f/***	Omission
	/w/**	/w/**	Omission
/ð/	/z/*	/z/*	Omission
	/d/****	/d/****	Omission

Blends
Addition of / / between consonants***
Omission of final consonant clusters****

Vowels
Shortening or lengthening of vowels (seat–sit, it–eat*)
Difficulty with /I/, /ɔ/, and /æ/, and substitution of /e/ for /æ/**
Difficulty with /I/, /æ/, /U/, and /ə/****

* Mandarin dialect of Chinese only
** Cantonese dialect of Chinese only
*** Mandarin, Cantonese, and Japanese
**** Vietnamese only
Source: Adapted from Cheng, L. (June, 1987). Cross-cultural and linguistic considerations in working with Asian populations. *Asha, 29*(6), 33–38.

TABLE B.8
Grammatical contrasts between Asian English and Standard American English

Asian English Grammatical Structure	SAE Grammatical Structure
Plural -s	
Not used with numerical adjective: *three cat*	Used regardless of numerical adjective: *three cats*
Used with irregular plural: *three sheeps*	Not used with irregular plural: *three sheep*
Auxiliaries *to be* and *to do*	
Omission: *I going home. She not want eat.*	Obligatory and inflected in the present progressive form: *I am going home.*
Uninflected: *I is going. She do not want eat.*	*She does not want to eat.*
Verb *have*	
Omission. *You been here.*	Obligatory and inflected: *You have been here. He has one.*
Uninflected. *He have one.*	
Past tense -ed	
Omission: *He talk yesterday.*	Obligatory, nonovergeneralization, and single-marking: *He talked yesterday. I ate yesterday. She didn't eat.*
Overgeneralization: *I eated yesterday.*	
Double-marking: *She didn't ate.*	
Interrogative	
Nonreversal: *You are late?*	Reversal and obligatory auxiliary: *Are you late? Do you like ice cream?*
Omitted auxiliary: *You like ice cream?*	
Perfect marker	
Omission: *I have write letter.*	Obligatory: *I have written a letter.*
Verb-noun agreement	
Nonagreement: *He go to school. You goes to school.*	Agreement: *He goes to school. You go to school.*
Article	
Omission: *Please give gift.*	Obligatory with certain nouns: Please give the gift. She went to school.
Overgeneralization: *She go the school.*	
Preposition	
Misuse: *I am in home.*	Obligatory specific use: *I am at home. He goes by bus.*
Omission: *He go bus.*	
Pronoun	
Subjective/objective confusion: *Him go quickly.*	Subjective/objective distinction *He gave it to her.*
Possessive confusion: *It him book.*	Possessive distinction: *It's his book.*

TABLE B.8 (continued)

Asian English Grammatical Structure	SAE Grammatical Structure
Demonstrative	
Confusion: *I like those horse.*	Singular/plural distinction: *I like that horse.*
Conjunction	
Omission: *You I go together.*	Obligatory use between last two items in a series: *You and I are going together. Mary, John, and Carol went.*
Negation	
Double-marking: *I didn't see nobody.*	Single obligatory marking: *I didn't see anybody. He didn't come.*
Simplified form: *He no come.*	
Word order	
Adjective following noun (Vietnamese): *clothes new.*	Most noun modifiers precede noun: *new clothes.*
Possessive following noun (Vietnamese): *dress her.*	Possessive precedes noun: *her dress.*
Omission of object with transitive verb: *I want.*	Use of direct object with most transitive verbs: *I want it.*

Source: Adapted from Cheng, L. (June, 1987). Cross-cultural and linguistic considerations in working with Asian populations. *Asha, 29*(6), 33–38.

TABLE B.9
Pragmatic and nonlinguistic contrasts between Asian English
and Standard American English

Asian English	Standard American English
• Considered impolite, especially for children, to interrupt in a conversation.	• Appropriate to interrupt in certain circumstances.
• Addressing others may be controlled by several hierarchies that govern social interactions. May be many forms of address.	• Forms of address less rigid, more informal. Limited number of forms.
• Social distance is a factor of age, sex, status, and marital status. Therefore, questions relative to these factors are considered appropriate.	• Standards of social distance are less rigid. Questions about age and status may be considered inappropriate.
• Kinship terms are very important in determining the relationship between two speakers and extend beyond the immediate and extended family to include nonfamily members.	• Kinship terms, such as aunt or uncle, occasionally extended beyond family. Have less rigid effect on speakers in a conversation.
• May keep composed when very emotional. May withhold facial expression.	• More emotive, expressive.
• Do not express public affection.	• Kiss and hug in public.
• May not maintain eye contact with a superior.	• Usually stare at a superior in conversation.
• Humility respected and may respond with embarrassment to praise.	• Acceptable, within bounds, to be personally boastful.
• Giggle when embarrassed or shy.	• Giggle when mocking or "making fun" of someone.
• Touching or hand-holding between members of the same sex is acceptable.	• Touching or hand-holding between members of the same sex is considered as a sign of homosexuality.
• Hand-holding/hugging/kissing between men and women in public looks ridiculous.	• Hand-holding/hugging/kissing between men and women in public is acceptable.
• A slap on the back is insulting.	• A slap on the back denotes friendliness.
• It is not customary to shake hands with persons of the opposite sex.	• It is customary to shake hands with persons of the opposite sex.
• Finger beckoning is only used by adults to call little children and not vice-versa.	• Finger beckoning is often used to call people.

Sources: Taylor, O. (in press). Clinical practice as a social occasion. In L. Cole & V. Deal (Eds.), *Communication disorders in multicultural populations.* Rockville, MD: American Speech-Language-Hearing Association. Reprinted with permission. Adapted from Cheng, L. (June 1987). Cross-cultural and linguistic considerations in working with Asian populations. *Asha, 29*(6), 33–38.

C
Language Tests for Bidialectal and Bilingual Children

TABLE C.1
Screening and diagnostic instruments

Name	Description	Cost	Publisher
ALL INDIA INSTITUTE OF MEDICAL SCIENCES Aphasia Diagnostic Test Battery Aphasia Screening Test Battery Test of Auditory Comprehension of Language Test of Articulation Subhash Bhatnagar	Test batteries developed to identify and diagnose language and speech impairments in the Hindi population. The Aphasia Diagnostic Test Battery is currently undergoing standardization. The tests for auditory comprehension and articulation are in experimental forms and are under revision.	Nominal cost for duplication	Subhash Bhatnagar Department of Speech Pathology and Audiology Marquette University Milwaukee, WI 53233 (414) 224–7349
Assessment of Phonological Processes—Spanish *Barbara Hodson*	An assessment instrument which identifies broad error patterns in unintelligible utterances while deemphasizing differences related to dialect or normal developmental variations.	Manual and lists $35.00	Los Amigos Research Associates 7035 Galewood, Suite D San Diego, CA 92120 (619) 225–0938

(continued)

TABLE C.1
Screening and diagnostic instruments

Name	Description	Cost	Publisher
Bilingual Aphasia Test *Michel Paradis*	An assessment measure for evaluating residual abilities in each of an aphasic patient's languages. The test has been transposed into 40 different languages and 60 language pairs.	Consult publisher for current price information.	L. Erlbaum Associates, Inc. 365 Broadway Hillsdale, NJ 07642 (201) 666–4110
Bilingual Health and Developmental History Questionnaire *Christina Gomez-Valdez*	A questionnaire for use when interviewing Spanish-speaking parents to obtain information about their child's acquisition of developmental milestones. Questions are listed in both English and Spanish.	Instruction booklet and 30 copies of questionnaire $16.00	Academic Communication Associates Publications Division, Dept. 2C P.O. Box 6044 Oceanside, CA 92056 (619) 758–9593
Bilingual Home Inventory	A bilingual instrument that special educators, psychologists, and other professionals can use to interview parents of handicapped children and youth in order to determine educational objectives appropriate for students' homes and communities. Available in English/Spanish, English/Portuguese, and English/Philipino.	$9.00	Dr. Herbert Grossman, Director Bilingual/Multicultural Special Education Programs Division of Special Education and Rehabilitation Services San Jose State University San Jose, CA 95192 (408) 277–9160
Bilingual Language Proficiency Questionnaire *Larry J. Mattes* *George Santiago*	A parent interview questionnaire which can be used to obtain information about bilingual children's development and functional use of a variety of speech and language skills. Items are listed in both English and Spanish.	Instruction booklet and 30 record forms $15.00	Academic Communication Associates Publications Division, Dept. 2C P.O. Box 6044 Oceanside, CA 92056 (619) 758–9593
Boehm Test of Basic Concepts-Revised *Ann E. Boehm*	A test designed to measure children's mastery of basic concepts. The test manual and instruments are available in Spanish.	Examination Kit $17.00 Components also available separately.	Order Service Center The Psychological Corporation P.O. Box 9954 San Antonio, TX 78204 (800) 228–0752

TABLE C.1 (*continued*)

Name	Description	Cost	Publisher
Brigance Diagnostic Assessment of Basic Skills, Portuguese Edition	A Portuguese bilingual adaptation of the Brigance Test.	$40.00	Dr. Herbert Grossman, Director Bilingual/Multicultural Special Education Programs Division of Special Education and Rehabilitation Services San Jose State University San Jose, CA 95192 (408) 277–9160
Cartoon Conservation Scales	A measure for assessing intellectual development in any language without bias. Designed to test for gifted or special education placement.	Complete Kit $79.00	CTB/McGraw Hill Del Monte Research Park Monterey, CA 93940 (800) 538–9547 (408) 649–8400
Chinese Oral Proficiency Test	An exam in Chinese/English for testing children in grades K–6 for oral comprehension and word associations.	Test Packet and 30 Answer Sheets $2.95	The National Hispanic University 255 East 14th Street Oakland, CA 94606 (415) 451–0511
El CIRCO Assessment Series	An instrument for assessing comprehension of simple mathematical concepts and basic linguistic structures in Spanish and English. An additional language check is available to screen facility in Spanish prior to administration. Test was developed expressly for Spanish-speaking children from Mexican-American, Puerto Rican, and Cuban backgrounds.	Test Booklets (30) $28.85 Language Check $10.00	CTB/McGraw Hill Del Monte Research Park Monterey, CA 93940 (800) 538–9547 (408) 649–8400
Comprehensive Identification Process (CIP)—Spanish Edition *R. Reid Zehrbach*	Designed to identify children aged 2 ½–5 ½ years who may be eligible for special preschool programming.	Screening Kit $84.00 Components also available separately.	Scholastic Testing Service, Inc. Dept. E. 480 Meyer Road P.O. Box 1056 Bensenville, IL 60106 (312) 766–7150

(*continued*)

TABLE C.1 *(continued)*

Name	Description	Cost	Publisher
Compton Phonological Assessment of Foreign Accent *Arthur J. Compton*	A step by step approach for analyzing the speech of non-native English speakers. Analysis is derived from a sampling of speech sounds on single words, phrases, sentences, oral reading and conversation.	Complete Set $45.00 Additional Response Booklets (25) $15.00	Carousel House P.O. Box 4480 San Francisco, CA 94101 (800) LANGUAGE (415) 921–0629
Compton Speech and Language Screening Evaluation: Spanish Adaptation *Arthur J. Compton* *Marlaine Kline*	Provides an estimate of speech and language development of Spanish-speaking children, ages 3 through 6 years. Assesses comprehension and production.	Complete Set $50.00 Additional Response Forms (25) $6.00	Carousel House P.O. Box 4480 San Francisco, CA 94101 (800) LANGUAGE (415) 921–0629
Developmental Assessment of Spanish Grammar (DASG) *Allen S. Toronto*	A language analysis procedure for Spanish-speaking children which is an adaptation from the Developmental Sentence Scoring (DSS) procedure in English. The procedure is detailed in a journal article: Toronto, A.S. (1976). Developmental assessment of Spanish grammar. Journal of Speech and Hearing Disorders, *41*(2), 150–171.	N/A	N/A
Dos Amigos Verbal Language Scale *Donald Britchlow*	Assesses cognitive levels of language functioning in both English and Spanish among individual students between the ages of 5 and 13 years.	Complete Set $14.95	United Educational Service Box 605 East Aurora, NY 14052 (716) 652–9131
Examines Para Diagnosticar Impedimentos de Afasia *Joseph S. Keenan* *Esther G. Brassell*	An adaptation of the Aphasia Language Performance Scale (ALPS) which can be used to assess 9 areas of language functioning in Spanish-speaking Individuals grade 7 through adult. Performance is evaluated and reported in terms of language competency, not grade-level ratings.	$30.00	Pinnacle Press P.O. Box 1122 Murfresboro, TN 37133–1122 (615) 893–4464

TABLE C.1 *(continued)*

Name	Description	Cost	Publisher
Expressive One-Word Picture Vocabulary Test—Spanish *Morrison F. Gardner*	Companion to the Receptive One-Word Picture Vocabulary Test. Estimates the quality and quantity of a child's vocabulary. Also attempts to provide an estimate of a bilingual child's fluency in English. Two levels are available: Lower level for children 2 through 11 years, and upper extension for children 12 through 16 years (which can also be administered in small groups for children who can write responses).	Lower Level Test Kit $44.95 Upper Extension Test Kit $40.95 Components also available separately.	Children's Hospital of San Francisco Publications Department OPR-110 P.O. Box 3805 San Francisco, CA 94119 (415) 750–6165 (415) 387–8700
Goodenough-Harris Drawing Test *Florence L. Goodenough* *Dale B. Harris*	A nonverbal assessment tool for evaluating cognitive ability in children 3–15 years. This measure can be used with non-English-speaking children and can be administered individually or in groups.	Complete Kit $31.00 Test Booklet (35) $24.00	Order Service Center The Psychological Corporation P.O. Box 9954 San Antonio, TX 78204 (800) 228–0752
Human Figures Drawing Test (HFDT) *Eloy Gonzales*	A measure of nonverbal conceptual ability of 5- through 10-year-olds which can be used when assessing non-English speakers. Cognitive maturity is evaluated by analyzing drawings of human figures.	Complete Kit $39.00	Pro-Ed 5341 Industrial Oaks Blvd. Austin, TX 78735–8898 (512) 892–3142
Language Assessment Scales	Test for determining oral language proficiency in English and Spanish. Available at three levels— PreLAS for preschoolers, LAS I for grades Kindergarten through 5, and LAS II for grades 6 through 12.	Complete Kit $69.00	CTB/McGraw Hill Del Monte Research Park Monterey, CA 93940 800) 538–9547 (408) 649–8400
Lindamood Auditory Conceptualization Test—Spanish *Charles H. Lindamood* *Patricia C. Lindamood*	Criterion-referenced test measures auditory perception and conceptualization of speech sounds. Spanish version of examiner's cue sheet is available for testing Spanish-speaking subjects.	Complete Program $42.00	DLM Teaching Resources One DLM Park Allen, TX 75002 (800) 527–4747

(continued)

TABLE C.1 (*continued*)

Name	Description	Cost	Publisher
Look Listen and Tell, a Language Screening Instrument for Indian Children	This instrument was developed for use as a language screening device for Native American children 3–7 years of age. It is designed to be used by child-care workers with no formal training in speech-language pathology. It is not yet formally standardized.	$3.00	Southwest Communication Resources, Inc. P.O. Box 788 Bernalillo, NM 87004 (505) 867–3396
Marysville Oral Language Assessment for Diagnosis and Planning	An assessment measure to evaluate expressive and receptive language as well as reading and written language in both English and Spanish. Limited quantities of the test remain available and it will not be reprinted.	Test is Free Oral Language Assessment Handbook $5.00	Marysville Joint Unified School District 1919 B Street Marysville, CA 95901 (916) 741–6000
Medida de Sintaxis Bilingue, I & II (Bilingual Syntax Measure, I and II) *Marina K. Burt Heidi C. Dulay Eduardo Hernandez Chavez*	Uses cartoon-type pictures and questions to elicit language samples which can then be analyzed to determine proficiency levels in English and Spanish. BSM is available at two levels: BSM I for grades K–2, BSM II for grades 3–12.	Complete Set BSM I $140.00 BSM II $152.00 Components also available separately.	Order Service Center The Psychological Corporation P.O. Box 9954 San Antonio, TX 78204 (800) 228–0752
Medida Espanola de Articulacion (Spanish Articulation Measure) *Marilyn Aldrich-Mason Blanche Figueroa-Smith Mary Martinez-Hinshaw*	Tool to assess early acquisition of phonemes in Spanish.	Consult publisher for current price.	Martha Lerma San Ysidro School District 4350 Otay Mesa Road San Ysidro, CA 92073 (619) 428–4476
Multicultural Vocabulary Test *Gerard Trudeau*	A test of expressive vocabulary in English and Spanish which uses body parts as stimulus items, for children aged 3 to 12 years.	$20.00	Los Amigos Research Associates 7035 Galewood, Suite D San Diego, CA 92120 (619) 225–0938

TABLE C.1 *(continued)*

Name	Description	Cost	Publisher
PAL Oral Language Dominance Measure *Rosa Apodaca*	Responses to pictures provide information for determining oral language proficiency in English and/or Spanish.	$9.00	Susie Snyder El Paso Public Schools P.O. Box 2100 El Paso, TX 79998 (915) 779–4056
Parent as a Teacher Inventory (PAAT)—Spanish Edition *Robert D. Strom*	For parents of children age 3–9 years to obtain information on the parent-child interactive system, and for use in parent-education curriculum.	Set $27.50 Components also available separately.	Scholastic Testing Service, Inc. 480 Meyer Road P.O. Box 1056 Bensenville, IL 60106 (312) 766–7150
Peabody Picture Vocabulary Test (Spanish Version)	A test of receptive vocabulary development in Spanish.	Complete Kit $42.00	American Guidance Publishers' Building Circle Pines, MN (800) 328–2560
Preschool Language Assessment Instrument (PLAI): The Language of Learning in Practice—Spanish Language Edition *Marian Blank* *Susan Rose* *Laura Berlin*	Assesses the ability of 3- to 6-year-olds to name, imitate, sequence, match, define, predict, remember information, problem solve, and describe. Information obtained is designed to provide insight into how children handle language demands and ways to effect appropriate programming.	Complete Kit $42.50 Extra Forms $22.50	The Speech Bin 231 Clarksville Road P.O. Box 218 Princeton Junction, NJ 08550–0218 (609) 799–3935
Preschool Language Scale (PLS)—Spanish *Irla Lee Zimmerman* *Violette G. Steiner* *Roberta Evatt Pond*	Diagnostic measure of receptive and expressive language, with items measuring grammar, vocabulary, memory, attention span, temporal/spatial relations, and self-image. Record forms are available in English or Spanish (Mexican-American).	PLS Starter Kit $49.00 Components also available separately.	Order Service Center The Psychological Corporation P.O. Box 9954 San Antonio, TX 78204 (800) 228–0752
Prueba De Lectura y Lenguaje Escrito (PLLE) *Donald D. Hammill* *Stephen C. Larsen* *J. Lee Weiderholt* *Joanna Fountain-Chambers*	A test of reading and writing in Spanish.	$62.00	Pro-Ed 5341 Industrial Oaks Blvd. Austin, TX 78735 (512) 892–3142

(continued)

TABLE C.1 (*continued*)

Name	Description	Cost	Publisher
Prueba Del Desarrollo Initial Del Lenguaje (PDIL) *Wayne P. Hresko* *D. Kim Reid* *Donald D. Hammill*	A test of spoken language in Spanish.	$30.00	Pro-Ed 5341 Industrial Oaks Blvd. Austin, TX 78735 (512) 892–3142
Pruebas de Expresion Oral y Percepcion de la Lengua Espanola (PEOPLE) *Sharon Mares*	A bilingual assessment tool intended to be administered by bilingual speech-language pathologists to children of Mexican descent between 6 and 10 years of age.	$5.00	Los Angeles County Office of Education Kit Carson School, Resource Room, Rm. 2 3530 W. 147th Street Hawthorne, CA 90250 (213) 676–0121 (213) 676–0122
Receptive One-Word Picture Vocabulary Test—Spanish *Morrison F. Gardner*	Companion to the Expressive One-Word Picture Vocabulary Test. Assesses the ability of children age 2 through 11 years to match an object or concept with its name for determining receptive vocabulary skills in Spanish and/or English.	Test Kit $44.95 Components also available separately.	Children's Hospital of San Francisco Publications Department OPR-110 P.O. Box 3805 San Francisco, CA 94119 (415) 750–6165 (415) 387–8700
Screening Test of Spanish Grammar *Allen S. Toronto*	A measure to identify Spanish-speaking children without grammatical proficiency and in need of further evaluation.	Test $29.95 Spanish Response Forms (100) $24.95	Northwestern University Press 1735 Benson Avenue Evanston, IL 60201 (312) 491–5313
Spanish Articulation Measures *Larry J. Mattes*	A criterion-referenced test which includes spontaneous and elicited tasks to assess production of speech sounds and use of phonological processes, such as stridency deletion, cluster reduction, velar fronting, and syllable deletion. For use with school-aged Spanish-speaking children.	Complete Kit $23.00 Record Forms (50) $8.50	The Speech Bin 231 Clarksville Road P.O. Box 218 Princeton Junction, NJ 08550–0218 (609) 799–3935

TABLE C.1 (*continued*)

Name	Description	Cost	Publisher
Spanish Language Assessment Procedures: A Communication Skills Inventory (Revised and Expanded) *Larry J. Mattes*	Twenty-six criterion-referenced measures to assess vocabulary development, speech sound production, sentence structure, listening, pragmatics, and other aspects of a child's communicative functioning.	Complete Kit $38.00 Components also available separately.	Academic Communication Associates Publications Division Department 2C P.O. Box 6044 Oceanside, CA 92056 (619) 758–9593
Spanish Language Synthetic Sentence Identification (SSI–S) Developed and recorded by: *Jerger*	Ten sets of synthetic sentences in Spanish, with accompanying instructions and response card (also in Spanish). Scoring forms provided are in English. Available with both contra- and ipsilateral competing messages.	Reel to Reel or Cassette Tapes $42.50	Auditec of St. Louis 330 Selma Avenue St. Louis, MO 63119 (314) 962–5890
Spanish Oral Language Screening Instrument	A Spanish screening instrument in Spanish/English for determining language skills in Spanish-speaking children, grades K–6.	$2.95	The National Hispanic University 255 East 14th Street Oakland, CA 94606 (415) 451–0511
Spanish/English Language Performance Test	A test for determining oral language proficiency. The test is out of print but still available as long as supplies last.	Classroom Kit (materials for administering test to entire class) $30.00	CTB/McGraw Hill Del Monte Research Park Monterey, CA 93940 800) 538–9547 (408) 649–8400
Spotting Language Problems: Pragmatic Criteria for Language Screening *Jack S. Damico* *John W. Oller*	A language screening instrument which uses a pragmatic approach; for use with English speaking, bilingual and/or limited English proficient children. In-service training suggestions for teachers are also provided.	$25.00	Los Amigos Research Associates 7035 Galewood, Suite D San Diego, CA 92120 (619) 225–0938
SRT and Discrimination Lists—French Recorded by: *Auditec*	Tapes of a list of words for speech reception threshold testing and four lists of words for speech discrimination testing in French.	Reel to Reel $38.00 Cassette $32.00	Auditec of St. Louis 330 Selma Avenue St. Louis, MO 63119 (314) 962–5890

(*continued*)

TABLE C.1 *(continued)*

Name	Description	Cost	Publisher
SRT and Discrimination Lists—Spanish Recorded by: *Auditec* SRT words developed by: *Pasco*	Tapes which consist of lists in Spanish for speech reception threshold and speech discrimination testing. One recording contains two forms of 36 trisyllable words for SRT, and four lists of bisyllable words for speech discrimination. Also included are two lists of monosyllables. The recordings are spoken by an audiologist from Mexico.	SRT & Discrimination (Reel to Reel) $38.00 Monosyllables (Reel to Reel) $34.00 SRT and Discrimination (Cassette) $32.00 Monosyllables (Cassette) $24.50	Auditec of St. Louis 330 Selma Avenue St. Louis, MO 63119 (314) 962–5890
Structured Photographic Expressive Language Test-II, Preschool *Ellen O'Hara Werner* *Janet Dawson* *Krescheck*	A test of expressive language for standard English or Black English or Spanish speakers, available for preschoolers or elementary age children.	Both Tests $46.00 Preschool only $37.00	Janelle Publications P.O. Box 12 Sandwich, IL 60548 (312) 552–7771
System of Multicultural Pluralistic Assessment (SOMPA) *Jane R. Mercer* *June F. Lewis*	A system for assessing cognitive and sensorimotor abilities and adaptive behavior of children age 5–11 years. Components of the SOMPA include a parent interview which can be conducted in English or Spanish, student assessment materials, and the Adaptive Behavior Inventory for Children (ABIC) which can also be used independently. Normative data are provided for Black, Hispanic and White children.	Complete SOMPA Kit (includes ABIC) $99.00 Components also available separately.	Order Service Center The Psychological Corporation P.O. Box 9954 San Antonio, TX 78204 (800) 228–0752
Test for Auditory Comprehension of Language: English and Spanish Forms (Revised)	This norm referenced test designed for use with children 3.0 to 6.11 measures receptive language problems in English or Spanish.	Complete TACL–R $99.00	DLM Teaching Resources One DLM Park Allen, TX 75002 (800) 527–4747

TABLE C.1 *(continued)*

Name	Description	Cost	Publisher
Texas-Acevedo Screening of Speech and Language *Mary Ann Acevedo*	An English/Spanish articulation and language screening test for English- or Spanish-speaking children 3 to 6 years of age.	Free-furnished only to Head Start programs, Preschools or others who provide screening services at no cost to clients.	Vision, Hearing and Speech Services Bureau of Maternal and Child Health Texas Department of Health 1100 West 49th Street Austin, TX 78756 (512) 458–7111
Woodcock Language Proficiency Battery (English and Spanish Form) *Richard W. Woodcock*	A battery which measures three components of language proficiency including oral, reading, and written language.	$66.00	DLM Teaching Resources One DLM Park Allen, TX 75002 (800) 527–4747
Zuni Articulation Test	A Zuni alphabet book has been adapted for use as a stimulus book for articulation testing by the Zuni Public School System. Picture and word stimuli for sounds in initial and medial positions are provided. Several pictures are presented for each sound. Some training is required in test administration procedures.	Contact the School District for current information on training and availability of the test.	Zuni Public School District Speech and Language Therapy Program P.O. Drawer A Zuni, NM 87327
Zuni Language Screening Instrument	A measure designed to quickly evaluate language proficiency in the Zuni language for children in grades kindergarten through 12. Both receptive and expressive language are measured, and a language sample can be obtained. Instructions have been taped in Zuni, and age appropriate language samples obtained from the test's picture sequence stories have also been taped to assist in the assessment of spontaneous speech. Some training is required in test administration procedures.	Contact the School District for current information on training and availability of the test.	Zuni Public School District Speech and Language Therapy Program P.O. Drawer A Zuni, NM 87327

Source: Deal, V., and Rodriguez, V. (1987). *Resource guide to multicultural tests and materials in communicative disorders.* Rockville, MD: American Speech-Language-Hearing Association. Reprinted with permission.

D
Language Analysis Methods

Assigning Structural Stage/Complex Sentence Development

In Assigning Structural Stage, Miller (1980) proposes a three-tiered analysis that includes MLU, percentage correct of Brown's 14 morphemes, and sentence analysis. These three measures enable the speech-language pathologist to determine the stage of development and to describe the forms used. Although less precise than Developmental Sentence Scoring (DSS), Assigning Structural Stage is more descriptive and prescriptive in nature. After determining the child's stage of language development, the speech-language pathologist can target linguistic forms in the next stage (Prutting, 1979).

Analysis begins by collecting a language sample. The speech-language pathologist collects 50 to 100 utterances or 15 minutes of conversation, whichever is larger, from the child for analysis. Unlike DSS, these utterances do not have to be sentences. First, she calculates MLU to determine the stage of development and the approximate language age of the child. MLU calculation is discussed in Chapter 4.

Once she has determined MLU, the speech-language pathologist decides on the analysis method to follow. She may choose Assigning Structural Stage and/or Complex Sentence Development. If the MLU of the child is below 3.0, the speech-language pathologist uses only Assigning Structural Stage. If the child's MLU is above 4.5, she uses only Complex Sentence Development. For MLUs of 3.0 to 4.5, she uses both procedures.

In Assigning Structural Stage, the speech-language pathologist calculates the percentage correct for Brown's 14 morphemes. A minimum number of occurrences or possibilities of occurrence are needed before the speech-language pathologist can decide on consistency or inconsistency of use or nonuse. The child should attempt a morpheme at least four times before a percentage correct figure is calculated.

The percentage correct value is determined by dividing the number of correct appearances by the total number of obligatory contexts. After calculating the percent correct, the speech-language pathologist can again attempt to describe the child's stage of language development.

Next, she analyzes each utterance within four possible categories of noun phrase, verb phrase, and negative and interrogative development. Utterances are divided into noun and verb phrases where applicable, and each phrase is assigned to the stage of development that best describes its structures. Negative or interrogative utterances are further assigned to stages representing their level of development.

The speech-language pathologist should be familiar with the information Miller (1980) presents for each stage of development. Some of this information is presented in Table 4.7, although Miller presents a great deal more. The analysis process is demonstrated here using some of the information in Table 4.7. Consider the child's utterance "Want a big doggie." The noun phrase, "a big doggie," has been expanded by the addition of an article and an adjective to the noun. This noun phrase occurs in the object position of the sentence. Expansion of the noun phrase only in the object position is an example of stage II (see intrasentence column). Therefore, this sentence represents noun phrase development characteristic of stage II. The verb phrase is unelaborated and no subject is present. This represents stage I development. No analysis is required for negative or interrogative forms.

Complex Sentence Development is used similarly, but different samples and categories are used for analysis. Analysis is based on a 15-minute sample of the child's communication rather than on 50 utterances. For children with MLUs between 3.0 and 4.5, these samples can overlap. Five aspects of complex sentences are noted: percentage of both conjoined and embedded sentences within the sample, type of embedding, conjoining, and conjunctions, and the number of different conjunctions. At each stage, Miller describes development by the forms exhibited by 50–90% and by greater than 90% of the children.

Limited data from Complex Sentence Development are incorporated in Table 4.7. By post-stage V, 90% of children should be using *and* within a 15-minute sample. To complete a full analysis, the speech-language pathologist should consult Complex Sentence Development (Miller, 1980).

Each sentence is analyzed using Assigning Structural Stage or Complex Sentence Development or both, and the data are summarized. Most likely, the child will exhibit language forms in each stage of development. Now, the speech-language pathologist must use her skill.

Even mature language users occasionally use language forms that are characteristic of less mature learning. Adults use many one-word utterances everyday. These forms are not the most characteristic forms, however, and the speech-language pathologist must gather a summary of overall language form to determine most accurately the user's abilities. It is the same with the language-impaired child. The speech-language pathologist determines those behaviors that are most characteristic of the child. These might be behaviors at a particular stage that the child uses most frequently or behaviors that represent the highest attainment level. The speech-language pathologist must make this determination.

All data from the two analysis methods—Assigning Structural Stage and Complex Sentence Development—are combined to place the child's language form within a stage or stages of development and to describe the child's language form. The child functioning well below age expectancy may need intervention.

Developmental Sentence Scoring

Developmental Sentence Scoring (Lee, 1974) is one of the most widely used and popular instruments for assessing children's syntactic and morphologic development. Even so, DSS requires considerable study by the speech-language pathologist to score language samples correctly. Although the instructions are explicit and straightforward, they require a thorough understanding of English syntax and morphology. Because the scale does not evaluate many aspects of children's language, it should only be one aspect of an evaluation battery.

The following section discusses the primary aspects of DSS and its most common problems. This survey cannot take the place of a thorough reading of DSS procedures and actual practice with the instrument.

To rate a sample of child language, the speech-language pathologist collects 50 different consecutive *sentences*. No speaker uses full sentences all the time. Therefore, utterances that do not qualify as sentences are simply omitted, and the remainder collected until 50 consecutive sentences are amassed. DSS analysis should not be undertaken if less than 50% of the child's utterances are sentences.

Because the sample should include 50 different consecutive sentences, repeated sentences are discarded unless there is some change. Run-on sentences of several independent clauses joined by conjunctions are segmented so that no more than two independent clauses are joined. For example, the following run-on should be divided as noted:

[We went to the zoo, and I saw monkeys,] [and we had a picnic, and I ate a hot dog,] [and I fed pigeons, and we came home on the bus.]

The *and* at the beginning of each sentence ("*and* we had . . ., *and* I fed . . .") would not be scored. A sentence may have more than one *and* if the word does not link clauses but is used for compound subjects, verbs, or objects, for example:

Tom, Mary, *and* John were throwing *and* kicking beach balls *and* soccer balls.

Sentences that begin with a conjunction, such as "Because I falled down," are included in the sample, but the conjunction itself should not be scored unless it links clauses, as in "Because I falled down, I finded a penny."

Each sentence is rated on the basis of eight grammatical categories and assigned a score of 1 to 8 points in the applicable categories. The categories and point values are given in Table D.1. Each structure demonstrated in the sentence is scored each time that it occurs. For example, sentence 1 in Table D.2, "I don't know what I like," contains the word *I* twice. Therefore, the word receives a score of 1 twice under personal pronouns, in addition to other points.

Sentences that would be acceptable mature forms are given an additional point called a *sentence point*. The sentence point should only be awarded when the sentence is syntactically and semantically correct by mature standards. The following would not receive a sentence point:

Carol and me went to the store.
Nobody didn't go.
I got six pencils in my desk.

In Table D.2, sentence 2, "What you like?," receives a score of 4; it does not receive a sentence point because it is not an acceptable mature sentence. Sentence 3, "I don't know," does receive the sentence point.

TABLE D.1
Developmental sentence scoring categories and point values

Score	Indefinite Pronouns or Noun Modifiers	Personal Pronouns	Main Verbs	Secondary Verbs
1	it, this, that	1st and 2nd person: I, me, my, mine, you, your(s)	A. Uninflected verb: I *see* you. B. copula, is or 's: *It's* red. C. is + verb + ing: He *is coming.*	
2		3rd person: he, him, his, she, her, hers	A. -s and -ed: *plays, played* B. irregular past: *ate, saw* C. Copula: *am, are, was, were* D. Auxiliary *am, are, was, were*	Five early-developing infinitives: I wan*na see* (want *to see*) I'm gon*na see* (going *to see*) I got*ta see* (got *to see*) Lem*me* [to] *see* (let me [*to*] *see*) Let's [to] play (let [us *to*] play)
3	A. no, some, more, all, lot(s), one(s), two (etc.), other(s), another B. something, somebody, someone	A. Plurals: we, us, our(s), they, them, their B. these, those		Non-complementing infinitives: I stopped *to play.* I'm afraid *to look.* It's hard *to do that.*
4	nothing, nobody, none, no one		A. can, will, may + verb: *may go* B. Obligatory do + verb: *don't go* C. emphatic do + verb: I *do see.*	Participle, present or past: I see a boy *running* I found the toy *broken.*
5		Reflexives: myself, yourself, himself, herself, itself, themselves		A. Early infinitival complements with differing subjects in kernels: I want you *to come.* Let him [*to*] *see.* B. Later infinitival complements: I had *to go.* I told him *to go.* I tried *to go.* He ought *to go.* C. Obligatory deletions: Make it [*to*] *go.* I'd better [*to*] *go.* D. Infinitive with wh-word: I know what *to get.* I know how *to do* it.

Negatives	Conjunctions	Interrogative Reversals	Wh Questions
it, this, that + copula or auxiliary is, 's, + not: It's *not* mine. This is *not* a dog. That *is not* moving.		Reversal of copula: *Isn't it* red? *Were they* there?	

			A. who, what, what + noun:
			    Who am I? *What is* he eating? *What book* are you reading?
			 B. where, how many, how much, what . . . do. what . . . for
			    Where did it go?
			    How much do you want?
			    What is he *doing*?
			    What is a hammer *for*?

	and		

can't, don't		Reversal of auxiliary be:
		    Is he coming? *Isn't he* coming? *Was he* going?
		    Wasn't he going?	

isn't, won't	A. but
	 B. so, and so, so that
	 C. or, if
			when, how, how + adjective
			    When shall I come?
			    How do you do it?
			    How big is it?

(continued)

TABLE D.1 *(continued)*

Score	Indefinite Pronouns or Noun Modifiers	Personal Pronouns	Main Verbs	Secondary Verbs
6		A. Wh-pronouns: who, which, whose, whom, what, that, how many, how much I know *who* came. That's *what* I said. B. Wh-word + infinitive: I know *what* to do. I know *who(m)* to take	A. could, would, should, might + verb: *might come, could be* B. Obligatory does, did + verb C. Emphatic does, did + verb	
7	A. any, anything. anybody, anyone B. every, everything, everybody, everyone C. both, few, many, each, several, most, least, much, next, first, last, second (etc.)	(his) own, one, oneself, whichever, whoever, whatever Take *whatever* you like.	A. Passive with *get*, any tense Passive with *be*, any tense B. must, shall + verb: *must come* C. have + verb + en: *I've eaten* D. have got: *I've got* it.	Passive infinitival complement: With *get*: I have *to get dressed.* I don't want to *get hurt.* With *be*: I want *to be pulled.* It's going *to be locked.*
8			A. have been + verb + ing had been + verb + ing B. modal + have + verb + en: *may have eaten* C. modal + be + verb + ing: *could be playing* D. Other auxiliary combinations: *should have been sleeping*	Gerund: *Swinging* is fun. I like *fishing.* He started *laughing.*

Source: Lee, L. (1974). *Developmental sentence analysis (pp. 134–135).* Evanston, IL: Northwestern University Press. Copyright © 1974 by Northwestern University. Reprinted with permission.

Negatives	Conjunctions	Interrogative Reversals	Wh Questions
	because	A. Obligatory do, does, did: *Do they* run? *Does it* bite? *Did*n't *it* hurt? B. Reversal of modal: *Can you* play? *Won't it* hurt? *Shall I* sit down? C. Tag question: It's fun, *isn't it?* It isn't fun, *is it?*	
All other negatives: A. Uncontracted negatives: I can *not* go. He has *not* gone. B. Pronoun-auxiliary or pronoun-copula contraction: I'm *not* coming. He's *not* here. C. Auxiliary-negative or copula-negative contraction: He *wasn't* going. He *hasn't* been seen. It *couldn't* be mine. They *aren't* big.			why, what if, how come, how about + gerund *Why* are you crying? *What if* I won't do it? *How come* he is crying? *How about* coming with me?
	A. where, when, how, while, whether (or not), till, until, unless, since, before, after, for, as, as + adjective + as, as if, like, that, than I know *where* you are. Don't come *till* I call. B. Obligatory deletions: I run faster *than* you [run]. I'm *as big as* a man [is big]. It looks *like* a dog [looks]. C. Elliptical deletions (score 0): That's *why* [I took it]. I know *how*. [*I can do it*]. D. *Wh-words* + infinitive: I know how to do it.	A. Reversal of auxiliary have: *Has he* seen you? B. Reversal with two or three auxiliaries: *Has he been* eating? *Couldn't he have* waited? *Could he have been* crying? *Wouldn't he have been* going?	whose, which, which + noun *Whose* cat is that? *Which book* do you want?

TABLE D.2
Language sample analysis using Developmental Sentence Scoring

Name:
D.O.B.:
D.O.K.:
C.A.:
Score

Developmental sentence scoring form

	Indefinite Pronouns	Personal Pronouns	Main Verbs	Secondary Verbs	Negatives	Conjunctions	Interrogative Reversals	Wh Questions	Sentence Point	Total
I don't know what I like	1, 1, 6	4, 1			4				1	18
What do you like?	1, 6	1								8
I don't know.	1	4			4			1		10
He bes happy	2	inc								2

Attempt markers and incomplete markers may also be awarded for structures. Attempt markers—a line or hyphen in place of a score—are awarded when a structure is attempted but incorrect. Naturally, as in sentence 4, "He bes happy," the sentence cannot receive a sentence point. Surface structures that are conversationally appropriate but incomplete receive the incomplete marker *inc* in place of a score. If the structure is conversationally acceptable, it receives a sentence point. For example, in the following exchange, the child's response would receive an incomplete for the main verb.

> CLINICIAN: Who let the guinea pig out?
> CHILD: I didn't. [I didn't (let him out).]

The point value of each sentence is totaled and added to the value for every other sentence. This overall total is divided by the number of sentences (usually 50) to yield a score. The speech-language pathologist must remember that this value is a DSS score and not an MLU. The two values are very different.

She then applies the DSS score to a table of ages and scores to compare the child's performance with that of other children at that age. Figure D.1 lists the average scores (50th percentile) for each age and the scores for the 10th, 25th, 75th, and 90th percentile. For example, an average score for a 4-year-old would be approximately 7.3. Only the highest 10% of 4-year-olds would receive a score of 9.0 (90th percentile).

According to the instructions, children whose scores place them below the 10th percentile should be considered for therapy. Therefore, a 4-year-old who scores below 4.7 should be considered for therapy.

An age equivalent for the child placing below the 10th percentile can be determined by noting the point at which the horizontal line for the child's score crosses the diagonal 50th-percentile line. At this age, the child's score is an average score. For example, the child age 5 ½ who receives an average score of 5.0 points is well below the 10th percentile for that age and needs intervention. The age equivalent would be found by following the 5.0 line to the left until it intersects the horizontal 50th-percentile line. This occurs at an age of 3 years. Thus, the child's age equivalent is approximately 3 years.

Age equivalent or functioning level, if needed, can be found in the same way for children, such as those with mental retardation, who may exceed the age norm ceiling of 6 ½ years. Obviously, the percentile values are not relevant.

Language delay in years can be determined by subtracting the age equivalent from the child's chronological age. In the previous example, the child's language delay is approximately 2 ½ years. Although this value means little for the direction of therapy, it does provide a score for those people, such as administrators, who demand such data and can be used as an index of change over time.

The most common problems encountered with DSS are associated with determination of grammatical units and with scoring (Lively, 1984). These problems are discussed briefly in the following section. Readers can refer to Lively (1984) for a more thorough discussion.

Scoring adverbs as indefinite pronouns/noun modifiers. Words, such as *first, last,* and *everywhere,* that tell the manner or place of an action are adverbs ("Let's do this *first.*") and should not be scored as indefinite pronoun/noun modifiers. In contrast, other words, especially numbers, should be scored when they do function as indefinite pronoun/noun modifiers, as in the following:

> Can I have *one*?
> I have *two* dolls.
> *No one* don't like me.

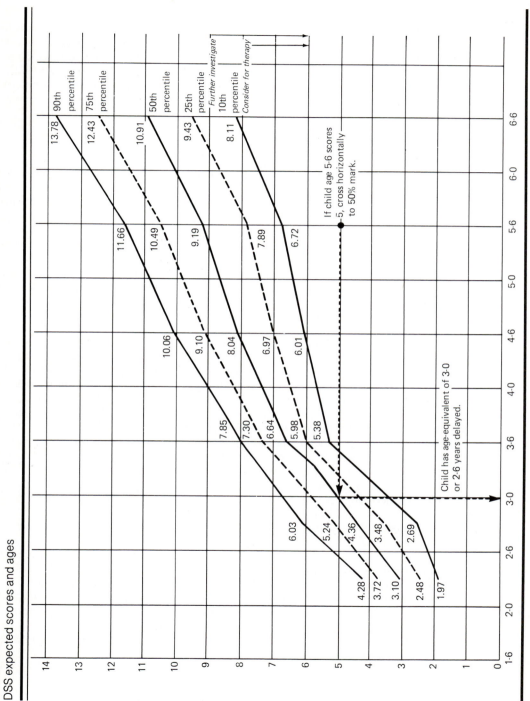

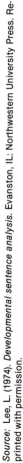

Source: Lee, L. (1974). *Developmental sentence analysis.* Evanston, IL: Northwestern University Press. Reprinted with permission.

Personal pronoun/wh- conjunction/wh- question confusion. *Wh-* words may be used as personal pronouns (score 6) or as conjunctions (score 8). The distinction can be clarified by remembering that a complete clause will follow the conjunction.

I want the one *that* talks.	(Pronoun, because ''talks'' is not a complete clause.)
He told us *that* we could shovel his driveway.	(Conjunction, because ''we could shovel his driveway'' is a complete clause.)
I know *what* you want.	(Pronoun, because ''you want'' is not a complete clause.)
What do you want?	(*Wh-* question)

Main verbs. All uninflected or unmarked verbs receive a score of 1. Regular or irregular inflected verbs receive some other score.

I *like* ice cream.	(Uninflected = 1)
She *likes* ice cream.	(Inflected = 2)
She *ate* ice cream.	(Inflected = 2)

Incorrect attempts, such as using *got* for *have,* receive an attempt score. The verb *do* as a main verb receives a 1 or 2. As an auxiliary, it receives a 4 if uninflected and a 6 if inflected. The modal auxiliary verbs *can, will,* and *may* are scored in the same manner.

Do it for me.	(Uninflected main verb = 1)
I *did* my homework.	(Inflected main verb = 2)
I *do* like ice cream.	(Uninflected auxiliary = 4)
I *did* like ice cream.	(Inflected auxiliary = 6)
He *does* like ice cream.	(Inflected auxiliary = 6)
I *can* swim.	(Uninflected modal = 4)
I *could* swim.	(Inflected modal = 6)

In contrast, the modal auxiliaries *must* and *shall* are always scored as 7. The perfect tense forms of *have* + *verb*(en) also receive a 7. All sentences with two or more auxiliaries, as in ''He could have gone,'' receive an 8.

Passive sentences present a special case, and speech-language pathologists should refer to Lee (1974).

Compound sentences can be very difficult, especially if material is omitted. With compound verbs, each is scored. If the auxiliary is omitted, both verbs should still receive the full score.

I *was singing* and *dancing.*	(The second ''was'' is omitted and understood, so each verb receives a score of 2.)

If, on the other hand, the main verb is omitted, only the complete form is scored and the other abbreviated or elliptical form receives an incomplete score.

I *did* complete my lesson, but Carol *didn't.*	(The second ''did'' receives an incomplete score, whereas the first receives a 6.)

Secondary verbs. The chief error in this category is in identifying the infinitive. Often the signal word *to* is omitted. If the child uses *gonna, wanna, gotta, lemme,* or *let's,* the infinitive is scored as 2. Other infinitives receive a 5, if the subject of the infinitive is different from the subject of the main verb.

I wanna go.	(Score as 2.)
I want to go.	(Score as 2.)
I want her to go.	(Different subjects = 5)
Make the car (to) go.	(The subject is understood to be ''you'' and car is ''to go,'' so score the infinitive as 5.)

Negatives. The only negative to receive a score of 1 is the *this/that/it* + *is/'s not* form. All other forms of this combination receive a higher score. Any other subject or auxiliary verb receives a score of 7.

It is not yours.	(''It is not'' = 1)
It's not yours.	(''It's not'' = 1)
It isn't yours.	(''It isn't'' = 5)
You *can't* do it.	(''Can't'' = 7)

Interrogative reversals. Speech-language pathologists often overlook interrogative reversals when scoring *wh-* questions. Tag questions, except those ending in *huh, okay, eh,* and the like, receive a score of 6.

Obviously, Developmental Sentence Scoring is a very complex analysis system, not to be attempted without a thorough knowledge of both English syntax and DSS procedures. Unfortunately, the child's score offers little direction for intervention, although Lee suggests appropriate places at which to begin intervention, based primarily on the percentage of correct production. The hierarchy presented in Table D.1 offers only limited guidance and omits many important structures. This type of problem seems inherent in any analysis system that reduces complex behavior to point values.

Language Assessment, Remediation, and Screening Procedure (LARSP)

The Language Assessment, Remediation, and Screening Procedure or LARSP (Crystal, Fletcher, & Garman, 1976, revised 1981) is more widely used in England, Canada, and Australia than in the United States. More psycholinguistic in nature than the other methods included in this appendix, LARSP analyzes language based on phrase and sentence structure and on the number of elements found in the child's utterances. These values relate to seven stages of language development, mostly in the preschool years.

The speech-language pathologist collects 30 minutes of the child's speech from two different 15-minute activities. In the first, the child plays with a familiar adult; in the second, the child and adult participate in a dialogue.

All utterances are included in the analysis, describing what the child can or cannot do. Therefore, all utterances are transcribed with intonations and pauses indicated. Important nonlinguistic information is also included to aid analysis. The speech-language pathologist uses the following markers when transcribing:

TABLE D.3

LARSP profile chart

Name   Age   Sample date   Type

A	**Unanalysed**			**Problematic**		
	1 Unintelligible	2 Symbolic Noise	3 Deviant	1 Incomplete	2 Ambiguous	3 Stereotypes

B Responses

				Normal Response						Abnormal		
					Major							
			Repetitions	Elliptical			Reduced	Full	Minor	Structural	∅	Problems
Stimulus Type		Totals		1	2	3+						
	Questions											
	Others											

C Spontaneous

D Reactions

	General	Structural	∅	Other	Problems

Stage I (0.9–1.6)	**Minor**		*Responses*		*Vocatives*	*Other*	*Problems*
	Major	*Comm.*	*Quest.*		*Statement*		
		·V·	·Q·	·V·	·N·	Other	Problems

Stage II (1.6–2.0)	Conn.			Clause				Phrase		Word
		VX	QX	SV	AX		DN	VV		
				SO	VO		Adj N	V part		-ing
				SC	VC		NN	Int X		
				Neg X	Other		PrN	Other		pl

Stage III (2.0–2.6)		X + S:NP	X + V:VP	X + C:NP		X + O:NP	X + A:AP		-ed
		VXY	QXY	SVC	VCA	D Adj N	Cop		-en
		let XY		SVO	VOA	Adj Adj N	Aux^M_O		
		do XY	VS(X)	SVA	VO_dO_i	Pr DN			3s
				Neg XY	Other	$Pron^P_O$	Other		gen

Stage IV (2.6–3.0)		XY + S:NP	XY + V:VP	XY + C:NP		XY + O:NP	XY + A:AP		n't
		+ S	QVS	SVOA	AAXY	NP Pr NP	Neg V		'cop
			QXY +	SVCA	Other	Pr D Adj N	Neg X		
		VXY +	VS(X +)	SVO_dO_i		cX	2 Aux		'aux
			tag	SVOC		XcX	Other		

Stage V (3.0–3.6)	*and*	Coord.	Coord.	Coord. 1 1 +		Postmod. 1 1 + clause		-est
	c	Other	Other	Subord. A 1 1 +				-er
	s			S C O		Postmod. 1 + phrase		-ly
	Other			Comparative				

	(+)				(−)		

Stage VI (3.6–4.6)	NP	VP	Clause	Conn.	Clause		Phrase					Word	
					Element	NP			VP			N	V
	Initiator	Complex	Passive	and	∅	D	Pr	$Pron^P$	Aux^M	Aux^O	Cop	*irreg*	
	Coord.		Complement.	c	⇄	D∅	Pr∅						
			how what	s	Concord	D⇄	Pr⇄		∅			*reg*	
	Other								Ambiguous				

Stage VII (4.6+)	*Discourse*		*Syntactic Comprehension*	
	A Connectivity	*it*		
	Comment Clause	*there*	*Style*	
	Emphatic Order	Other		

Total No. Sentences	Mean No. Sentences Per Turn	Mean Sentence Length

Source: Crystal, D., Fletcher, P., and Garman, M. (1976, revised 1981). *The grammatical analysis of language disability.* New York: Elsevier. Reprinted with permission. Revised 1981.

( )   Parentheses, placed around unintelligible speech, may be left blank, may signal the possible number of syllables, or may guess at the unintelligible portion by placing words within.

?   A question mark is placed before any word for which the transcriptional accuracy is in doubt. This occurs when two listeners disagree.

*   Asterisks are placed around speakers' words that overlap.

(())   Double parentheses are placed around interjections or repairs that do not disturb the flow of communication.

Analysis is accomplished on a worksheet and transferred to the Profile Chart shown in Table D.3. First, synchronic analysis is accomplished in sections A, B, and C. In-depth analysis is accomplished using the developmental stage portion of the chart. The authors recommend that the total analysis be completed using eight separate scans of the transcript.

In scan 1, the speech-language pathologist removes for later analysis all utterances that cannot be analyzed. There are two types: unanalyzed and problematic. Unanalyzed utterances may be wholly unintelligible, may consist of symbolic noise, such as truck or airplane sounds, or may be *deviant* sentences. Deviant sentences are utterances that are structurally inadmissible in adult grammar and are not part of the expected grammatical development of nonimpaired children. Problematic utterances include incomplete sentences that do not represent expected grammatical development and ambiguous sentences that may be interpreted in two different ways, based on the communication situation. The number of utterances within each category is tallied and placed in section A of the Profile Chart. With these utterances identified, the subsequent scans are less problematic.

The second scan, recorded in sections B and C, establishes the proportion of spontaneous to responsive utterances and analyzes the type of each. The type of response depends on the type of stimulus sentence. LARSP distinguishes between question stimuli and others.

Normal responses may be classified as *elliptical major sentences,* in which shared information is omitted; *full major sentences;* or *minor sentences* consisting of single word answers, such as *yes/no.* In addition, elliptical sentences are rated by the number of elements included in each. Abnormal responses may demonstrate either *structural deviance,* in which there is a mismatch between the expected structural pattern of the response and the one produced, or *zero response,* in which a response is expected but not received. Other responses are classified as *repetitions* of the other speaker or *problems.* The problems category is an *other* category for those utterances that do not fit anywhere else. The number of each type of response is recorded in section B in the type of response column and in the stimulus row.

Spontaneous utterances are divided into *novel* sentences and *full self-repetitions.* The number of utterances within each category are recorded in the appropriate space on the Profile Chart.

Scan 3 is for sentence connectivity. Each type is tabulated and counted. The four types include *intonation,* in which emphasis or stress indicates old or contrasting information; *vocabulary replacement,* in which another word other than a pronoun replaces the old information; *common sense semantic connection,* in which sequencing provides connectivity; and *grammatical links,* such as adverbs, cross-referenced articles and pronouns, and ellipsis.

Scans 4 through 7 are more grammatical in nature and include coordination and subordination, clause structure, phrase structure, and word structure, respectively. Scans 5, 6, and 7 provide the most information on structure. Information regarding the number of each type of structure is recorded under the most appropriate stage next to the structures

TABLE D.4
LARSP clausal and phrasal structure coding

V	Verb
Q	Question word (*What, where*)
N	Noun
X	All elements that may co-occur with another element
S	Subject
C/O	Complement/object
A	Adverb (Usually location)
Neg	Negative word (*No, not*)
D	Demonstrative (Including possessive pronouns)
Adj	Adjective
Pr	Preposition
Part	Particle (*Out* as in *Come out*)
Y	Used with X to indicate any **two** elements of clause structure
NP	Noun phrase
VP	Verb phrase
Cop	Copula
Aux	Auxiliary verb (Not just *be*)
Pron	Pronoun
O_d	Direct object
O_i	Indirect object
Z	Use with X and Y to indicate any **three** elements of clause structure
c	Coordinating conjunction
s	Subordinating conjunction

listed. Clausal and phrasal structure coding is listed in Table D.4. The stages represent seven theoretical levels of development of syntax and should not be confused with Brown's stages of development. Approximate ages for each stage are given in Table D.5. Crystal et al. (1976) provide descriptions and examples of each stage.

Morphological markers or *word-structure patterns* are also recorded on the right side of the Profile Chart. These are not related to any specific stage. The coding for these markers is given in Table D.6.

Scan 8 involves only the utterances that are problems because of structural abnormalities. These may provide a key to disordered language.

Finally, three additional items of information are computed: the total number of sentences, the mean number of sentences per turn, and the mean sentence length in words.

TABLE D.5
LARSP stages and approximate ages

Stage I	9 mos.—1 yr. 6 mos.
Stage II	1 yr. 6 mos.—2 yrs.
Stage III	2 yrs.—2 yrs. 6 mos.
Stage IV	2 yrs. 6 mos.—3 yrs.
Stage V	3 yrs.—3 yrs. 6 mos.
Stage VI	3 yrs. 6 mos.—4 yrs. 6 mos.
Stage VII	4 yrs. 6 mos.—9 yrs.

TABLE D.6
LARSP word-structure pattern codes

-ing	Present progressive -*ing*
pl	Plural -*s* marker
-ed	Past tense -*ed*
-en	Past participle -*en*
3s	Third person singular -*s*
gen	Possessive -*s*
n't	Contracted negative (is*n't*)
'cop	Contracted form of the copula (She*'s* happy)
'aux	Contracted form of the auxiliary *be* (He*'s* eating)
-est	Superlative -*est*
-er	Comparative -*er*
-ly	Adverbial suffix -*ly*

The total number of sentences includes all utterances, even repetitions, except for unanalyzed and problem utterances. The mean number of utterances per turn is found by combining the totals in sections B and C and dividing this amount by the total of the conversational partner's stimulus types, found in section B.

Conclusion

Although somewhat more specific than Assigning Structural Stage/Complex Sentence Development (Miller, 1980), LARSP is more theoretical and based on older, more psycholinguistic models of language development. While LARSP avoids the pitfalls of phrase structure-based grammars, it still adheres to the notion of elements added one at a time. It might be best to ignore the stage information but incorporate a portion of the analysis methodology, especially the phrasal and sentential structures. Responsive versus spontaneous data and the mean number of sentences per turn are also valuable.

Crystal et al. (1976) provide some interpretation of the results with regard to specific language impairments. Sketchy intervention programs are suggested for the patterns exhibited in the samples.

Systematic Analysis of Language Transcripts (SALT)

Systematic Analysis of Language Transcripts, or SALT (Miller & Chapman, 1985), is one of the most promising computer analysis methods available. Based on Assigning Structural Stage/Complex Sentence Development (Miller, 1981), SALT is designed for use with the IBM PC or the Apple II series computers. Within limits, SALT analyzes morphemic, pragmatic, and semantic aspects of a language sample.

The transcript is typed using standard English orthography. Time is critical for calculation of duration and pause times. Each feature to be analyzed is signaled with a different marker. Therefore, it takes approximately 7 minutes for the skilled user to enter each minute of conversation into the transcription format.

The speech-language pathologist can accomplish several types of analyses using SALT. These types include utterance type; turn overlap and distribution; pause duration and number; utterances per minute and words per utterance; frequency of verbal and nonverbal data of interest, such as past tense; utterance length; type-token ratio; MLU;

Brown's stages of development; expected age range of development; word and category lists; and other user-designated analysis.

Conclusion

SALT is a very promising and versatile analysis method that is easy for the speech-language pathologist to use after she becomes familiar with entering the transcript into the computer. As with other computer analysis methods, however, it is not the great panacea. At present, most results are a calculation of those features signaled by the speech-language pathologist when she enters the data. Thus, special care is required to ensure that features are signaled accurately.

E
Selected English Morphological Prefixes and Suffixes

Derivational		Inflectional
Prefixes	**Suffixes**	
a- (in, on, into, in a manner)	-able (ability, tendency, likelihood)	-ed (past)
bi- (twice, two)	-al (pertaining to, like, action, process)	-ing (at present)
de- (negative, descent, reversal)	-ance (action, state)	-s (plural)
	-ation (denoting action in a noun)	-s (third person marker)
ex- (out of, from, thoroughly)	-en (used to form verbs from adjectives)	-'s (possession)
inter- (reciprocal between, together)	-ence (action, state)	
mis- (ill, negative, wrong)	-er (used as an agentive ending)	
out- (extra, beyond, not)	-est (superlative)	
over- (over)	-ful (full, tending)	
post- (behind, after)	-ible (ability, tendency, likelihood)	
pre- (to, before)	-ish (belonging to)	
pro- (in favor of)	-ism (doctrine, state, practice)	
re- (again, backward motion)	-ist (one who does something)	
semi- (half)	-ity (used for abstract nouns)	
super- (superior)	-ive (tendency or connection)	
trans- (across, beyond)	-ize (action, policy)	
tri- (three)	-less (without)	
un- (not, reversal)	-ly (used to form adverbs)	
under- (under)	-ment (action, product, means, state)	
	-ness (quality, state)	
	-or (used as an agentive ending)	
	-ous (full of, having, like)	
	-y (inclined to)	

F
Indirect Elicitation Techniques

There is an infinite variety of indirect elicitation techniques, although we tend to rely on two old favorites:

Tell me what you see.
Tell me in a whole sentence.

Here are a few conversational techniques that came to mind one day. The list is not exhaustive, merely illustrative.

Technique	Target	Example	
The emperor's new clothes	Negative statements	CLINICIAN:	Oh Shirley what beautiful yellow boots.
		CLIENT:	I'm not wearing boots!
Pass it on	Requests for information	CLINICIAN:	John, do you know where Linda's project is?
		CLIENT:	No.
		CLINICIAN:	Oh, see if she does?
		CLIENT:	Linda, where's you project?
Violating routines ("Silly rabbit")	Imperatives, directives	CLINICIAN:	Here's your sandwich.
		CLIENT:	Nothing in it.
		CLINICIAN:	Oh you must like different sandwiches than I do. What do you want?
		CLIENT:	Peanut butter.
		CLINICIAN:	How do I do it (there's your opener)

Technique	Target	Example
Nonblabbermouth	Requests for information	CLINICIAN: (Place interesting object in front of child) Boy, is this neat. CLIENT: What is it? CLINICIAN: A flibbideejibbit (Now *STOP*. Don't give anymore info.) CLIENT: What's it do?
What I have	Request for action	CLINICIAN: Oh I can't wait to show you what I have in this bag. It's really neat. (Wait client out)
Guess what I did	Request for information Past tense verbs	CLINICIAN: Guess what I did yesterday in the park. CLIENT: Jogged? Picked flowers? Had a picnic?
Mumble	Contingent query	At height of an interesting story or punchline of a joke, clinician should mumble so that child does not receive message. If needed, increase pressure by asking questions on what was just said.
Ask someone else	Request for information	CLINICIAN: What do you need? CLIENT: Sugar. CLINICIAN: I don't know where it is. Why don't you ask Sally where the sugar is.
Rule giving	Request for objects	CLINICIAN: I have the athletic equipment for recess. If you need some, just ask me. CLIENT: I want jump rope.
Request for assistance	Initiating conversation	CLINICIAN: John, can you ask Keith to help me.
Modeling with meaningful intent	I want _____	CLINICIAN: We have lots of colored paper for our project. Now let's see who needs some. I want a green one. (Take one and wait) CLIENT: I want blue.
"Screw up" #1	Locatives Prepositions	CLINICIAN: Can you help me dress this doll. (Place shoe on doll's head) How's that? CLIENT: No. The shoe goes *on* the doll's foot. CLINICIAN: But now the foots all gone. CLIENT: No. Its *in* the shoe.
"Screw up" #2	Negative statements	CLINICIAN: Here's your snack. (Give child a pencil) CLIENT: That's not a snack.
Request for topic	Statements	CLINICIAN: Now let's talk about your birthday party. (Not shared information)
Expansion of child utterance into desired form	Infinitives	CLIENT: I want paste crayon. CLINICIAN: You want crayon to *sing with?* CLIENT: No, to color. CLINICIAN: What? CLIENT: I want crayon to color.

G
Intervention Activities and Language Targets

Targets

Activities	Vocabulary	Word association	Auditory processing and memory	Variety of pragmatic features	Conversational repair	Presupposition	Register	Categorization	Topic introduction and maintenance	Turn taking	Sequencing	Giving directions	Following directions	Interrogatives	Negatives	Requests for information	Requests for assistance	Requests for objects	Prepositions/spatial terms	Articles and/or demonstratives	Pronouns	Adverbs	Adjectives/descriptive words	Verb tensing	Plurals	Nouns
Barrier tasks			X			X					X	X	X													
Body tracing	X										X	X	X				X		X				X	X		
Colorforms								X											X	X			X	X		
*Cooking	X											X	X	X		X	X	X					X	X	X	X
Describing pictures that others can not see						X														X			X			X
Dolls, clothing, and furniture	X						X												X				X		X	X
Dressing												X	X					X	X	X	X		X	X	X	X
Dress-up				X			X												X				X		X	
Explaining "how-to"					X	X		X	X		X	X			X							X	X			
Farm or zoo play	X					X			X		X	X	X		X										X	X
Guiding others through an activity						X						X	X						X							
Treasure Hunt- "You're getting warmer..."																										
Interviewing					X		X		X	X				X		X										
"I see something that's..."		X												X		X			X				X			
Jeopardy		X												X	X	X										
Kitchen play	X			X					X	X							X	X					X			

*See page 378.

Activity																			
*Making things	X	X	X	X	X	X	X	X	X	X	X	X	X	X					X
Map following	X			X	X	X	X												
Mime				X	X	X	X	X	X	X	X					X			
My "ME" book	X	X													X	X			
Music and action songs								X	X										
Nature or science activity	X		X	X	X	X	X	X	X	X	X	X	X	X	X			X	X
Obstacle course	X	X				X	X	X			X								
Planning an activity	X	X	X	X	X	X					X	X	X					X	X
Planting seeds	X	X	X	X	X	X		X										X	X
Playhouse	X	X			X														
Playing teacher				X	X	X		X	X	X	X	X	X					X	
Pretend shopping	X	X				X	X	X	X	X	X	X		X				X	
Puppet show			X						X	X		X							X
Putting objects in order	X		X							X		X		X					
"Safety Town" (Safety curriculum for preschool and kindergarten)			X	X	X	X	X		X	X	X		X					X	
Simon says					X	X	X	X			X							X	
Simulated restaurant			X	X	X	X	X	X										X	
Sorting clothing	X	X	X	X	X														
Story-telling (true or make-believe)			X	X	X	X	X	X			X	X	X					X	X
Telephone play			X	X	X	X	X				X	X	X	X		X		X	X
TV commercials	X			X	X	X	X	X			X	X	X	X	X	X	X		
"Twenty questions" variations	X		X	X	X	X												X	
Washing dishes	X	X	X	X	X	X	X	X			X	X	X					X	
"What am I?"	X		X	X	X	X	X	X		X	X	X	X	X					X
"What did you do when. . . ?"	X		X	X	X	X	X	X		X	X	X	X	X				X	X

*See page 378.

* Possible cooking activities:

1. Cookies, cupcakes, muffins
2. Cornbread and butter
3. Edible honeybees - Mix 1/2 cup peanut butter, 1 T. plus 1/3 cup honey, 2 T. sesame seeds, and 2 T. toasted wheat germ. Roll into balls. Make stripes on the bee by dipping a toothpick in cocoa powder and pressing into ball. Use slivered almonds for wings.
4. English muffin pizzas
5. Fruit salad - Use a few vegetables just to confuse the issue and to elicit some language.
6. Ice cream sundaes
7. Instant pudding
8. Milkshakes - Lots of variations here, such as vanilla, chocolate, and banana (use real ones in the blender).
9. Peanut butter and jelly sandwiches
10. Peanut butter balls - Mix 1/2 cup honey, 1/2 cup peanut butter, 1 cup dry milk, and 1 cup oatmeal. Roll into balls. Refrigerate.
11. Peanut butter "face" sandwiches - Make faces on the bread with a peanut butter base using raisins (eyes), peanut (nose), chocolate chips (mouth), and carrot slivers or coconut (hair).
12. Picnic lunch
13. Popcorn and popcorn balls

** Things to make:

1. Cereal box instrument - Use a strong cereal box with a circular hole cut in the face similar to the hole in a guitar. Stretch various size rubber bands around the box and tack them into wooden blocks that act as bridges.
2. Costumes from grocery bags - Cut eye holes or a hole for face. Cut arm holes if desired. Decorate bag. Slip over child.
3. Cowgirl and cowboy outfits from grocery bags - Bags can easily be cut to resemble vests and yokes. Be sure to fringe them. Add a bandana and you have the outfit.
4. Decorate a shoebox "room" with scraps of wallpaper.
5. Food sculptures - Use shredded coconut or lettuce, raisins, peanuts, M & Ms, hot cinnamon candies, cheese strips, fruit halves, celery and carrot sticks, olives, marshmallows, gum drops, and toothpicks.
6. Holiday cards
7. Kites
8. Paper bag puppets
9. Paper butterflies
10. Paper flowers
11. Playdough - Mix 2 cups flour, 1 cup water, 1 T. salad oil, 1 cup salt, and food coloring.
12. Potato and sponge prints
13. Sachets - Cloves and crumbled bay leaves and cinnamon sticks in square of cloth. Pull ends of cloth together and tie with a ribbon.
14. Snowmen and snowwomen - Use styrofoam balls, pipecleaners, cloves, and toothpicks.
15. Stained glass windows - Cut out a cardboard mold. Tape aluminum foil over one side of the cut-out sections. Place this side down. Fill the holes with Elmer's glue. Swirl in food coloring. Allow to dry thoroughly. Peel foil. Hang in sunny window.

Note: A variety of language features can be elicited within these activities by using the indirect elicitation techniques in Appendix F and the nonlinguistic strategies in Chapter 8.

H
Analyzing Classroom Communication Breakdown

The following questions can serve as a guideline to the teacher in determining where students are failing in formal communicative interactions in the classroom. Several different interactions should be analyzed to get an overall perspective of the child's linguistic abilities, cognitive status, and communicative competence.

Language

Phonologic System

- [ ] Has the child acquired the rules that govern the sounds of the language being used? (e.g., Does Jim make different articulation errors each time he speaks?)
- [ ] How successful is the child in understanding spoken utterances? (e.g., Does Mary know that *cat* and *rat* are two different words?)
- [ ] How successful is the child in producing spoken utterances? (e.g., To what degree is the child unintelligible?)

Semantic System

- [ ] Is the child familiar with the vocabulary being used by the teacher? Has he or she heard these words before in similar situations? in different situations? (e.g., Does Joan know this is an angle without someone pointing to it?)
- [ ] Do the vocabulary items have meaning for the child? Do the words have meaning only in specific contexts or does the child understand the word in all contexts? (e.g., Does Joan know what an angle is?)
- [ ] Does the child have word-finding difficulties for familiar vocabulary items? for new words? (e.g., Are there hesitations or word substitutions when Jackie speaks?)

Syntactic System

- ☐ Has the child acquired the rules that govern word order and other aspects of grammar? (e.g., Does Mary understand subject-verb agreement?)
- ☐ Is the child familiar with the grammatical form being used by the teacher? Has he or she heard this form in similar situations? in different situations? (e.g., Does Dan know who is doing the hitting in the sentence ''Mary was hit by Tom''?)
- ☐ Is the grammatical form that is being used meaningful to the child? Does the child understand the relationships that exist among the lexical items in the utterance? (e.g., Does Marie know why the sentence ''The desk stepped on my toes'' is anomalous?)
- ☐ Does the child have access to the grammatical form needed to express his or her response? (e.g., How adequately does Tommy express himself on a topic of his interest?)

Pragmatics—Functional Use or Intent?

- ☐ Does the child know the rules for communicative intent that govern social interactions at home? at school? (e.g., Who talks when and under what conditions?)
- ☐ Does the child know the rules for politeness?
- ☐ Does the child know when to make eye contact?
- ☐ Does the child know how close it is permissible to stand when talking to another person?
- ☐ Does the child know when to raise his or hand for recognition?
- ☐ Does the child know that it is helpful to the learning process to request clarification of new information?
- ☐ Does the child know how to interpret both direct and indirect requests?

Thinking

Information Processing

- ☐ Is the child's attention span long enough to attend to a stimulus utterance or event? (e.g., Does Bobbie watch the teacher when he or she holds a pencil up?)
- ☐ Does the child attend to so many environmental stimuli that he or she is unable to focus on a single one? (e.g., Is Mary constantly turning to look when noises or movements occur?)
- ☐ Is the child's sensory input reduced or distorted?
- ☐ What is the length of the child's short-term memory? Is it long enough for the child to hold the utterance to decode it? (e.g., Can Georgia remember a list of things to buy at the play store?)
- ☐ Does the child spontaneously rehearse or use mnemonic devices to aid short-term memory? If the child does not rehearse spontaneously, can he or she be taught to use such strategies?
- ☐ Does the child have a backlog of experiences against which to judge new information? (e.g., ''Kay, have ever been to a farm to see a cow?'')

☐ Is the child's long-term memory functionally accessible? (e.g., ''Do you remember your phone number, Tim?'')

☐ Does the child form associations between new and previously stored information? Is the new information integrated with the old? (e.g., ''What does this new ball look like? Isn't it just like the one we saw at the soccer game?'')

☐ Is retrieval from long-term memory impaired?

☐ Does the child spontaneously evaluate the quality of the information received and the response being formulated?

Conceptual information

☐ Has the child had enough previous experience to interpret conceptual notions correctly? (e.g., Has the child had experience with blocks of different shapes before being asked to classify them?)

☐ If not, has the previous experience been deficient in the quantity of experiences or in the appropriateness or variety of concept instances?

☐ Does the child have difficulty in expressing the conceptual relationships required by the situation? (e.g., Has the child been given the language to use to talk about squares and rectangles?)

Integration and association of information

☐ Is the child able to integrate new information into old, previously stored information?

☐ Is the child able to make use of integrated or associated information provided by the teacher? (e.g., Can the child use analogies provided by the teacher?)

☐ Is the child able to formulate a response that demonstrates that integration of information has taken place?

The consequence of going through an analysis of this sort is having the information needed to modify classroom interactions to make them better situations for learning. Modifications might be in teacher language, topics or content, and the context of the interaction. The assessment by the teacher can be developed into an ongoing activity that provides continuing feedback on the success of interactions as learning situations. For children with language disorders, such interactive assessment in the classroom setting provides the opportunity for linguistic experience appropriate to the level of functioning and in an amount that is not possible under traditional models of intervention.

Source: Vetter, D. (1982) Language Disorders and Schooling. Reprinted from *Topics in Language Disorders*, Vol. 2, No. 4 (pp. 17–19), with permission of Aspen Publishers, Inc., © 1982.

I
Definitions of Illocutionary and Semantic Functions

Functions	Examples
Semantic	
Nomination—naming a person or object using a single- or multiword name or a demonstrative-plus as a name	Doggie, Choo-choo This horsie
Location—marking spatial relationships Utterances may contain single location words or two-word utterances containing an agent, action, or object plus a location word. The function can be demonstrated in response to *where* questions.	PARTNER: Where's Doggie? CLIENT: Chair. Ball table, Doggie chair, Throw me, Throw here (*X* + locative)
Negation—marking of nonexistence, rejection, and denial using single negative words or a negative followed by another word (negative + *X*)	
Nonexistence generally develops first and marks the absence of a once-present object.	All gone (count as a single word), Away, No milk (client drank it), All gone car (the ride is over), No
Rejection marks an attempt to prevent or to stop an event.	PARTNER: Time for bed. CLIENT: No (or No bed) Stop it. No milk (pushes glass away)
Denial marks rejection of a proposition	PARTNER: See the bear? CLIENT: No bear.

(continued)

Functions	Examples

Modification

    Possession—appreciating that an object belongs to or is frequently associated with someone. Single-word utterances signal the owner's name. In two-word utterances, stress is usually on the initial word, the possessor. — Mine, My dollie, Johnnie bike (modifier + head) Dollie (client clutches doll)

    Attribution—using descriptors for properties not inherently part of the object — Yukky, Big doggie, Little baby (modifier + head)

    Recurrence—understanding that an object can reappear or an event can be reenacted — More, More milk, 'Nuther cookie (modifier + head)

Notice—signaling that an object has appeared, an event has happened, or an attempt to gain attention — Hi Mommy, Bye-bye, Look Jim

Action—marking an activity

    Action—single-action words — Jump, Eat

    Agent + Action—two-word signal that an animate initiated an activity — Mommy throw, Doggie eat, Baby sleep

    Action + Object—two-word signal that an animate or inanimate object was the recipient of action — Eat cookie, Throw ball

Illocutionary

Answer—client responds to questions. The questioner's behaviors are a cue for the client's response; the response probably would not be produced without this cue. The client's responses are cognitively related to the question, although they may be incorrect.

    PARTNER (*holding doll*): What's this?
    CLIENT: Baby

    PARTNER: Is this a mirror?
    CLIENT: No

Question—client asks for information or verification by addressing the other person verbally. The client's behavior is a stimulus or cue and indicates that he expects an answer. The client can ask himself questions when engaged in egocentric play.

    CLIENT (*picks up toy telephone*): Phone?
    CLIENT: What this?

Reply—client makes meaningful response to the content of the other speaker's previous utterance, a verbal cue external to the client. The client may continue to build on the content and ignore the form of the utterance, such as responding to a word or thought in a question without answering the question. In many cases, the client will build on the content *and* respond with an appropriate form. This category does not include mere repetition.

    PARTNER: Johnny, bring me the scissors. (command)
    CLIENT: No.

    PARTNER: May I have the keys? (request)
    CLIENT: In a minute.

    PARTNER: This is a cute dog. (declaration)
    CLIENT: My doggie.

Functions	Examples
Elicitation—client self-repeats in response to a request for repetition or clarification or in response to "Say *x*."	CLIENT: Kitty go. (declaration) PARTNER: What? CLIENT: Kitty go. PARTNER: Mary, say "ball." CLIENT: Ball.
Continuant—client signals that he is listening and wants to continue the interchange, or that he missed what was said.	Uh-huh, Okay. I see, yes. What? Huh?
Declaration—client makes a statement that is situationally related and for communication but is not in response to another speaker. The utterance is more like a commentary. Cues are internal or situational but not verbal. This category also includes situationally related phonemic exclamations.	CLIENT (*playing game with mother and glances out*): It raining out. CLIENT (*playing with car*): Car go up. PARTNER: This is a cute doggie. CLIENT: My doggie. (reply) He lives in a house. (declaration) PARTNER: This is a cute doggie. CLIENT: My doggie. (reply) I have kitty, too. (declaration)
Practice—client repeats or imitates in whole or part what he or another person says with no change in intonation that would indicate a change of intent. In addition, internal replay without added new information is considered *practice*. This category also includes counting, singing, babbling, or rhyming behaviors in which the client seems to be experimenting or rehearsing.	PARTNER: Ball. CLIENT: Ball. PARTNER: See the red ball. CLIENT: Red ball. PARTNER: See the red ball. CLIENT: See ball. (practice) Ball, ball, ball. (practice)
Perseverative responses, even if the other person interjects an utterance between them, are considered *practice* as long as they do not mark discrete events or objects.	
Name—client labels an object or event that is present, but the label is not in response to a question. This verbal behavior is usually accomplished by pointing or nodding.	CLIENT (*picks up ball*): Ball. CLIENT (*points to ball*): That ball.
Suggestion, Command, Demand, Request—The primary function of the client's utterance is to influence another person's behavior by getting that person to do something or to give the client permission. The form may be imperative, declarative, or interrogative.	CLIENT: Gimmie cookie. CLIENT: Stop that. CLIENT: Mommy. CLIENT: Throw ball. (*parent throws ball*) Throw ball. (*parent throws ball*) Throw ball.

Source: Owens, R. (1982). From the manual for the *Program for the acquisition of language with the severely impaired*. Copyright © 1982 by The Psychological Corporation. Adapted by permission. All rights reserved.

Glossary

Assimilation Phonological process in which a child changes one syllable to make it more like another, as in *doddie* (/d di/) for *doggie*.

Augmentative communication Communication other than verbal that may complement or supplement verbal means.

Construct validity Accuracy with which or extent to which a measure describes or measures some trait or construct.

Content generalization Carryover of the learned entity to untrained content.

Content validity Faithfulness with which a sample or measure represents some attribute or behavior.

Context generalization Carryover of the learned entity to novel situations.

Contingency Relatedness of an utterance to the previous utterance. Contingency may relate to meaning (semantic contingency) and/or intention or purpose (pragmatic contingency) of the previous utterance.

Contingent query Request for clarification.

Contrast training Training method that teaches a child to discriminate between structures and situations that obligate use of the feature being trained and those features that do not.

Copula Verb *to be* used as a main verb.

Criterion validity Effectiveness or accuracy with which a measure predicts success.

Deixis Process of using the speaker's perspective as a reference.

Discriminative stimulus (S^D) A stimulus in the presence of which the trainee will be reinforced for a correct response. For example, in the presence of the phone ringing, one is reinforced for answering it by the party on the other end.

Ellipsis Omission of known or shared information in subsequent utterances in which it would be redundant.

Generalization Carryover of learning to untrained content and/or novel situations; an interaction of the learner, the learned content, and the context or environment.

Illocutionary function Intention(s) of a speaker.

Incidental teaching   Training within everyday activities and contexts with everyday partners as teachers.

Internal consistency   Degree of relationship among items and the overall test.

Linguistic context   Verbal features of the context that precede, accompany, and follow a verbalization.

Minimal pairs   Two words that differ by only one phoneme that signals a difference of meaning.

Minimally symbolic   Highest level of functioning is the use of symbols singularly or in limited combinations.

Modal   Auxiliary or helping verb that expresses mood or a feeling toward the main verb. Examples include *may, might, must, will, should, could,* and *would.*

Nonlinguistic context   Features of the context, other than linguistic ones, that precede, accompany, and follow a verbalization. The non-linguistic context of an utterance or verbalization is what is happening in the environment at the time of the verbalization.

Presupposition The speaker's assumption about the knowledge level of the listener or what the listener knows and needs to know.

Presymbolic   Prior to the use of symbols in the form of words, signs, pictures, and the like.

Reduplication   A phonological process in which a child changes one syllable in a two-syllable word to repeat another syllable, as in *mama* or *wawa* (water).

Referential communication Speaker selects and verbally identifies attributes of an entity, thereby enabling the listener to identify the entity accurately.

Reliability   Repeatability of a measure based on the accuracy or precision with which a sample, at one time, represents performance based on either a different but similar sample or the same sample at a different time.

Representativeness   Degree to which a sample reflects the general feature being measured.

Script   Basic sequential notion of familiar events.

Semantic function   Meaning(s) of a speaker.

Standard error of measure (SEm)   The statistical error inherent in a score, representing the range that a score may indicate.

Story grammar   Organizational pattern of narratives.

Strategy-based intervention Training that teaches the child information processing and problem-solving strategies.

Systems model   Intervention that targets the child's interactive systems or contexts.

Transparency   "Guessability" of an augmentative symbol.

T-units (Minimal terminal units)   A main clause plus any attached or embedded subordinate clause or nonclausal structure.

Turnabout   Contingent utterance(s) that acknowledges the partner's previous utterance and cues the partner for the next response.

Validity   Effectiveness of a test in representing, describing, or predicting an attribute. A test's ability to assess what it purports to measure.

References

Adler, S. (1973). The non-verbal child (3rd ed.). Springfield, IL: Charles C Thomas.

Adler, S. (1988). A new job description and a new task for the public school clinician: Relating effectively to the nonstandard dialect speaker. *Language, Speech, and Hearing Services in Schools, 19*, 28–33.

Alley, G., & Deshler, D. (1979). *Teaching the learning disabled adolescent: Strategies and methods.* Denver: Love Publishing.

Alpert, C., & Rogers-Warren, A. (1984). *Mothers as incidental language trainers of their language-disordered children.* Unpublished manuscript, University of Kansas, Lawrence.

Ames, L. (1966). Children's stories. *Genetic Psychological Monographs, 73*, 307–311.

Anderson, G., & Nelson, N. (1988). Integrating language intervention and education in an alternate adolescent language classroom. *Seminars in Speech and Language, 9*, 341–353.

Andrews, J., Andrews, M., & Shearer, W. (1989). Parents' attitudes toward involvement in speech-language services. *Language, Speech, and Hearing Services in Schools, 20*, 391–399.

Andrews, N., & Fey, M. (1986). Analysis of the speech of phonologically impaired children in two sampling conditions. *Language, Speech, and Hearing Services in Schools, 17*, 187–198.

Anselmi, D., Tomasello, M., & Acunzo, M. (1986). Young children's responses to neutral and specific contingent queries. *Journal of Child Language, 13*, 135–144.

Applebee, A. (1978). *The child's concept of story.* Chicago: University of Chicago Press.

Argyle, M., & Cook, M. (1976). *Gaze and mutual gaze.* Cambridge, MA: Harvard University Press.

Arwood, E. (1983). *Pragmaticism: Theory and application.* Rockville, MD: Aspen.

Atkins, C., & Cartwright, L. (1982). An investigation of the effectiveness of three elicitation procedures on Head Start children. *Language, Speech, and Hearing Services in Schools, 13*, 33–36.

Baer, R., Williams, J., Osnes, P., & Stokes, T. (1984). Delayed reinforcement as an indiscriminable contingency in verbal/nonverbal correspondence training. *Journal of Applied Behavior Analysis, 17*, 29–44.

Baggett, P. (1979). Structurally equivalent stories in movies and text and the effect of medium on recall. *Journal of Verbal Learning and Verbal Behavior, 18*, 333–356.

Baker, B. (1976). Parent involvement in programming for the developmentally disabled child. In L. Lloyd (Ed.), *Communication assessment and intervention* (pp. 691–733). Baltimore: University Park Press.

Baker, B., Murphy, D., Heifitz, L., & Brightman, A. (1975). *Parents as teachers: Followup after 18 months.* Cambridge, MA: Behavioral Education Projects.

Bankson, N. (1977). Bankson Language Screening Test. Baltimore: University Park Press.

Barnes, S., Gutfreund, M., Satterly, D., & Wells, G. (1983). Characteristics of adult speech which predict children's language development. *Journal of Child Development, 10,* 65–84.

Barrett, M. (1983). The early acquisition and development of the meanings of action-related words. In T. Seiler & W. Wannenmacher (Eds.), *Concept development and development of word meaning.* New York: Springer-Verlag.

Bashir, A. (1987). Language and curriculum. Paper presented at the Language Learning Disabilities Institute, Emerson College, Boston.

Bates, E. (1976). Pragmatics and sociolinguistics in child language. In D. Morehead & A. Morehead (Eds.), *Normal and deficient child language* (pp. 411–463). Baltimore: University Park Press.

Bates, E. (1979). *The emergence of symbols.* New York: Academic Press.

Bates, E., Bretherton, I., Shore, C., & McNew, S. (1983). Names, gestures, & objects: The role of context in the emergence of symbols. In K. Nelson (Ed.), *Children's language: Vol. 4* (pp. 59–123). Hillsdale, NJ: Erlbaum.

Bates, E., & MacWhinney, B. (1982). Functionalist approaches to grammar. In E. Wanner & L. Gleitman (Eds.), *Language acquisition: The state of the art.* New York: Cambridge University Press.

Bateson, M. (1975). Mother-infant exchanges: The epigenesis of conversational interaction. *Annals of the New York Academy of Sciences, 263,* 101–113.

Battles, D. (1990, March). *Black dialects.* Paper presented at the Spring Workshop of the Genesee Valley Speech-Language-Hearing Association, Rochester, NY.

Bayley, N. (1969). The Bayley Scales of Infant Development. San Antonio: Psychological Corporation, Harcourt Brace Jovanovich.

Beckwith, L., Cohen, S., Kopp, C., Parmelee, A., & Marcy, T. (1976). Caregiver-infant interaction and early cognitive development in preterm infants. *Child Development, 47,* 579–587.

Bedrosian, J. (1982). A sociolinguistic approach to communication skills: Assessment and treatment methodology for mentally retarded adults. Unpublished doctoral dissertation, University of Wisconsin.

Bedrosian, J. (1984). Conversational development. In W. Perkins (Ed.), *Current therapy in communication disorders: Language handicaps in children* (pp. 95–103). New York: Thieme-Stratton.

Bedrosian, J. (1985). An approach to developing conversational competence. In D. Ripich & F. Spinelli (Eds.), *School discourse problems.* San Diego: College Hill Press.

Bedrosian, J. (1988). Adults who are mildly to moderately mentally retarded: Communicative performance, assessment, and intervention. In S. Calculator & J. Bedrosian (Eds.), *Communication assessment and intervention for adults with mental retardation* (pp. 265–307). San Diego: College-Hill.

Bedrosian, J., & Willis, T. (1987). Effects of treatment on the topic performance of a school-age child. *Language, Speech, and Hearing Services in Schools, 18,* 158–167.

Benedict, H. (1979). Early lexical development: Comprehension and production. *Journal of Child Language, 6,* 183–200.

Berko Gleason, J. (1971). Berko's Test of the Child's Learning of English Morphology. In A. Bar-Adon & W. Leopold (Eds.), *Child language: A book of readings* (pp. 153–167). Englewood Cliffs, NJ: Prentice-Hall.

Bernstein, D. (1989). Assessing children with limited English proficiency: Current prospectives. *Topics in Language Disorders, 9*(3), 15–20.

Beukelman, D., Jones, R., & Rowan, M. (1989). Frequency of word usage by nondisabled peers in integrated preschool classrooms. *Augmentative and Alternative Communication, 5,* 243–248.

Beukelman, D., Yorkston, K., & Dowden, P. (1985). *Communication augmentation: A casebook of clinical management.* San Diego: College-Hill.

Biber, D. (1986). Spoken and written textual dimensions in English: Resolving the contradictory findings. *Language, 62,* 384–414.

Bishop, D., & Edmundson, A. (1987). Language-impaired 4-year-olds: Distinguishing transient from persistent impairment. *Journal of Speech and Language Disorders, 52,* 156–173.

Bjorkland, D., Ornstein, P., & Haig, J. (1975, April). Development of organizational patterns in free recall: The effects of training in categorization. Paper presented at the biennial meeting of the Society for Research in Child Development, Denver.

Blache, S., & Parsons, C. (1980). A linguistic approach to distinctive feature training. *Language, Speech, and Hearing Services in Schools, 4,* 203–207.

Blache, S., Parsons, C., & Humphreys, J. (1981). A minimal word-pair model for teaching the linguistic significance of distinctive feature properties. *Journal of Speech and Hearing Disorders, 46,* 291–295.

Blake, I. (1984). Language development in working-class black children: An examination of form, content, and use. Unpublished doctoral dissertation, Columbia University, New York City.

Blank, M. (1980). Cognitive functions of language in the preschool years. *Developmental Psychology, 10,* 229–245.

Blank, M., & Franklin, E. (1980). Dialogue with preschoolers: A cognitively-based system of assessment. *Applied Psycholinguistics, 1,* 127–150.

Blank, M., Gessner, M., & Esposito, A. (1979). Language without communication. *Journal of Child Language, 6,* 329–352.

Blank, M., & Marquis, A. (1987). *Directing discourse: 80 situations for teaching meaningful conversations to children.* Tucson, AZ: Communication Skill Builders.

Blank, M., Rose, S., & Berlin, L. (1978). *The language of learning.* New York: Grune & Stratton.

Blau, A. (1983). Vocabulary selection in augmentative communication: Where do we begin? In H. Winitz (Ed.), *Treating language disorders: For clinicians by clinicians.* Baltimore: University Park Press.

Blau, A., Lahey, M., & Oleksiuk-Velez, A. (1984). Planning goals for intervention: Language testing or language sampling? *Exceptional Children, 51,* 78–79.

Blaxley, L., Clinker, M., & Warr-Leeper, G. (1983). Two language screening tests compared with Developmental Sentence Scoring. *Language, Speech, and Hearing Services in Schools, 14,* 38–46.

Bliss, L. (1987). "I can't talk anymore; my mouth doesn't want to." The development and clinical applications of modal auxiliaries. *Language, Speech, and Hearing Services in Schools, 18,* 72–79.

Bloom, L., & Lahey, M. (1978). *Language development and language disorders.* New York: Wiley.

Bloom, L., Lahey, M., Hood, L., Lifter, K., & Fiess, K. (1980). Complex sentences: Acquisition of syntactic connectives and the semantic relations they encode. *Journal of Child Language, 7,* 235–261.

Bloom, L., Rocissano, L., & Hood, L. (1976). Adult-child discourse: Developmental interaction between information processing and linguistic knowledge. *Cognitive Psychology, 8,* 521–522.

Bonderman, I. (1987). *Handbook for phonological preschool.* Fountain Valley, CA: Fountain Valley School District, Rush Printing.

Bowman, S. (1984). A review of referential communication skills. *Australian Journal of Human Communication Disorders, 12,* 93–112.

Boyd, R., Stauber, K., & Bluma, S. (1977). *The portage parent program: Instructor's manual.* Portage, WI: Cooperation Educational Service Agency 12.

Bracken, B. (1988). Rate and sequence of positive and negative poles in basic concept acquisition. *Language, Speech, and Hearing Services in Schools, 19,* 410–417.

Bradley, R., & Caldwell, B. (1976). The relation of infants' home environments to mental test performance at 54 months: A follow-up study. *Child Development, 47,* 1172–1174.

Bray, C. (1982). *The learning disabled child and how relative is the relative pronoun in embedded sentence constructions.* Unpublished manuscript, Psycholinguistics Research Seminar, Boston University.

Bray, C., & Wiig, E. (1987). *Let's talk inventory for children.* San Antonio, TX: Psychological Corporation.

Bretherton, I. & Beeghly, M. (1982). Talking about internal states: The acquisition of an explicit theory of mind. *Developmental Psychology, 18,* 906–921.

Bricker, W., & Bricker, D. (1974). An early language training strategy. In R. Schiefelbusch &

L. Lloyd (Eds.), *Language perspectives-acquisition, retardation, and intervention* (pp. 431–468). Baltimore: University Park Press.

Brinton, B., & Fujiki, M. (1982). A comparison of request-response sequences in the discourse of normal and language-disordered children. *Journal of Speech and Hearing Disorders, 47,* 57–62.

Brinton, B., & Fujiki, M. (1989). *Conversational management with language-impaired children.* Rockville, MD: Aspen.

Brinton, B., Fujiki, M., & Sonnenberg, E. (1988). Responses to requests for clarification by linguistically normal and language-impaired children in conversation. *Journal of Speech and Hearing Disorders, 53,* 383–391.

Brinton, B., Fujiki, M., Winkler, E., & Loeb, D. (1986). Responses to requests for clarification in linguistically normal and language-impaired children. *Journal of Speech and Hearing Disorders, 51,* 370–378.

Brown, A., & Campione, J. (1984). Three faces of transfer: Implication for early competence, individual difference, and instruction. In M. Lamb, A. Brown, & B. Rogoff (Eds.), *Advances in developmental psychology: Vol. 3* (pp. 143–192). Hillsdale, NJ: Erlbaum.

Brown, A., Kane, M., & Echols, C. (1986). Young children's mental models determine analogical transfer across problems with a common goal structure. *Cognitive development, 1,* 103–125.

Brown, J. (1989). The truth about scores children achieve on tests. *Language, Speech, and Hearing Services in Schools, 20,* 366–371.

Brown, L., Branston, M., Hamre-Nietupski, S., Pumpian, I., Certo, N., & Gruenewald, L. (1979). A strategy for developing chronological age appropriate and functional curricular content for severely handicapped adolescents and young adults. *Journal of Special Education, 13,* 81–90.

Brown, L., Nietupski, J., & Hamre-Nietupski, S. (1976). Criterion of ultimate functioning. In M. Thomas (Ed.), *Hey, don't forget about me! Education's investment in the severely, profoundly and multiply handicapped* (pp. 16–35). Reston, VA: Division of Mental Retardation, The Council for Exceptional Children.

Brown, L., Shiraga, B., Rogan, P., York, J., Zanella Albright, K., McCarthy, E., Loomis, R., & Van-

Deventer, P. (1988). The "why" question in instruction programs for people who are severely intellectually disabled. In S. Calculator & J. Bedrosian (Eds.), *Communication assessment and intervention for adults with mental retardation* (pp. 139–153). San Diego: College-Hill.

Brown, L., Sweet, M., Shiraga, B., York, J., Zanella, K., & Rogan, P. (1984). *Educational programs for students with severe handicaps: Vol. 14.* Madison, WI: Madison Metropolitan School District.

Brown, R. (1973). *First language.* Cambridge, MA: Harvard University Press.

Bruner, J. (1975). The ontogenesis of speech acts. *Journal of Child Language, 2,* 1–20.

Bruner, J. (1978). Acquiring the uses of language. Paper presented as Berlyne Memorial Lecture, University of Toronto.

Bryan, T., Donahue, M., & Pearl, R. (1981). Learning disabled children's peer interaction during a small group problem-solving task. *Learning Disability Quarterly, 4,* 13–22.

Bryan, T., Donahue, M., Pearl, R., & Herzog, A. (1981). *Mother-learning disabled child conversational interactions during a problem-solving task.* Chicago: Chicago Institute for the Study of Learning Disabilities.

Bryen, D., & Joyce, D. (1985). Language intervention with the severely handicapped: A decade of research. *The Journal of Special Education, 19,* 7–39.

Buium, N., Rynders, J., & Turnure, J. (1974). Early maternal linguistic environment of normal and Down's syndrome language-learning children. *American Journal of Mental Deficiency, 79,* 52–58.

Bullowa, M. (1979). Introduction; Prelinguistic communication: A field for scientific research. In M. Bullowa (Ed.), *Before speech* (pp. 1–62). New York: Cambridge University Press.

Bunce, B. (1989). Using a barrier game format to improve children's referential communication skills. *Journal of Speech and Hearing Disorders, 54,* 33–43.

Bunce, B., Ruder, K., & Ruder, C. (1985). Using the miniature linguistic system in teaching syntax: Two case studies. *Journal of Speech and Hearing Disorders, 50,* 247–253.

Buttrill, J., Niizawa, J., Biemer, C., Takahashi, C., & Hearn, S. (1989). Serving the language learning disabled adolescent: A strategies-based model. *Language, Speech, and Hearing Services in Schools, 20,* 185–204.

Buzolich, M., & Wiemann, J. (1988). Turn-taking in atypical conversations: The case of the speaker/augmented communicator dyad. *Journal of Speech and Hearing Research, 31,* 3–18.

Bzoch, K., & League, R. (1971). *Assessing language skills in infancy.* Baltimore: University Park Press.

Cairns, H., & Hsu, J. (1978). Who, why, when and how: A developmental study. *Journal of Child Language, 5,* 478–488.

Calculator, S. (1985). Describing and treating discourse problems in mentally retarded children: The myth of mental retardese. In D. Ripich & F. Spinelli (Eds.), *School discourse problems* (pp. 125–147). San Diego: College-Hill.

Calculator, S. (1988a). Exploring the language of adults with mental retardation. In S. Calculator & J. Bedrosian (Eds.), *Communication assessment and intervention for adults with mental retardation* (pp. 95–106). San Diego: College-Hill.

Calculator, S. (1988b). Promoting the acquisition and generalization of conversational skills by individuals with severe disabilities. *Augmentative and Alternative Communication, 4,* 94–103.

Calculator, S. (1988c). Teaching functional communication skills to nonspeaking adults with mental retardation. In S. Calculator & J. Bedrosian (Eds.), *Communication assessment and intervention for adults with mental retardation* (pp. 309–338). San Diego: College-Hill.

Calculator, S., & D'Altilio-Luchko, C. (1983). Evaluating the effectiveness of a communication board training program. *Journal of Speech and Hearing Disorders, 48,* 185–192.

Calculator, S., & Delaney, D. (1986). Comparison of nonspeaking and speaking mentally retarded adults clarification strategies. *Journal of Speech and Hearing Research, 51,* 252–259.

Calculator, S., & Dollaghan, C. (1982). The use of communication boards in a residential setting. *Journal of Speech and Hearing Disorders, 14,* 281–287.

Camarata, S. (1989). Final consonant repetition: A linguistic perspective. *Journal of Speech and Hearing Disorders, 54,* 159–162.

Camarata, S., Hughes, C., & Ruhl, K. (1988). Mild/moderate behaviorally disordered students: A population at risk for language disorders. *Language, Speech, and Hearing Services in Schools, 19,* 191–200.

Campbell, T., & Shriberg, L. (1982). Associations among pragmatic functions, linguistic stress, and natural phonological processes in speech-delayed children. *Journal of Speech and Hearing Research, 4,* 547–553.

Caramazza, A., Grober, E., Garvey, C., & Yates, J. (1977). Comprehension of anaphoric pronouns. *Journal of Verbal Learning and Verbal Behavior, 16,* 601–609.

Cardoso-Martins, C., Mervis, C., & Mervis, C. (1985). Early vocabulary acquisition by children with Downs syndrome. *American Journal of Mental Deficiency, 90,* 255–265.

Carlson, F., (1981). A format for selecting vocabulary for the nonspeaking child. *Language, Speech, and Hearing Services in Schools, 12,* 240–245.

Carpenter, A., & Strong, J. (1988). Pragmatic development in normal children: Assessment of a testing protocol. *National Student Speech-Language-Hearing Associational Journal, 12,* 40–49.

Carr, E. (1979). Teaching autistic children to use sign language: Some research issues. *Journal of Autism and Developmental Disorders, 9,* 345–359.

Carr, E., & Durand, V. (1985). Reducing behavior problems through functional communication training. *Journal of Applied Behavior Analysis, 18,* 111–126.

Carr, E., & Kologinsky, E. (1983). Acquisition of sign language by autistic children II: Spontaneity and generalization. *Journal of Applied Behavior Analysis, 16,* 297–314.

Carr, E., & Lovaas, O. (1982). Contingent electric shock as a treatment for severe behavior problems. In S. Axelrod & J. Apsche (Eds.), *The effects of punishment on human behavior* (pp. 221–246). New York: Academic Press.

Carr, E., Newson, C., & Binkhoff, J.(1980). Escape as a factor in the aggressive behavior of two retarded children. *Journal of Applied Behavior Analysis, 13,* 101–117.

Carrow, E. (1973). Test for Auditory Comprehension of Language. Austin, TX: Urban Research Group.

Carrow, E. (1974). Carrow Elicited Language Inventory. Austin, TX: Learning Concepts.

Carson, J. (1987). *Tell me about your picture: Art ac-*

tivities to help children communicate. Englewood Cliffs, NJ: Prentice Hall.

Catts, H., & Kamhi, A. (1986). The linguistic basis of reading disorders: Implications for the speech-language pathologist. *Language, Speech, and Hearing Services in Schools, 17,* 329–341.

Catts, H., & Kamhi, A. (1987). Intervention for reading disabilities. *Journal of Childhood Communication Disorders, 2*(1), 67–80.

Cazden, C. (1972). *Child language and education.* New York: Holt, Rinehart & Winston.

Chafe, W. (1970). *Meaning and the structure of language.* Chicago: University of Chicago Press.

Channell, R., & Peek, M. (1989). Four measures of vocabulary ability compared in older preschool children. *Language, Speech, and Hearing Services in Schools, 20,* 407–417.

Chapman, R. (1981). Exploring childrens' communicative intents. In J. Miller, *Assessing language production in children* (pp. 22–25). Baltimore: University Park Press.

Chapman, R., & Miller, J. (1980). Analyzing language and communication in the child. In R. Schiefelbusch (Ed.), *Nonspeech language and communication: Assessment and intervention* (pp. 159–195). Baltimore: University Park Press.

Chapman, R., Miller, J., MacKenzie, H., & Bedrosian, J. (1981, August). Development of discourse skills in the second year of life. Paper presented at the Second International Congress for the Study of Child Language, Vancouver.

Chapman, K., & Terrell, B. (1988). "Verb-alizing": Facilitating action word usage in young language-impaired children. *Topics in Language Disorders, 8*(2), 1–13.

Chappell, G. (1980). Oral language performance of upper elementary school students obtained via story reformulation. *Language, Speech, and Hearing Services in Schools, 11,* 236–250.

Charhop, M., Schreibman, L., & Thebodeau, M. (1985). Increasing spontaneous verbal responding in autistic children using time delay. *Journal of Applied Behavior Analysis, 18,* 155–166.

Cheng, L. (1987). *Assessing Asian language performance.* Rockville, MD: Aspen.

Cheng, L. (1987, June). Cross-cultural and linguistic considerations in working with Asian populations. *Asha, 29*(6), 33–38.

Cheseldine, S., & McConkey, R. (1979). Parental speech to young Down's syndrome children: An intervention study. *American Journal on Mental Deficiency, 83,* 612–620.

Cheung, D. (Forthcoming). *The Toa of learning: Socialization of Chinese American children.* Unpublished doctoral dissertation, Stanford University.

Christie, D., & Schumacher, G. (1975). Developmental trends in the abstraction and recall of relevant vs. irrelevant thematic information from connected verbal material. *Child Development, 46,* 598–602.

Cimorell, J. (1983). *Language facilitation, a complete cognitive therapy program.* Baltimore: University Park Press.

Cirrin, F., & Rowland, C. (1985). Communication assessment of nonverbal youths with severe/profound mental retardation. *Mental Retardation, 23,* 52–62.

Clancy, P., Jacobsen, T., & Silva, M. (1976). The acquisition of conjunction: A cross-linguistic study. *Papers and reports in child language development, 13,* 71–80. Stanford University Committee on Linguistics.

Clark, C. (1981). Learning words using traditional orthography and the symbols of Rebus, Bliss, and Carrier. *Journal of Speech and Hearing Disorders, 46,* 191–196.

Clark, E. (1973). Non-linguistic strategies and the acquisition of word meanings. *Cognition, 2,* 161–182.

Clark, E., & Andersen, E. (1979). Spontaneous repairs: Awareness in the process of acquiring language. *Papers and Reports on Child Language Development, 16,* 1–12.

Clark, G., & Seifer, R. (1982). Facilitating mother-infant communication: A treatment model for high risk and developmentally delayed infants. *Infant Mental Health Journal, 4*(2), 67–81.

Cochrane, R. (1983). Language and the atmosphere of delight. In H. Winitz (Ed.), *Treating language disorders: For clinicians by clinicians* (pp. 143–162). Baltimore: University Park Press.

Coggins, T., Olswang, L., & Guthrie, J. (1987). Assessing communicative intents in young children: Low structured observation or elicitation tasks? *Journal of Speech and Hearing Disorders, 52,* 44–49.

Cole, D., Vandercook, T., & Rynders, J. (1987). Dyadic interactions between children with and without mental retardation: Effect of age discrepancy. *American Journal of Mental Deficiency, 92,* 194–202.

Cole, K., & Dale, P. (1986). Direct language instruction and interactive language instruction with language delayed preschool children: A comparison study. *Journal of Speech and Hearing Research, 29,* 206–217.

Cole, K., Mills, P., & Dale, P. (1989). Examination of test-retest and split-half reliability for measures derived from language samples of young handicapped children. *Language, Speech, and Hearing Services in Schools, 20,* 259–268.

Cole, M., & Cole, J. (1981). *Effective intervention with the language impaired child.* Rockville, MD: Aspen.

Cole, P. (1982). *Language disorders in preschool children.* Englewood Cliffs, NJ: Prentice Hall.

Cole, P., Harbert, W., Herman, G., & Sridhar, S. (1980). The acquisition of subjecthood. *Language, 56,* 719–743.

Collins, W. (1983). Social antecedents, cognitive processing, and comprehension of social portrayals on television. In E. Higgins, D. Ruble, & W. Hartup (Eds.), *Social cognition and social development* (pp. 110–133). New York: Cambridge University Press.

Collins, W., Wellman, H., Keniston, A., & Westby, S. (1978). Age-related aspects of comprehension and inference from a television dramatic narrative. *Child Development, 49,* 389–399.

Comrie, B. (1976). *Aspects.* New York: Cambridge University Press.

Connell, P. (1982). On training language rules. *Language, Speech, and Hearing Services in Schools, 13,* 231–240.

Connell, P. (1986). Teaching subjecthood to language-disordered children. *Journal of Speech and Hearing Research, 29,* 481–492.

Connell, P. (1987a). An effect of modeling and imitation teaching procedures on childen with and without specific language impairment. *Journal of Speech and Hearing Research, 30,* 105–113.

Connell, P. (1987b). Teaching language rules as solutions to language problems: A baseball analogy. *Language, Speech, and Hearing Services in Schools, 18,* 194–205.

Connell, P. (1988). Induction, generalization, and deduction: Models for defining language generalization. *Language, Speech, and Hearing Services in Schools, 19,* 282–291.

Connell, P., Gardner-Gletty, D., Dejewski, J., & Parks-Reinick, L. (1981). Response to Courtright and Courtright. *Journal of Speech and Hearing Research, 24,* 146–148.

Connell, P., & Myles-Zitler, C. (1982). An analysis of elicited imitation as a language evaluation procedure. *Journal of Speech and Hearing Disorders, 47,* 390–396.

Constable, C. (1983). Creating communicative context. In H. Winitz (Ed.), *Treating language disorders: For clinicians by clinicians* (pp. 97–120). Baltimore: University Park Press.

Constable, C. (1986). The application of scripts in the organization of language intervention contexts. In K. Nelson (Ed.), *First knowledge: Structure and function in development.* Hillsdale, NJ: Erlbaum.

Cook-Gumperz, J. (1977). *Situated instructions: Language socialization of school-age children.* New York: Academic Press.

Cook-Gumperz, J., & Corsaro, W. (1976). *Socioecological constraints on children's communicative strategies.* Papers on language and context. Berkeley Language Behavior Research Laboratory, Working Paper, 46.

Cook-Gumperz, J., & Gumperz, J. (1978). Context in children's speech. In N. Waterson & C. Snow (Eds.), *The development of communication* (pp. 3–23). New York: Wiley.

Cooper, J., & Flowers, C. (1987). Children with a history of acquired aphasia: Residual language and academic impairments. *Journal of Speech and Hearing Disorders, 52,* 251–262.

Cooper, J., Moodley, M., & Reynell, J. (1978). *Helping language development.* New York: St. Martin's Press.

Cooper, J., Moodley, M., & Reynell, J. (1979) The developmental language programme: Results from a five year study. *British Journal of Disorders of Communication, 14,* 57–69.

Corrigan, R. (1975). A scalogram analysis of the development of the use and comprehension of "because" in children. *Child Development, 46,* 195–201.

Cosaro, J. (1989). Activities to enhance listening skills. *Language, Speech, and Hearing Services in Schools, 20,* 433–435.

Costello, J. (1983). Generalization across settings:

Language intervention with children. In J. Miller, D. Yoder, & R. Schiefelbusch (Eds.), *Contempory issues in language intervention* (ASHA Report No. 12) (pp. 275–297). Rockville, MD: American Speech-Language-Hearing Association.

Courtright, J., & Courtright, I. (1976). Imitative modeling as a theoretical base for instructing language-disordered children. *Journal of Speech and Hearing Research, 19,* 655–663.

Courtright, J., & Courtright, I. (1979). Imitative modeling as a language intervention strategy: The effects of two mediating variables. *Journal of Speech and Hearing Research, 22,* 389–402.

Cox, M., & Richardson, J. (1985). How do children describe spatial relationships. *Journal of Child Language, 12,* 611–620.

Craig, H. (1979). A comparison of three-party and two-party conversations of normal children: An examination of increased social complexity. Unpublished doctoral dissertation, University of Michigan, Ann Arbor.

Craig, H. (1983). Applications of pragmatic language models for intervention. In T. Gallagher & C. Prutting (Eds.), *Pragmatic assessment and intervention issues in language* (pp. 101–127). San Diego: College-Hill.

Craig, H., & Evans, J. (1989). Turn exchange characteristics of SLI children's simultaneous and nonsimultaneous speech. *Journal of Speech and Hearing Disorders, 54,* 334–347.

Craig, H., & Washington, J. (1986). Children's turn-taking behaviors: Social-linguistic interactions. *Journal of Pragmatics, 10,* 173–197.

Crais, E., & Chapman, R. (1987). Story recall & inferencing skills in language-learning disabled and nondisabled children. *Journal of Speech and Hearing Disorders, 52,* 50–55.

Creaghead, N. (1984). Strategies for evaluating and targeting pragmatic behaviors in young children. *Seminars in Speech and Language, 5,* 241–251.

Creaghead, N., & Donnelly, K. (1982). Comprehension of superordinate and subordinate information by good and poor readers. *Language, Speech, and Hearing Services in Schools, 13,* 177–186.

Cross, T. (1977). Mothers' speech adjustments: The contribution of selected listener variables. In C. Snow & C. Ferguson (Eds.), *Talk-ing to children: Language input and acquisition* (pp. 151–188). New York: Cambridge University Press.

Cross, T. (1978). Mothers' speech and its association with rate of language acquisition in young children. In N. Waterson & C. Snow (Eds.), *The development of communication* (pp. 199–216). London: Wiley.

Cross, T. (1981). The linguistic experience of slow language learners. In A. Nesdale, C. Pratt, R. Grieve, J. Field, D. Illingworth, & J. Hogben (Eds.), *Advances in child development.* Proceedings of the First National Conference on Child Development, University of Western Australia, Nedlands.

Cross, T. (1984). Habilitating the language-impaired child: Ideas from studies of parent-child interaction. *Topics in Language Disorders, 4*(4), 1–14.

Cross, T., Johnson-Morris, J., & Nienhuys, T. (1980). Linguistic feedback and maternal speech: Comparisons of mothers addressing hearing and hearing-impaired children. *First Language, 1,* 163–189.

Crystal, D., Fletcher, P., & Garman, P. (1976). *The grammatical analysis of language disability.* New York: Elsevier North-Holland.

Culatta, B., & Horn, D. (1982). A program for achieving generalization of grammatical rules to spontaneous discourse. *Journal of Speech and Hearing Disorders, 47,* 174–180.

Culatta, B., Page, J., & Ellis, J. (1983). Story retelling as a communicative performance screening tool. *Language, Speech, and Hearing Services in Schools, 14,* 66–74.

Cunningham, C., Glenn, S., Wilkinson, P., & Sloper, P. (1985). Mental ability, symbolic play and receptive and expressive language of young children with Down's syndrome. *The Journal of Child Psychology and Psychiatry and Applied Disciplines, 26,* 255–265.

Curcio, F., & Paccia-Cooper, J. (1982). Strategies in evaluating autistic children's communication. *Topics in Language Disorders, 3*(1), 43–49.

Dale, P. (1980). Is early pragmatic development measurable? *Journal of Child Development, 7,* 1–12.

Dale, P., & Henderson, V. (1987). An evaluation of the Test of Early Language Development as a measure of receptive and expressive language.

Language, Speech, and Hearing Services in Schools, 18, 179–187.

Damico, J. (1987). Addressing language concerns in the schools: The SLP as a consultant. *Journal of Childhood Communication Disorders, 11*(1), 17–40.

Damico, J. (1988). The lack of efficacy in language therapy: A case study. *Language, Speech, and Hearing Services in Schools, 19,* 51–66.

Daniloff, R., & Moll, K. (1968). Coarticulation of lip rounding. *Journal of Speech and Hearing Research, 11,* 707–721.

Darley, F. (1979). *Evaluation of appraisal techniques in speech and language pathology.* Reading, MA: Addison-Wesley.

Davis, A. (1972). *English problems of Spanish speakers.* Urbana, IL: National Council of Teachers of English.

Deal, V., and Rodriguez, V. (1987). *Resource guide to multicultural tests and materials in communicative disorders.* Rockville, MD: American Speech-Language-Hearing Association.

DeLemos, C. (1981). International processes in the child's construction of language. In W. Deutsch (Ed.), *The child's construction of language* (pp. 57–76). New York: Academic Press.

DeMaio, L. (1984). Establishing communication networks through interactive play: A method for language programming in the clinic setting. *Seminars in Speech and Language, 5,* 199–211.

Denckla, M., & Rudel, R. (1976). Naming of object drawings by dyslexic and other learning disabled children. *Brain and Language, 3,* 1–15.

Dennis, M., Sugar, J., & Whitaker, H. (1982). The acquisition of tag questions. *Child Development, 53,* 1254–1257.

Desher, D., Alley, G., Warner, M., & Schumaker, J. (1981). Instructional practices for promoting skill acquisition and generalization in severely learning disabled adolescents. *Learning Disability Quarterly, 4,* 145–152.

DeSpain, A., & Simon, C. (1987). Alternative to failure: A junior high school language development-based curriculum. *Journal of Childhood Communication Disorders, 11*(1), 139–179.

Dever, R. (1978). *Talk: Teaching the American language to kids.* Columbus, OH: Merrill.

deVilliers, J., & deVilliers, P. (1978). *Language acquisition.* Cambridge, MA: Harvard University Press.

Dewey, M., & Everard, M. (1974). The near normal autistic adolescent. *Journal of Autism and Childhood Schizophrenia, 4,* 348–356.

Diana v. State Board of Education. (1970). C-70-37 (RFP District N., California).

Dik, S. (1980). *Studies in functional grammar.* New York: Academic Press.

DiSegna, D., & Liles, B. (1987). Story grammar in children with and without language disorder: Story generation, story retelling, and story comprehension. *Journal of Speech and Hearing Research, 30,* 539–551.

Dollaghan, C. (1987a). Comprehension monitoring in normal and language-impaired children. *Topics in Language Disorders, 7*(2), 45–60.

Dollaghan, C. (1987b). Fast mapping in normal and language-impaired children. *Journal of Speech and Hearing Disorders, 52,* 218–222.

Dollaghan, C., & Kaston, N. (1986). A comprehension monitoring program for language-impaired children. *Journal of Speech and Hearing Disorders, 51,* 264–271.

Dollaghan, C. & Miller, J. (1986). Observational methods in the study of communicative competence. In R. Schiefelbusch (Ed.), *Language competence: Assessment and intervention* (pp. 99–129). San Diego: College-Hill.

Donahue, M. (1983). Language-disabled children as conversational partners. *Topics in Language Disorders, 4,* 15–27.

Donahue, M. (1984). Learning disabled children's conversational competence: An attempt to activate an inactive listener. *Applied Psycholinguistics, 5,* 21–36.

Donahue, M. (1985). Communicative style in learning disabled children: Some implications for classroom discourse. In D. Ropich & F. Spinelli (Eds.), *School discourse problems* (pp. 97–124). San Diego: College-Hill.

Donahue, M., Pearl, R., & Bryan, T. (1980). Learning disabled children's conversational competence: Responses to inadequate messages. *Applied Psycholinguistics, 1,* 387–403.

Donnellan, A., Mirenda, P., Mesaros, R., & Fassbender, L. (1984). Analyzing the communicative functions of aberrant behavior. *Journal of the Association for Persons with Severe Handicaps, 9,* 210–222.

Dore, J. (1974). A pragmatic description of early

language development. *Journal of Psycholinguistic Research, 3,* 343–350.

Dore, J. (1975). Holophrases, speech acts and language universals. *Journal of Child Language, 2,* 21–40.

Dore, J. (1976). Children's illocutionary acts. In R. Freedle (Ed.), *Discourse production and comprehension,* Vol. 1. Hillsdale, NJ: Erlbaum.

Dore, J. (1977). Oh them sheriff: A pragmatic analysis of children's responses to questions. In S. Ervin-Tripp & C. Mitchell-Kernan (Eds.), *Child discourse* (pp. 139–163). New York: Academic Press.

Dore, J. (1986). The development of conversational competence. In R. Schiefelbusch (Ed.), *Language competence: Assessment and intervention.* San Diego: College-Hill.

Downing, J. (1987). Conversational skills training: Teaching adolescents with mental retardation to be verbally assertive. *Mental Retardation, 25,* 147–155.

Downing, J., & Siegel-Causey, E. (1988). Enhancing the nonsymbolic communicative behavior of children with multiple impairments. *Language, Speech, and Hearing Services in Schools, 19,* 338–348.

Dubois, E., & Bernthal, J. (1978). A comparison of three methods of obtaining articulatory responses. *Journal of Speech and Hearing Disorders, 43,* 295–305.

Duchan, J. (1982a). Forward. *Topics in Language Disorders, 3*(1), ix–xiv.

Duchan, J. (1982b). The elephant is soft and mushy: Problems in assessing children's language. In N. Lass, L. McReynolds, J. Northern, & D. Yoder (Eds.), *Speech, language, and hearing: Vol. 2. Pathologies of speech and language* (pp. 741–760). Philadelphia: W. B. Saunders.

Duchan, J. (1983a). Autistic children are noninteractive: Or so we say. *Seminars in Speech and Language, 4,* 53–61.

Duchan, J. (1983b). Language processing and geodesic domes. In T. Gallagher & C. Prutting (Eds.), *Pragmatic assessment and intervention issues in language* (pp. 83–100). San Diego: College-Hill.

Duchan, J. (1984). Clinical interactions with autistic children: The role of theory. *Topics in Language Disorders, 4*(4), 62–71.

Duchan, J. (1986a). Language intervention

through sensemaking and fine tuning. In R. Schiefelbusch (Ed.), *Language competence: Assessment and intervention* (pp. 187–212). San Diego: College-Hill.

Duchan, J. (1986b). Learning to describe events. *Topics in Language Disorders, 6*(4), 27–36.

Duchan, J. (1987). Special education for the non-handicapped: How to interact with those who are different. In P. Knoblock (Ed.), *Understanding exceptional children* (pp. 163–199). Boston: Little, Brown.

Duchan, J., & Weitzner-Lin, B. (1987). Nurturant-naturalistic intervention for language-impaired children: Implications for planning lessons and tracking progress. *Asha, 29*(7), 45–49.

Dudley-Marling, C. (1987). The role of SLP's in literacy learning. *Journal of Childhood Communication Disorders, 2*(1), 81–90.

Dudley-Marling, C., & Rhodes, L. (1987). Pragmatics and literacy. *Language, Speech, and Hearing Services in Schools, 18,* 41–52.

Duncan, S. (1974). On the structure of speaker-auditor interaction during speaker turns. *Language and Society, 2,* 161–180.

Duncan, S., & Fiske, D. (1977). *Face-to-face interaction: Research, methods, and theory.* Hillside, NJ: Erlbaum.

Dunham, J. (1989). The transparency of manual signs in a linguistic and an environmental nonlinguistic context. *Augmentative and Alternative Communication, 5,* 214–225.

Dunn, C., & Barron, C. (1982). A treatment program for disordered phonology: Phonetic and linguistic considerations. *Language, Speech, and Hearing Services in Schools, 13,* 100–109.

Dunn, L., & Dunn, L. (1981). Peabody Picture Vocabulary Test—revised. Circle Pines, MN: American Guidance Service.

Dunst, C. (1980). *Clinical and educational manual for use with the Uzgiris and Hunt scales of infant psychological development.* Baltimore: University Park Press.

Durand, J. (1982). Analysis of intervention of self-injurious behavior. *Journal of the Association for Persons with Severe Handicaps, 7,* 44–53.

Durand, V., & Kishi, G. (1986). *Reducing severe behavior problems among persons with dual sensory impairments: An evaluation of a technical assistance model.* Unpublished manuscript, State University of New York at Albany.

Dyer, K., Santarcangelo, S., & Luce, S. (1987). Developmental influences in teaching language forms to individuals with developmental disabilities. *Journal of Speech and Hearing Disorders, 52,* 335–347.

Dyson, A., & Robinson, T. (1987). The effect of phonological analysis procedure on the selection of potential remediation targets. *Language, Speech, and Hearing Services in Schools, 18*(4), 364–377.

Ecklund, S., & Reichle, J. (1987). A comparison of normal children's ability to recall symbols from two logographic systems. *Language, Speech, and Hearing Services in Schools, 18,* 34–40.

Edmonston, N., & Thane, N. (1990, April). *Children's concept comprehension: Acquisition, assessment, intervention.* Paper presented at the annual convention of the New York State Speech-Language-Hearing Association, Kiamesha Lake.

Edwards, M. (1983). Selection criteria for developing therapy goals. *Journal of Childhood Communication Disorders, 7,* 36–45.

Edwards, M. (1984, April). Phonological analysis. Presentation for Genesee Valley Speech-Language-Hearing Association, Rochester, NY.

Elbert, M., & Gierut, J. (1986). *Handbook of clinical phonology: Approaches to assessment and training.* San Diego: College-Hill.

Elbert, M., Rockman, B., & Saltzman, D. (1980). *Contrasts: The use of minimal pairs in articulation training.* Austin, TX: Exceptional Resources.

Ellis, R., & Wells, G. (1980). Enabling factors in adult-child discourse. *First language, 1,* 46–82.

Emerick, L., & Haynes, W. (1986). *Diagnosis and evaluation in speech pathology* (3rd ed.). Englewood Cliffs, NJ: Prentice Hall.

Ervin-Tripp, S. (1966). Language development. In L. Hoffman & M. Hoffman (Eds.), *Review of Child Development Research, 2,* 55–105. New York: Russell Sage Foundation.

Ervin-Tripp, S. (1977). Wait for me roller skate. In S. Ervin-Tripp & C. Mitchell-Kernan (Eds.), *Child discourse* (pp. 165–188). New York: Academic Press.

Evesham, M. (1977). Teaching language skills to children. *British Journal of Disorders of Communication, 12,* 23–29.

Falvey, M., Bishop, K., Grenot-Scheyer, M., & Coots, J. (1988). Issues and trends in mental retardation. In S. Calculator & J. Bedrosian (Eds.), *Communication assessment and intervention for adults with mental retardation* (pp. 45–65). San Diego: College-Hill.

Farrier, L., Yorkston, K., Marriner, N., & Beukelman, D. (1985). Conversational control in nonimpaired speakers using an augmentative communication system. *Augmentative and Alternative Communication, 1,* 65–73.

Fasold, R., & Wolfram, W. (1970). Some linguistic features of Negro dialect. In R. Fasold & R. Shuy (Eds.), *Teaching standard English in the inner city.* Washington, D.C.: Center for Applied Linguistics.

Fay, W., & Schuler, A. (1980). *Emerging language in autistic children.* Baltimore: University Park Press.

Feagans, L., & Short, E. (1986). Referential communication and reading performance in learning disabled children over a 3-year period. *Developmental Psychology, 22,* 177–183.

Ferguson, C. (1978). Learning to pronounce: The earliest stages of phonological development in the child. In F. Minifie & L. Lloyd (Eds.), *Communication and cognitive abilities—Early behavioral assessment.* Baltimore: University Park Press.

Ferguson, C., Peizer, D., & Weeks, T. (1973). Model-and-replica phonological grammar of a child's first words. *Lingua, 31,* 35–39.

Ferrier, E., & Davis, M. (1973). A lexical approach to the remediation of final sound omissions. *Journal of Speech and Hearing Disorders, 38,* 126–130.

Fey, M. (1986). *Language intervention with young children.* San Diego: College-Hill.

Fey, M. (1987, April). Is natural always best? Paper presented at the New York State Speech-Language-Hearing Association annual convention, Liberty.

Fey, M. (1988). Generalization issues facing language interventionists: An introduction. *Language, Speech, and Hearing Services in Schools, 19,* 272–281.

Fey, M., & Leonard, L. (1983). Pragmatic skills of specific language impairment. In T. Gallagher & C. Prutting (Eds.), *Pragmatic assessment and intervention issues in language* (pp. 65–82). San Diego: College-Hill.

Fey, M., Leonard, L., & Wilcox, K. (1981). Speech-style modifications of language-impaired children. *Journal of Speech and Hearing Disorders, 46,* 91–97.

Fey, M., & Stalker, C. (1986). A hypothesis-testing approach to treatment of a child with an idiosyncratic (morpho)phonological system. *Journal of Speech and Hearing Disorders, 51,* 324–336.

Fey, M., Warr-Leeper, G., Webber, S., & Disher, L. (1988). Repairing children's repairs: Evaluation and facilitation of children's clarification requests and responses. *Topics in Language Disorders, 8*(2), 63–84.

Fillmore, C. (1968). The case for case. In E. Bach & R. Harmas (Eds.), *Universals in linguistic theory* (pp. 1–90). New York: Holt, Rinehart & Winston.

Fillmore, C., Kempler, D., & Wang, W. (Eds.). (1979). *Individual differences in language ability and language behavior.* New York: Academic Press.

Fisher, H., & Logemann, J. (1987). The Fisher-Logemann test of Articulation Competence. Boston: Houghton-Mifflin.

Fletcher, P. (1979). The development of the verb phrase. In P. Fletcher & M. Garman (Eds.), *Language acquisition.* New York: Cambridge University Press.

Fletcher, P. (1978). Review of D. Major, The acquisition of modal auxiliaries in the language of children. *Journal of Child Language, 2,* 318–322.

Fluharty, N. (1978). Fluharty Preschool Speech and Language Screening Test. Boston: Teaching Resources Corp.

Fokes, J. (1976). *Fokes sentence builder.* Boston, MA: Teaching Resources Corp.

Folger, J., & Chapman, R. (1978). A pragmatic analysis of spontaneous imitations. *Journal of Child Language, 5,* 25–38.

Foster, R., Giddan, J., & Stark, J. (1973). *Assessment of children's language comprehension.* Palo Alto, CA: Consulting Psychologists Press.

Foster, S. (1985). The development of discourse topic skills in infants and young children. *Topics in Language Disorders, 5*(2), 31–45.

Francik, E., & Clark, H. (1985). How to make requests that overcome obstacles to compliance. *Journal of Memory and Language, 24,* 560–568.

Frankel, R. (1982). Autism for all practical purposes: A microinteractional view. *Topics in Language Disorders, 3*(1), 33–43.

Fredricks, H., Baldwin, D., & Grove, D. (1974). A home-center based parent-training model. In J. Grim (Ed.), *Training parents to teach: Four models.* Chapel Hill, NC: Technical Assistance Development Systems.

Friedman, P., & Friedman, K. (1980). Accounting for individual differences when comparing the effectiveness of remedial language teaching methods. *Applied Psycholinguistics, 2,* 151–170.

Fried-Oken, M. (1984). The development of naming skills in normal and language deficient children. Unpublished doctoral dissertation, Boston University.

Fried-Oken, M. (1987). Qualitative examination of children's naming skills through test adaptations. *Language, Speech, and Hearing Services in Schools, 18,* 206–216.

Friend, T., & Channell, R. (1987). A comparison of two measures of receptive vocabulary. *Language, Speech, and Hearing Services in Schools, 18,* 231–237.

Fudala, J. (1970). Arizona Articulation Proficiency Scale: Revised. Los Angeles: Western Psychological Services.

Fujiki, M., & Brinton, B. (1984). Supplementing language therapy: Working with the classroom teacher. *Language, Speech, and Hearing Services in Schools, 15,* 98–109.

Fujiki, M., & Brinton, B. (1987). Elicited imitation revisited: Comparison with spontaneous language production. *Language, Speech, and Hearing Services in Schools, 18*(4), 301–311.

Fujiki, M., & Willbrand, M. (1982). A comparison of four informal methods of language evaluation. *Language, Speech, and Hearing Services in Schools, 13,* 42–52.

Furrow, D., Nelson, K., & Benedict, H. (1979). Mothers' speech to children and syntactic development: Some simple relationships. *Journal of Child Language, 6,* 423–442.

Gallagher, T. (1981). Contingent query sequences within adult-child discourse. *Journal of Child Language, 8,* 51–62.

Gallagher, T. (1983). Pre-assessment: A procedure for accommodating language use variability. In T. Gallagher & C. Prutting (Eds.), *Pragmatic assessment and intervention issues in language* (pp. 1–28). San Diego: College-Hill.

Gallagher, T., & Craig, H. (1982). An investigation of overlap in children's speech. *Journal of Psycholinguistic Research, 11,* 63–75.

Gallagher, T., & Prutting, C. (1983). *Pragmatic assessment and intervention issues in language.* San Diego: College-Hill.

Garcia, E. (1974). The training generalization of conversational speech form in nonverbal retardates. *Journal of Applied Behavior Analysis, 7,* 137–149.

Gardner, M. (1979). Expressive One-word Picture Vocabulary Test. Novato, CA: Academic Therapy.

Gardner, M. (1985). Receptive One-word Picture Vocabulary Test. Novato, CA: Academic Therapy.

Garnett, K. (1986). Telling tales: Narratives and learning disabled children. *Topics in Language Disorders, 6*(2), 44–56.

Garvey, C. (1975). Requests and responses in children's speech. *Journal of Child Language, 2,* 41–59.

Garvey, C. (1977). The contingent query: A dependent act in conversation. In M. Lewis & L. Rosenblum (Eds.), *Interaction, conversation, and the development of language* (pp. 63–93). New York: Wiley.

Geffner, D., & Freeman, L. (1980). Assessment of language comprehension of 6-year-old deaf children. *Journal of Communication Disorders, 13,* 455–470.

German, D. (1982). Word-finding substitutions in children with learning disabilities. *Language, Speech, and Hearing Services in Schools, 13,* 223–230.

German, D. (1987). Spontaneous language profiles of children with word-finding problems. *Language, Speech, and Hearing Services in Schools, 18,* 217–230.

Gierut, J. (1989). Maximal opposition approach to phonological treatment. *Journal of Speech and Hearing Disorders, 54,* 9–19.

Gierut, J., Elbert, M., & Dinnsen, D. (1987). A functional analysis of phonological knowledge and generalization learning in misarticulating children. *Journal of Speech and Hearing Research, 30,* 462–479.

Girolametto, L. (1988). Improving the social-conversational skills of developmentally delayed children: An intervention study. *Journal of Speech and Hearing Disorders, 53,* 156–167.

Glenn, C., & Stein, N. (1980). *Syntactic structures and real world themes in stories generated by children* (Technical report). Urbana: University of Illinois Center for the Study of Reading.

Glennen, S., & Calculator, S. (1985). Training functional communication board use: A pragmatic approach. *Augmentative and Alternative Communication, 1,* 134–142.

Gobbi, L., Cipani, E., Hudson, C., & Lapenta-Neudeck, R. (1986). Developing spontaneous requesting among children with severe mental retardation. *Mental Retardation, 24,* 357–364.

Goetz, L., Gee, K., & Sailor, W. (1985). Using a behavior chain interruption strategy to teach communication skills to students with severe disabilities. *Journal of the Association of Persons with Severe Handicaps, 10,* 21–30.

Goetz, L., & Sailor, W. (1988). New directions: Communication development in persons with severe disabilities. *Topics in Language Disorders, 8*(2), 41–52.

Goldberg, S. (1977). Social competence in infancy: A model of parent-infant interaction. *Merrill-Palmer Quarterly, 23,* 163–177.

Goldman, R., & Fristoe, M. (1986). The Goldman-Fristoe Test of Articulation. Circle Pines, MN: American Guidance Service.

Goldstein, H. (1984). Effects of modeling and corrected practice on generative language learning in preschool children. *Journal of Speech and Hearing Disorders, 49,* 389–398.

Goldstein, H., & Ferrell, D. (1987). Augmentative communication interaction between handicapped and nonhandicapped preschool children. *Journal of Speech and Hearing Disorders, 52,* 200–211.

Golinkoff, R. (1981). The case for semantic relations. *Journal of Child Language, 8,* 413–437.

Goosens, C., & Kraat, A. (1985). Technology as a tool for conversation and language learning for the physically disabled. *Topics in Language Disorders, 6,* 56–70.

Gordon, C., & Braun, C. (1983). Using story schema as an aid to reading and writing. *The Reading Teacher, 37,* 116–121.

Gordon, C., & Braun, C. (1985). Metacognitive processes: Reading and writing narrative discourse. In D. Forrest-Pressley, G. MacKinnon, & T. Waller (Eds.), *Metacognition, cognition, and human performance* (Vol. 2) (pp. 1–75). New York: Academic Press.

Goss, R. (1970). Language used by mothers of

deaf children and mothers of hearing children. *American Annals of the Deaf, 115*, 93–96.

Gottesleben, R., Tyack, D., & Buschini, G. (1974). Three case studies in language learning: Applied linguistics. *Journal of Speech and Hearing Disorders, 39*, 213–224.

Graham, L. (1976). Language programming and intervention. In L. Lloyd (Ed.), *Communication assessment and intervention strategies* (pp. 371–422). Baltimore: University Park Press.

Graves, D. (1981). Research update: Writing research for the 80's: What is needed? *Language Arts, 58*, 197–206.

Gray, B., & Ryan, B. (1973). *A language program for the non-language child*. Champaign, IL: Research Press.

Graybeal, C. (1981). Memory for stories in language-impaired children. *Applied Psycholinguistics, 2*, 269–283.

Greenberg, J. (1966). *Language universals*. The Hague: Mouton.

Greene, L., & Jones-Bamman, L. (1985). *Getting smarter: Simple strategies for better grades*. Belmont, CA: David S. Lake.

Grice, H. (1975). Logic and conversation. In D. Davidson and G. Harmon (Eds.), *The logic of grammar* (pp. 64–74). Encino, CA: Dickenson Press.

Griffith, P., & Sanford, A. (1975). Learning Accomplishment Profile for Infants. Winston-Salem, NC: Kaplan School Supply Corp.

Grimm, H. (1982). On the interrelation of internal and external factors in the development of language structures in normal and dysphasic preschoolers: A longitudinal study. Paper presented at the Kamehameha Educational Research Institute, Hawaii.

Grunwell, P. (1982) *Clinical phonology*. Rockville, MD: Aspen.

Guess, D., Benson, H., & Siegel-Causey, E. (1985). Concepts and issues related to choice-making and autonomy among persons with severe disabilities. *Journal of the Association for Persons with Severe Handicaps, 10*, 79–86.

Guess, D., & Helmstetter, E. (1986). Skill cluster instruction and the individualized curriculum sequencing model. In R. Horner, L. Meyer, & H. Fredericks (Eds.), *Education of learners with severe handicaps: Exemplary service strategies*. Baltimore: Brookes.

Guess, D., Sailor, W., & Baer, D. (1974). To teach language to retarded children. In R. Schiefelbusch & L. Lloyd (Eds.), *Language perspectives—Acquisition, retardation, and intervention* (pp. 529–563). Baltimore: University Park Press.

Guess, D., & Siegel-Causey, E. (1985). Behavioral control education of severely handicapped students: Who's doing what to whom? Why? In D. Bricker & J. Filler (Eds.), *Severe mental retardation: From theory to practice* (pp. 230–244). Reston, VA: Division on Mental Retardation of the Council for Exceptional Children.

Guevremont, D., Osnes, R., & Stokes, T. (1986a). Preparation for effective self-regulation: The development of generalized verbal control. *Journal of Applied Behavior Analysis, 19*, 99–104.

Guevremont, D., Osnes, R., & Stokes, T. (1986b). Programming maintenance after correspondence training interventions with children. *Journal of Applied Behavior Analysis, 19*, 215–219.

Gullo, D., & Gullo, J. (1984). An ecological language intervention approach with mentally retarded adolescents. *Language, Speech, and Hearing Services in Schools, 15*, 182–191.

Haas, A., & Owens, R. (1985). Preschoolers' pronoun strategies: You and me make us. Paper presented at the American Speech-Language-Hearing Association annual convention, Washington, D.C.

Haelsig, P., & Madison, C. (1986). A study of phonological processes exhibited by 3-, 4-, and 5-year-old children. *Language, Speech, and Hearing Services in Schools, 17*, 107–114.

Hale-Haniff, M., & Siegel, G. (1981). The effect of context on verbal elicited imitation. *Journal of Speech and Hearing Disorders, 45*, 27–30.

Halle, J. (1987). Teaching language in the natural environment: An analysis of spontaneity. *The Journal of the Association for Persons with Severe Handicaps, 12*, 28–37.

Halle, J. (1988). Adopting the natural environment as the context of training. In S. Calculator & J. Bedrosian (Eds.), *Communication assessment and intervention for adults with mental retardation*. San Diego: College-Hill.

Halle, J. (1989). Identifying stimuli in the natural environment that control verbal responses. *Journal of Speech and Hearing Disorders, 54*, 500–504.

Halle, J., Baer, D., & Spradlin, J. (1981). Teacher's

generalized use of delay as a stimulus control procedure to increase language use in handicapped children. *Journal of Applied Behavior Analysis, 14,* 389–409.

Halle, J., Marshall, A., & Spradlin, J. (1979). Time delay: A technique to increase language use and facilitate generalization in retarded children. *Journal of Applied Behavior Analysis, 12,* 431–439.

Halliday, M. (1974). *Language and social man.* Schools Council Programme in Linguistics and English Teaching. Papers series II, Vol. 3. London: Longman for the Schools Council.

Halliday, M., & Hasan, R. (1976). *Cohesion in English.* London: Longman.

Hammill, D., Brown, V., Larsen, S., & Wiederholt, J. (1980). *Test of adolescent language: A multidimensional approach to assessment.* Austin, TX: Pro-Ed.

Hammill, D., & Newcomer, P. (1982). The Test of Language Development—Primary. Austin, TX: Empiric Press.

Hanna, R., Lippert, E., & Harris, A. (1982). Developmental Communication Curriculum Inventory. San Antonio, TX: Psychological Corporation.

Hannah, E., & Gardner, J. (1974). Preschool Language Screening Test. Northridge, CA: Joyce Publications.

Hansen, C. (1978). Story retelling used with average and learning disabled readers as a measure of reading comprehension. *Learning Disability Quarterly, 1,* 62–69.

Harris, P., & Folch, L. (1985). Decrement in the understanding of big among English- and Spanish-speaking children. *Journal of Child Language, 12,* 685–690.

Harris, P., Morris, J., & Terwogt, M. (1986). The early acquisition of spatial adjectives: A cross-linguistic study. *Journal of Child Language, 13,* 335–352.

Hart, B. (1985). Naturalistic language training techniques. In S. Warren & A. Rogers-Warren (Eds.), *Teaching functional language* (pp. 63–88). Baltimore: University Park Press.

Hart, B., & Risley, T. (1968). Establishing the use of descriptive adjectives in the spontaneous speech of disadvantaged preschool children. *Journal of Applied Behavior Analysis, 1,* 109–120.

Hart, B., & Risley, T. (1974). Using preschool materials to modify the language of disadvantaged children. *Journal of Applied Behavior Analysis, 7,* 243–256.

Hart, B., & Risley, T. (1975). Incidental teaching of language in the preschool. *Journal of Applied Behavior Analysis, 8,* 411–420.

Hart, B., & Risley, T. (1980). In vivo language training: Unanticipated and general effects. *Journal of Applied Behavior Analysis, 12,* 407–432.

Hart, B., & Risley, T. (1986). Incidental strategies. In R. Schiefelbusch (Ed.), *Language competence: Assessment and intervention* (pp. 213–226). San Diego: College-Hill.

Hart, B., & Rogers-Warren, A. (1978). A milieu approach to teaching language. In R. Schiefelbusch (Ed.), *Language intervention strategies* (pp. 193–236). Baltimore: University Park Press.

Hasenstab, M., & Laughton, J. (1982). *Reading, writing, and the exceptional child: A psycho-sociolinguistic approach.* Rockville, MD: Aspen.

Haynes, W., Haynes, M., & Jackson, J. (1982). The effects of phonetic context and linguistic complexity on /s/ misarticulation in children. *Journal of Communication Disorders, 15,* 287–297.

Haynes, W., & Moran, M. (1989). A cross-sectional developmental study of final consonant production in southern Black children from preschool through third grade. *Language, Speech, and Hearing Services in Schools, 20,* 400–406.

Haynes, W., & Steed, S. (1987). Multiphonemic scoring of articulation in imitative sentences: Some preliminary data. *Language, Speech, and Hearing Services in Schools, 18,* 4–14.

Heath, S. (1983). *Ways with words: Language, life and work in communities and classrooms.* Cambridge: Cambridge University Press.

Heath, S. (1986a). Separating ''things of the imagination'' from life: Learning to read and write. In W. Teale & E. Sulzby (Eds.), *Emergent literacy* (pp. 156–172). Norwood, NJ: Ablex.

Heath, S. (1986b). Taking a cross-cultural look at narratives. *Topics in Language Disorders, 7*(1), 84–94.

Hedberg, N., & Fink, R. (1985, November). Surface and deep structure characteristics of language disordered children's narratives. Paper presented at the American Speech-Language-Hearing Association annual convention, Washington, DC.

Hedberg, N., & Stoel-Gammon, C. (1986). Narrative analysis: Clinical procedures. *Topics in Language Disorders, 7*(1), 58–69.

Hegde, M. (1980). An experimental-clinical analysis of grammatical and behavioral distinctions between verbal auxiliary and copula. *Journal of Speech and Hearing Research, 23,* 864–877.

Hegde, M., Noll, M., & Pecora, R. (1979). A study of some factors affecting generalization of language training. *Journal of Speech and Hearing Disorders, 44,* 301–320.

Heifetz, L. (1980). From consumer to middleman: Emerging roles for parents in the network of services for retarded children. In R. Abidin (Ed.), *Parent education and intervention handbook* (pp. 349–384). Springfield, IL: Charles C Thomas.

Helmstetter, E., & Guess, D. (1987). Application of individualized curriculum sequencing model to learners with severe sensory impairments. In L. Goetz, D. Guess, & K. Stremel-Campbell (Eds.), *Innovative program design for individuals with sensory impairments* (pp. 255–282). Baltimore: Brookes.

Hendrick, D., Prather, E., & Tobin, A. (1975). The Sequenced Inventory of Communication Development. Seattle: University of Washington Press.

Hess, C., Haug, H., & Landry, R. (1989). The reliability of type-token ratios for the oral language of school age children. *Journal of Speech and Hearing Research, 32,* 536–540.

Hess, C., Sefton, K., & Landry, R. (1986). Sample size and type-token ratios for oral language of preschool children. *Journal of Speech and Hearing Research, 29,* 129–134.

Hester, P., & Hendrickson, J. (1977). Training functional expressive language: The acquisition and generalization of five-element syntactic responses. *Journal of Applied Behavior Analysis, 10,* 316.

Higginbotham, D., & Yoder, D. (1982). Communication within natural conversational interaction: Implications for severely communicatively impaired persons. *Topics in Language Disorders, 2,* 1–19.

Hirst, W., & Weil, J. (1982). Acquisition of epistemic and deontic meanings of modals. *Journal of Child Language, 9,* 659–666.

Hodson, B. (1980). *The assessment of phonological processes.* Danville, IL: Interstate.

Hodson, B., & Paden, E. (1981). Phonological processes which characterize unintelligible speech and intelligible speech in early childhood. *Journal of Speech and Hearing Disorders, 46,* 369–373.

Hodson, B., & Paden, E. (1983). *Targeting intelligible speech.* San Diego: College-Hill.

Hoffman, P., Norris, J., & Monjure, J. (1990). Comparison of process targeting and whole language treatments for phonologically delayed preschool children. *Language, Speech, and Hearing Services in Schools, 21,* 102–109.

Hood, L., & Bloom, L. (1979) What, when, and how about why: A longitudinal study of expressions of causality in the language development of two-year-old children. *Monographs of the Society for Research in Child Development, 6* (Serial No. 181).

Horner, R., & Budd, C. (1983). *Teaching manual sign language to a nonverbal student: Generalization of sign use and collateral reduction of maladaptive behavior.* Eugene: University of Oregon Center on Human Development.

Horner, R., & Budd, C. (1985, March). Acquisition of manual sign use: Collateral reduction of maladaptive behavior, and factors limiting generalization. *Education and Training of the Mentally Retarded, 20,* 39–47.

Horner, R., McDonnell, J., & Bellamy, G. (1986). Teaching generalized skills: General case instruction in simulation and community settings. In R. Horner, L. Meyer, & H. Fredericks (Eds.), *Education of learners with severe handicaps* (pp. 289–314). Baltimore: Brookes.

Horstmeier, D., & MacDonald, J., (1978a). *Ready, set, go—Talk to me.* San Antonio: Psychological Corporation.

Horstmeier, D., & MacDonald, J. (1978b). Environmental Pre-language Battery. San Antonio: Psychological Corporation.

Hoskins, B. (1987). *Conversations: Language intervention for adolescents.* Allen, TX: DLM Teaching Resources.

Houghton, J., Bronicki, G., & Guess, D. (1987). Opportunities to express preferences and make choices among students with severe disabilities in classroom settings. *The Journal of the Association for Persons with Severe Handicaps, 12,* 18–27.

House, L., & Rogerson, B. (1984). *Comprehensive screening tool for determining the optimal communi-*

cation mode. East Aurora, NY: United Educational Services, Inc.

Hresko, W., Reid, D., & Hammill, D. (1981). Test of Early Language Development. Los Angeles: Western Psychological Services.

Hunt, J. (1961). *Intelligence and experience.* New York: Ronald Press.

Hunt, K. (1970). Syntactic maturity in school children and adults. *Monologues of the Society for Research in Child Development, 35* (Serial No. 134).

Hurlbut, B., Iwata, B., & Green, J. (1982). Nonvocal language acquisition in adolescents with severe physical disabilities: Blissymbolics versus iconic stimulus formats. *Journal of Applied Behavior Analysis, 15,* 241–258.

Huttenlocker, J., Smiley, P., & Charney, R. (1983). The emergence of action categories in the child: Evidence of verb meanings. *Psychological Review, 90,* 72–93.

Iglesias, A. (1986, May). The cultural-linguistic minority student in the classroom: Management decisions. Workshop presented at the State University College at Buffalo, NY.

Ingram, D. (1976). *Phonological disabilities in children.* New York: Elsevier.

Ingram, D. (1981). *Procedures for the phonological analysis of children's language.* Baltimore: University Park Press.

Ingram, D. (1983). The analysis and treatment of phonological disorders. *Seminars in Speech and Language, 4,* 375–388.

Iwata, B., Dorsey, M., Slifer, K., Bauman, K., & Richman, G. (1982). Toward a functional analysis of self-injury. *Analysis and Intervention in Developmental Disabilities, 2,* 3–20.

James, S. (1989). Assessing children with language disorders. In D. Bernstein & E. Tiegerman (Eds.), *Language and communication disorders in children* (2nd ed.) (pp. 157–207). Columbus, OH: Merrill.

Jimenez, B., & Iseyama, D. (1987). A model for training and using communication assistants. *Language, Speech, and Hearing Services in Schools, 18,* 168–171.

Johnson, A., Johnston, E., & Weinrich, B. (1981, November). I say yes—but I mean no: Pragmatic therapy ideas. Paper presented at the American Speech-Language-Hearing annual convention, Los Angeles.

Johnson, A., Johnston, E., & Weinrich, B. (1984).

Assessing pragmatic skills in children's language. *Language, Speech, and Hearing Services in Schools, 15,* 2–9.

Johnson, D., & Myklebust, H. (1967). *Learning disabilities: Educational principles and practices.* New York: Grune & Stratton.

Johnson, H., & Hood, S. (1988). Teaching chaining to unintelligible children: How to deal with open syllables. *Language, Speech, and Hearing Services in Schools, 19,* 211–220.

Johnson, J., Winney, B., & Pederson, O. (1980). Single word versus connected speech articulation testing. *Language, Speech, and Hearing Services in Schools, 11,* 169–174.

Johnston, J. (1982). Narratives: A new look at communication problems in older language disordered children. *Language, Speech, and Hearing Services in Schools, 13,* 144–145.

Johnston, J. (1983). What is language intervention? The role of theory. In J. Miller, D. Yoder, & R. Schiefelbusch (Eds.), *Contemporary issues in language intervention* (pp. 52–57). Rockville, MD: American Speech-Language-Hearing Association.

Johnston, J. (1984). Acquisition of locative meanings: Behind and in front of. *Journal of Child Language, 11,* 407–422.

Johnston, J. (1988). Generalization: The nature of change. *Language, Speech, and Hearing Services in Schools, 19,* 314–329.

Johnston, J., & Kamhi, A. (1984). Syntactic and semantic aspects of the utterances of language-impaired children: The same can be less. *Merrill-Palmer Quarterly, 30,* 65–86.

Johnston, J., & Slobin, D. (1979). The development of locative expressions in English, Italian, Serbo-Croatian, and Turkish. *Journal of Child Language, 6,* 529–545.

Johnston, J., & Smith, L. (1989). Dimensional thinking in language impaired children. *Journal of Speech and Hearing Research, 32,* 33–38.

Johnston, J., Trainor, M., Casey, P., & Hagler, P. (1981 November). *Effect of interview style and materials on language samples.* Paper presented at the annual convention of the American Speech-Language-Hearing Association, Los Angeles.

Jorm, A. (1983). *The psychology of reading and spelling disabilities.* Boston: Routledge & Kegan Paul.

Kahn, J. (1982, May). *Cognitive training and its rela-*

tionship to language of profoundly retarded children.
Paper presented at the American Association
on Mental Deficiency annual convention, Boston.

Kail, R., Hale, C., Leonard, L., & Nippold, M.
(1984). Lexical storage and retrieval in language-impaired children. *Applied Psycholinguistics, 5,* 37–49.

Kail, R., & Leonard, L. (1986). Word-finding abilities in language-impaired children. *ASHA Monographs, 25.*

Kail, R., & Marshall, C. (1978). Reading skill and memory scanning. *Journal of Educational Psychology, 70,* 808–814.

Kamhi, A. (1984). Problem solving in child language disorders: The clinician as clinical scientist. *Language, Speech, and Hearing Services in Schools, 15,* 226–234.

Kamhi, A. (1987). Metalinguistic abilities in language-impaired children. *Topics in Language Disorders, 7*(2), 1–12.

Kamhi, A. (1988). A reconceptualization of generalization and generalization problems. *Language, Speech, and Hearing Services in Schools, 19,* 304–313.

Kamhi, A., Catts, H., & Davis, M. (1984). The management of sentence processing demands. *Journal of Speech and Hearing Research, 27,* 329–338.

Kamhi, A., Gentry, B., & Mauer, D. (1987). Analogical learning and transfer in language-impaired children. Paper presented at the Wisconsin Symposium for Research in Child Language Disorders, Madison.

Kamhi, A., & Nelson, L. (1988). Early syntactic development: Simple clause types and grammatical morphology. *Topics in Language Disorders, 8*(2), 26–43.

Kangas, K., & Lloyd, L. (1988). Early cognitive skills as prerequisites to augmentative and alternative communication use: What are we waiting for? *Augmentative and Alternative Communication, 4,* 211–221.

Karmiloff-Smith, A. (1981). The grammatical marking of thematic structure in the development of language production. In W. Deutsch (Ed.), *The child's construction of language* (pp. 121–148). New York: Academic Press.

Kaye, K. (1979). Thickening thin data: The maternal role in developing communication and language. In M. Bullowa (Ed.), *Before speech* (pp. 191–206). New York: Cambridge University Press.

Kaye, K., & Charney, R. (1981). Conversational asymetry between mothers and children. *Journal of Child Language, 8,* 35–49.

Keefe, K., Feldman, H., & Holland, A. (1989). Lexical learning and language abilities in preschoolers with perinatal brain damage. *Journal of Speech and Hearing Disorders, 54,* 395–402.

Keenan, E. (1976). Towards a universal definition of "subject." In C. Li (Ed.), *Subject and topic* (pp. 303–333). New York: Academic Press.

Keenan, E., & Schieffelin, B. (1976). Topics as a discourse notion: A study of topic in the conversations of children and adults. In C. Li (Ed.), *Subject and topic* (pp. 335–383). New York: Academic Press.

Kelly, C., & Dale, P. (1989). Cognitive skills associated with the onset of multiword utterances. *Journal of Speech and Hearing Research, 32,* 645–656.

Kelly, D., & Rice, M. (1986). A strategy for language assessment of young children: A combination of two approaches. *Language, Speech, and Hearing Services in Schools, 17,* 83–94.

Kemper, S. (1984). The development of narrative skills: Explanations and entertainments. In S. Kuczaj (Ed.), *Discourse development: Progress in cognitive development research.* New York: Springer-Verlag.

Kemper, S., & Edwards, L. (1986). Children's expression of causality and their construction of narratives. *Topics in Language Disorders, 7*(1), 11–20.

Keogh, W. J., & Reichle, J. (1985). Communication and intervention for the "difficult-to-teach" severely handicapped. In S. Warren & A. Rogers-Warren (Eds.), *Teaching functional language: Generalization and maintenance of language skills* (pp. 157–194). Baltimore: University Park Press.

King, D. (1976). An innovative language habilitative program for preschool age children. In S. Adler (Ed.), *Early identification and intensive remediation of language retarded children* (pp. 133–162). Springfield, IL: Charles C. Thomas.

Kirk, S., McCarthy, J., & Winifred, K. (1968) Illinois Test of Psycholinguistic Abilities. Urbana: University of Illinois Press.

Klecan-Aker, J. (1984, November). The syntax of

normal and learning disabled school-age children. Paper presented at the American Speech-Language-Hearing Association annual convention, San Francisco.

Klecan-Aker, J. (1985). Syntactic abilities in normal and language deficient middle school children. *Topics in Language Disorders, 5*(3), 46–54.

Klecan-Aker, J., & Hedrick, D. (1985). A study of the syntactic language skills of normal school-aged children. *Language, Speech, and Hearing Services in Schools, 16,* 187–198.

Klee, T., & Fitzgerald, M. (1985). The relation between grammatical development and mean length of utterance in morphemes. *Journal of Child Language, 12,* 251–269.

Klee, T., Schaffer, M., May, S., Membrino, I., & Mougey, K. (1981). A comparison of the age-MLU relation in normal and specially language-impaired preschool children. *Journal of Speech and Hearing Disorders, 54,* 226–232.

Klein, H. (1981). Productive strategies for the pronunciation of early polysyllabic lexical items. *Journal of Speech and Hearing Research, 24,* 389–405.

Klein, H. (1984). Procedure for maximizing phonological information from single-word responses. *Language, Speech, and Hearing Services in Schools, 15,* 267–274.

Klein, M., Wulz, S., Hall, M., Walso, L., Carpenter, S., Lathan, D., Meyers, S., Fox, T., & Marshall, A. (1981). *Comprehensive communication curriculum guide.* Kansas Early Childhood Institute (ECI Document No. 902), University of Kansas, Lawrence.

Klima, E., & Bellugi, U. (1973). Syntactic regularities in the speech of children. In C. Ferguson & D. Slobin (Eds.), *Studies in child language* (pp. 333–353). New York: Holt, Rinehart & Winston.

Knight-Arest, I. (1984). Communicative effectiveness of learning disabled and normally achieving 10-to-13-year-old boys. *Learning Disability Quarterly, 7,* 237–245.

Knoblauch, C. (1980). Intentionality in the writing process: A case study. *College Composition and Communication, 31,* 153–159.

Koenig, L., & Biel, C. (1989). A delivery system of comprehensive language services in a school district. *Language, Speech, and Hearing Services in Schools, 20,* 338–365.

Kohl, F. (1981). Effects of motoric requirements on the acquisition of manual sign responses by severely handicapped students. *American Journal of Mental Deficiency, 85,* 396–403.

Kohler, F., & Fowler, S. (1985). Training prosocial behaviors to young children: An analysis of reciprocity with untrained peers. *Journal of Applied Behavior Analysis, 18,* 187–200.

Kopchick, G., & Lloyd, L. (1976). Total communication for the severely language impaired: A 24-hour approach. In L. Lloyd (Ed.), *Communication assessment and intervention strategies* (pp. 501–521). Baltimore: University Park Press.

Kouri, T. (1988). Effects of simultaneous communication in a child-directed treatment approach with preschoolers with severe disabilities. *Augmentative and Alternative Communication, 4,* 222–232.

Kouri, T. (1989). How manual sign acquisition relates to the development of spoken language: A case study. *Language, Speech, and Hearing Services in Schools, 20,* 50–62.

Kraat, A. (1985). *Communication interaction between aided and natural speakers: A state of the art report.* Toronto: Canadian Rehabilitation Council for the Disabled.

Kresheck, J., & Nicolosi, L. (1973). A comparison of black and white children's scores on the Peabody Picture Vocabulary Test. *Language, Speech, and Hearing Services in Schools, 4,* 37–40.

Kuczaj, S. (1982). Old and new forms, old and new meanings: The form-function hypotheses revisited. *First Language, 3,* 55–61.

Kuhn, D., & Phelps, H. (1976). The development of children's comprehension of causal direction. *Child Development, 47,* 248–251.

Kunze, L., Lockhart, S., Didow, S., & Caterson, M. (1983). Interactive model for the assessment and treatment of the young child. In H. Winits (Ed.), *Treating language disorders: For clinicians by clinicians* (pp. 19–96). Baltimore: University Park Press.

Labov, W. (1972). *Language in the inner city.* Philadelphia: University of Pennsylvania Press.

Lahe, M., & Silliman, E. (1987). *In other words, how do you put it? Narrative development and disorders.* Paper presented at the annual convention of the New York State Speech-Language-Hearing Association, Kiamesha Lake.

Lakoff, R. (1973). The logic of politeness; or minding your p's and q's. In C. Corum, T. Smith-

Stark, & A. Weiser (Eds.), *Papers from the ninth regional meeting of the Chicago Linguistic Society.* Chicago: University of Chicago Department of Linguistics.

LaMarre, J., & Holland, J. (1985). The functional independence of mands and tacts. *Journal of Experimental Analysis of Behavior, 43,* 5–19.

Lange, G. (1978). Organization-related processes in children's recall. In P. Ornstein (Ed.), *Memory development in children* (pp. 101–128). Hillsdale, NJ: Erlbaum.

Larry P. v. Riles. (1972, June 21). USLW 2033 (US).

Larson, V., & McKinley, N. (1987). *Communication assessment and intervention strategies for adolescents.* Eau Claire, WI: Thinking Publications.

Lasky, E., & Klopp, K. (1982). Parent-child interactions in normal and language-disordered children. *Journal of Speech and Hearing Disorders, 47,* 7–18.

Laughton, J., & Hasenstab, M. (1986). *The language learning process: Implications for management of disorders.* Rockville, MD: Aspen.

Launer, P., & Lahey, M. (1981). Passages: From the fifties to the eighties in language assessment. *Topics in Language Disorders, 1*(3), 11–29.

Lazar, R., Warr-Leeper, G., Nicholson, C., & Johnson, S. (1989). Elementary school teachers' use of multiple meaning expressions. *Language, Speech, and Hearing Services in Schools, 20,* 420–430.

Lee, L. (1971). Northwestern Syntax Screening Test. Evanston, IL: Northwestern University Press.

Lee, L. (1974). *Developmental sentence analysis.* Evanston, IL: Northwestern University Press.

Lee, L., Koenigsknecht, R., & Mulhern, S. (1975). *Interactive language development teaching.* Evanston, IL: Northwestern University Press.

Lee, R., Kamhi, A., & Nelson, L. (1983, November). *Communicative sensitivity in language-impaired children.* Paper presented at the annual convention of the American Speech-Language-Hearing Association, Cincinnati.

Leifer, J., & Lewis, M. (1984). Acquisition of conversational response skills by young Down syndrome and nonretarded children. *American Journal of Mental Deficiency, 88,* 610–618.

Lemme, M., Hedberg, N., & Bottenberg, D. (1984). Cohesion in narratives of aphasic adults. In R. Brookshire (Ed.), *Proceedings of*

clinical aphasiology conference. Minneapolis: BRK Press.

Lempers, J., & Elrod, M. (1983). Children's appraisal of different sources of referential communicative inadequacies. *Child Development, 54,* 509–515.

Leonard, L. (1975). Modeling as a clinical procedure in language training. *Language, Speech, and Hearing Services in Schools, 6,* 72–85.

Leonard, L. (1981). Facilitating language skills in children with specific language impairment: A review. *Applied Psycholinguistics, 2,* 89–118.

Leonard, L. (1985). The contribution of phonetic context to an unusual phonological pattern: A case study. *Language, Speech, and Hearing Services in Schools, 16,* 110–118.

Leonard, L., Bolders, J., & Miller, J. (1976). An examination of the semantic relations reflected in the language usage of normal and language-disordered children. *Journal of Speech and Hearing Research, 19,* 371–392.

Leonard, L., Prutting, C., Perozzi, J., & Berkley, R. (1978). Non-standardized approaches to the assessment of language behaviors. *American Speech and Hearing Association, 20,* 371–379.

Leonard, L., Schwartz, R., Allen, G., Swanson, L., & Loeb, D. (1989). Unusual phonological behavior and the avoidance of homonymy in children. *Journal of Speech and Hearing Research, 32,* 583–590.

Leonard, L., Schwartz, R., Chapman, R., Rowan, L., Prelock, P., Terrell, B., Weiss, A., & Messick, C. (1982). Early lexical acquisition in children with specific language impairment. *Journal of Speech and Hearing Research, 25,* 554–564.

Leonard, L., Steckol, D., & Panther, K. (1983). Returning meaning to semantic relations: Some clinical implications. *Journal of Speech and Hearing Disorders, 48,* 25–35.

Levinson, S. (1978). Activity types and language. *Pragmatics Microfiche, 3,* D1–G5.

Lewis, L., Duchan, J., & Lubinski, R. (1985, November). Assessing aspect through videotape procedures. Paper presented at the American Speech-Language-Hearing Association annual convention, Washington, DC.

Li, C., & Thompson, S. (1976). Subject and topic: A new typology of language. In C. Li (Ed.), *Subject and topic* (pp. 457–490). New York: Academic Press.

Lieberman, R., Heffron, A., West, S., Hutchinson, E., & Swem, T. (1987). A comparison of four adolescent language tests. *Language, Speech, and Hearing Services in Schools, 18,* 250–266.

Lieberman, R., & Michael, A. (1986). Content relevance and content coverage in tests of grammatical ability. *Journal of Speech and Language Disorders, 51,* 71–81.

Lieberman, R., Moore, S., & Hutchinson, E. (1984). What's the difference between language impaired and learning disabled children? Paper presented at the American Speech-Language-Hearing Association annual convention, San Francisco.

Lieven, E. (1978). Conversations between mothers and young children: Individual differences and their possible implications for the study of language learning. In C. Snow & C. Ferguson (Eds.), *Talking to children: Language input and acquisition* (pp. 173–187). Cambridge: Cambridge University Press.

Lieven, E. (1982). Context, process and progress in young children's speech. In M. Beveridge (Ed.), *Children thinking through language* (pp. 7–26). London: Edward Arnold.

Lieven, E. (1984). Interactional style and children's language learning. *Topics in Language Disorders, 4*(4), 15–23.

Light, J., Collier, B., & Parnes, P. (1985). Communication interaction between young nonspeaking physically disabled children and their caregivers: Part I—Discourse patterns. *Augmentative and Alternative Communication, 1,* 74–83.

Liles, B. (1985). Cohesion in the narrative of normal and language-disordered children. *Journal of Speech and Hearing Research, 28,* 123–133.

Liles, B. (1987). Episode organization and cohesion conjunctions in narratives of children with and without language disorder. *Journal of Speech and Hearing Research, 30,* 185–196.

Liles, B. (1990, April). *Clinical implications for narrative production.* Paper presented at the annual convention of the New York State Speech-Language-Hearing Association, Kiamesha Lake.

Litt, M., & Schreibman, L. (1982). Stimulus specific reinforcement in the acquisition of receptive labels by autistic children. *Analysis and Intervention in Developmental Disabilities, 1,* 171–186.

Lively, M. (1984). Developmental sentence scoring: Common scoring errors. *Language, Speech, and Hearing Services in Schools, 15,* 154–168.

Lloyd, P., Baker, E., & Dunn, J. (1984). Children's awareness of communication. In C. Garvey, L. Feagans, & R. Golinkoff (Eds.), *The origins and growth of communication* (pp. 281–296). Norwood, NJ: Ablex.

Loban, W. (1976). *Language development: Kindergarten through grade twelve,* Research report no. 18. Champaign, IL: National Council of Teachers of English.

Loban, W. (1979). Relationships between language and literacy. *Language Arts, 56,* 485–486.

Longacre, R. (1983). *The grammar of discourse.* New York: Plenum Press.

Longhurst, T. (1984). The scope of normative language assessment. In K. Ruder & M. Smith (Eds.), *Developmental language intervention: Psycholinguistic applications* (pp. 21–55). Baltimore: University Park Press.

Longhurst, T., & Grubb, S. (1974). A comparison of language samples collected in four situations. *Language, Speech, and Hearing Services in Schools, 5,* 71–78.

Looney, P. (1980). Instructional intervention with language-disordered learners. *Directive Learner, 2,* 30–31.

Louko, L., & Edwards, M. (1990, April). *Enhancing generalization for more efficient and effective phonological remediation.* Paper presented at the annual convention of the New York State Speech-Language-Hearing Association, Kiamesha Lake.

Lovaas, O. (1977). *The autistic child: Language development through behavior modification.* New York: Wiley.

Loveland, K., Landry, S., Hughes, S., Hall, S., & McEvoy, R. (1988). Speech acts and the pragmatic deficits of autism. *Journal of Speech and Hearing Research, 31,* 593–604.

Lovett, M., Dennis, M., & Newman, J. (1986). Making reference: The cohesive use of pronouns in the narrative discourse of hemidecorticate adolescents. *Brain and Language, 29,* 224–251.

Low, G., Newman, P., & Ravsten, M. (1989). Pragmatic considerations in treatment: Communication-centered instruction. In N. Craighead, P. Newman, & W. Secord (Eds.), *Assessment and remediation of articulatory and phonological disorders* (pp. 217–242). Columbus, OH: Merrill.

Lowe, R. (1986). Phonological process analysis using three position tests. *Language, Speech, and Hearing Services in Schools, 17,* 72–79.

Lucas, E. (1980). *Semantic and pragmatic language disorders.* Rockville, MD: Aspen.

Lund, N., & Duchan, J. (1988). *Assessing children's language in naturalistic contexts.* Englewood Cliffs, NJ: Prentice Hall.

Lust, B., & Mervis, C. (1980). Development of co-ordination in the natural speech of young children. *Journal of Child Language, 7,* 279–304.

Lyngaas, K., Nyberg, B., Hoekenga, R., & Gruenewald, L. (1983). Language intervention in the multiple contexts of the public school setting. In J. Miller, D. Yoder, & R. Schiefelbusch (Eds.), *Contemporary issues in language intervention, ASHA reports 12* (pp. 239–252). Rockville, MD: American Speech-Language-Hearing Association.

MacDonald, J. (1978a). Environmental Language Inventory. San Antonio: Psychological Corporation.

MacDonald, J. (1978b). OLIVER: Parent-administered Communication Inventory. San Antonio: Psychological Corporation.

MacDonald, J. (1985). Language through conversation: A model for intervention with language-delayed persons. In S. Warren & A. Rogers-Warren (Eds.), *Teaching functional language* (pp. 89–122). Baltimore: University Park Press.

MacDonald, J., Blott, J., Gordon, K., Spiegal, B., & Hartmann, M. (1974). An experimental parent-assisted treatment program for language-disordered children. *Journal of Speech and Hearing Disorders, 39,* 295–315.

MacDonald, J., & Gillette, Y. (1982). *A conversational approach to language delay: Problems and solutions.* Columbus, OH: Nisonger Center.

MacDonald, J., & Gillette, Y. (1986). Communicating with persons with severe handicaps: Roles of parents and professionals. *The Journal of the Association for Persons with Severe Handicaps, 11,* 255–265.

MacLachlan, B., & Chapman, R. (1988). Communication breakdown in normal and language learning-disabled children's communication and narration. *Journal of Speech and Hearing Disorders, 53,* 2–7.

Mahoney, G., & Powell, A. (1986). *Transactional intervention program: Teacher's guide.* Farmington, CT: Pediatric Research and Training Center, Health Center, University of Connecticut.

Mahoney, G., & Weller, E. (1980). An ecological approach to language intervention. *New Directions for Exceptional Children, 2,* 17–32.

Major, D. (1974). *The acquisition of modal auxiliaries in the language of children.* The Hague: Mouton.

Mandler, J., & Johnson, N. (1977). Remembrance of things parsed: Story structure and recall. *Cognitive Psychology, 9,* 111–151.

Manolson, A. (1983). *It takes two to talk.* Toronto: Hanen Early Language Resource Center.

Marion, K. (1983). Data-based language programs: A closer look. In H. Winits (Ed.), *Treating language disorders* (pp. 11–24). Baltimore: University Park Press.

Markman, E. (1981). Comprehension monitoring. In W. Dickson (Ed.), *Children's oral communication skills* (pp. 61–84). New York: Academic Press.

Marshall, N., Hegrenes, J., & Goldstein, S. (1973). Verbal interactions: Mothers and their retarded children vs. mothers and their nonretarded children. *American Journal of Mental Deficiency, 77,* 415–419.

Martin, J. (1972). Rhythmic (hierarchical) versus serial structure in speech and other behaviors. *Psychological Review, 79,* 487–509.

Marvin, C. (1987). Consultation services: Changing roles for SLP's. *Journal of Childhood Communication Disorders, 11*(1), 1–16.

Matsuda, M. (1989). Working with Asian parents: Some communication strategies. *Topics in Language Disorders, 9*(3), 45–53.

Mattes, L. (1982). The elicited language analysis procedure: A method for scoring sentence imitation tasks. *Language, Speech, and Hearing in Schools, 13,* 37–41.

McCabe, A., & Peterson, C. (1985). A naturalistic study of the production of causal connectives by children. *Journal of Child Language, 12,* 145–160.

McCabe, P., & Prizant, B. (1985). Encoding of new versus old information by autistic children. *Journal of Speech and Hearing Disorders, 50,* 230–240.

McCartney, K., & Nelson, K. (1981). Children's use of scripts in story recall. *Discourse Processes, 4,* 59–70.

McCauley, R., & Swisher, L. (1983, November). Uses and misuses of norm-referenced tests in language assessment. Paper presented at the American Speech-Language-Hearing Association annual convention, Cincinnati.

McCauley, R., & Swisher, L. (1984a). Psychometric review of language and articulation tests for preschool children. *Journal of Speech and Hearing Disorders, 49,* 34–42.

McCauley, R., & Swisher, L. (1984b). Use and misuse of norm-referenced tests in clinical assessment: A hypothetical case. *Journal of Speech and Hearing Disorders, 49,* 338–348.

McConkey, R., & O'Connor, M. (1982). A new approach to parental involvement in language intervention programmes. *Child: Care, Health, and Development, 8,* 163–176.

McCormick, L. (1986). Keeping up with language intervention trends. *Teaching Exceptional Children, 18,* 123–129.

McCormick, L., & Goldman, R. (1984). Designing an optimal learning program. In L. McCormick & R. Schiefelbusch (Eds.), *Early language intervention: An introduction* (pp. 201–241). Columbus, OH: Merrill.

McCune-Nicolich, L., & Carroll, S. (1981). Development of symbolic play: Implications for the language specialist. *Topics in Language Disorders, 2,* 1–16.

McDade, H., & Varnedoe, D. (1987). Training parents to be language facilitators. *Topics in Language Disorders, 7*(3), 19–30.

McDermott, R., Gospodinoff, K., & Aram, L. (1976). Criteria for an ethnographically adequate description of activities and their contexts. Paper presented at the American Anthropological Association annual meeting, Washington, DC.

McDermott, R., & Hood, L. (1982). Institutionalized psychology and the ethnography of schooling. In P. Gilmore & A. Glatthorn (Eds.), *Children in and out of school* (pp. 232–249). Washington, DC: Center for Applied Linguistics.

McDonald, J., & Gillette, Y. (1982). *ECO II: Ecological communication system.* Columbus, OH: Nisonger Center, Ohio State University.

McDonald, L., & Pien, D. (1982). Mother conversational behavior as a function of interactional intent. *Journal of Child Language, 9,* 337–358.

McGee, G., Krantz, P., Mason, D., & McClannahan, L. (1983). A modified incidental-teaching procedure for autistic youth: Acquisition and generalization of receptive object labels. *Journal of Applied Behavior Analysis, 16,* 329–338.

McGivern, A., Reiff, M., & Vender, B. (1978). *Language stories: Teaching language to developmentally disabled children.* New York: Day.

McGregor, K., & Leonard, L. (1989). Facilitating word-finding skills of language-impaired children. *Journal of Speech and Hearing Disorders, 54,* 141–147.

McKinley, N., & Lord-Larson, V. (1985). Neglected language-disordered adolescent: A delivery model. *Language, Speech, and Hearing Services in Schools, 16,* 2–15.

McKinley, N., & Schwartz, L. (1987). *Referential communication: Barrier activities for speakers and listeners, part 2.* Eau Claire, WI: Thinking Publications.

McLean, J., & Snyder-McLean, L. (1978). *A transactional approach to early language training.* Columbus, OH: Merrill.

McLean, J., & Snyder-McLean, L. (1988, September). Assessment and treatment of communicative competencies among clients with severe/profound developmental disabilities. Workshop presented for Craig Developmental Disabilities Service Office and State University of New York, Geneseo.

McLoughlin, C., & Gullo, D. (1984). Comparison of three formal methods of preschool language assessment. *Language, Speech, and Hearing Services in Schools, 15,* 146–153.

McNaughton, D., & Light, J. (1989). Teaching facilitators to support the communication skills of an adult with severe cognitive disabilities: A case study. *Augmentative and Alternative Communication, 5,* 35–41.

Mecham, M. (1974). *Motivation and learning-centered training programs for language delayed children.* Salt Lake City: Word Making Productions.

Mecham, M., Jex, J., & Jones, J. (1967). Utah Test of Language Development. Salt Lake City: Communication Research Associates.

Mele-McCarthy, J. (1990, April). *What's the meta*

with phonology? Paper presented at the annual convention of the New York State Speech-Language-Hearing Association, Kiamesha Lake.

Meline, T. (1988). The encoding of novel referents by language-impaired children. *Language, Speech, and Hearing Services in Schools, 19,* 119–127.

Meline, T., & Brackin, S. (1987). Language-impaired children's awareness of inadequate messages. *Journal of Speech and Hearing Disorders, 52,* 263–270.

Menn, L. (1971). Phonotactic rules in beginning speech. *Lingua, 26,* 225–251.

Menyuk, P., & Looney, P. (1972). A problem of language disorders: Length versus structure. *Journal of Speech and Hearing Research, 15,* 264–279.

Merritt, D., & Liles, B. (1985, November). Story recall and comprehension in older language disordered children. Paper presented at the American Speech-Language-Hearing Association annual convention, San Francisco.

Merritt, D., & Liles, B. (1987). Story grammar ability in children with and without language disorder: Story generation, story retelling, and story comprehension. *Journal of Speech and Hearing Research, 30,* 539–552.

Merritt, D., & Liles, B. (1989). Narrative analysis: Clinical applications of story generation and story retelling. *Journal of Speech and Hearing Disorders, 54,* 438–447.

Messick, C. (1988). Ins and outs of the acquisition of spatial terms. *Topics in Language Disorders, 8*(2), 14–25.

Messick, S. (1980). Test validity and the ethics of assessment. *American Psychologist, 35,* 1012–1027.

Meyer, L., & Evans. (1986). Modification of excess behavior: An adaptive and functional approach for educational and community settings. In R. Horner, L. Meyer, & H. Fredericks (Eds.), *Education of learners with severe handicaps* (pp. 315–350). Baltimore: Brookes.

Miller, J. (1978). Assessing children's language behavior: A developmental process approach. In R. Schiefelbusch (Ed.), *Bases of language intervention* (pp. 269–318). Baltimore: University Park Press.

Miller, J. (1981). *Assessing language production in children.* Baltimore: University Park Press.

Miller, J., & Chapman, R. (1981). The relation between age and mean length of utterance in morphemes. *Journal of Speech and Hearing Research, 24,* 154–161.

Miller, J., & Chapman, R. (1984). Disorders of communication: Investigating the development of language of mentally retarded children. *American Journal of Mental Deficiency, 88,* 536–545.

Miller, J., & Chapman, R. (1985). *Systematic analysis of language transcripts.* [Computer program.] Madison, WI: Language Analysis Laboratory, Weisman Center on Mental Retardation and Human Development.

Miller, J., & Yoder, D. (1972). The Miller-Yoder Test of Grammatical Comprehension (experimental edition). Madison: University of Wisconsin Bookstore.

Miller, J., & Yoder, D. (1974). An ontogenetic language teaching strategy for retarded children. In R. Schiefelbusch & L. Lloyd (Eds.), *Language perspectives—Acquisition, retardation, and intervention* (pp. 505–528). Baltimore: University Park Press.

Miller, L. (1989). Classroom-based language intervention. *Language, Speech, and Hearing Services in Schools, 20,* 153–169.

Miller, P. (1982). *Amy, Wendy, and Beth.* Austin: University of Texas Press.

Milosky, L., & Wilkinson, L. (1984, November). Requests for information and responses obtained in classroom learning groups. Paper presented at the American Speech-Language-Hearing Association annual convention, San Francisco.

Mire, S., & Chisholm, R. (1990). Functional communication goals for adolescents and adults who are severely and moderately mentally handicapped. *Language, Speech, and Hearing Services in Schools, 21,* 57–58.

Mirenda, P., & Donnellan, A. (1986). Effects of adult interaction style on conversational behavior in students with severe communication problems. *Language, Speech, and Hearing Services in Schools, 17,* 126–141.

Mirenda, P., & Locke, P. (1989). A comparison of symbol transparency in nonspeaking persons with intellectual disabilities. *Journal of Speech and Hearing Disorders, 54,* 131–140.

Mishler, E. (1975). Studies in dialogue and discourse: Types of discourse initiated by and sustained through questioning. *Journal of Psycholinguistic Research, 4,* 99–121.

Mishler, E. (1979). Meaning in context: Is there any other kind? *Harvard Educational Review, 49,* 1–19.

Mistry, J., & Lange, G. (1985). Children's organization and recall of information in scripted narratives. *Child Development, 56,* 953–961.

Mizuko, M. (1987). Transparency and ease of learning of symbols represented by Blissymbolics, PCS, & Picsyms. *Augmentative and Alternative Communications, 3,* 129–136.

Moeller, M., & McConkey, A. (1984). Language intervention with preschool deaf children: A cognitive/linguistic approach. In W. Perkins (Ed.), *Current therapy of communication disorders: Hearing disorders* (pp. 11–25). New York: Thieme-Stratton.

Moeller, M., Osberger, M., & Eccarius, M. (1986). Cognitively based strategies for use with hearing-impaired students with comprehension deficits. *Topics in Language Disorders, 6*(4), 37–50.

Moerk, E. (1975). Verbal interactions between children and their mothers during the preschool years. *Journal of Developmental Psychology, 11,* 788–794.

Moerk, E. (1977). *Pragmatic and semantic aspects of early language development.* Baltimore: University Park Press.

Monahan, D. (1984). *Remediation of common phonological processes.* Tigard, OR: C. C. Publications.

Monahan, D. (1986). Remediation of common phonological processes: Four case studies. *Language, Speech, and Hearing Services in Schools, 17,* 199–206.

Montgomery, J., & Bonderman, I. (1989). Serving preschool children with severe phonological disorders. *Language, Speech, and Hearing Services in Schools, 20,* 76–83.

Morehead, D., & Ingram, D. (1976). The development of base syntax in normal and linguistically deviant children. In D. Morehead & A. Morehead (Eds.), *Normal and deficient child language* (pp. 209–238). Baltimore: University Park Press.

Morris, S. (1982). *Pre-speech assessment scale.* Clifton, NJ: Preston.

Morris, S., & Klein, M. (1987). *Pre-feeding skills.* Tucson, AZ: Therapy Skill Builders.

Moses, N., & Maffei, L. (1989, April). Classroom language intervention for communication oriented preschools. Paper presented at the New York State Speech-Language-Hearing Association annual conference, Liberty.

Mulac, A., & Tomlinson, C. (1977). Generalization of an operant remediation program for syntax with language-delayed children. *Journal of Communication Disorders, 10,* 231–244.

Muma, J. (1978). *Language handbook.* Englewood Cliffs, NJ: Prentice Hall.

Muma, J. (1983). Speech-language pathology: Emerging clinical expertise in language. In T. Gallagher & C. Prutting (Eds.), *Pragmatic assessment and intervention issues in language* (pp. 195–205). San Diego: College-Hill.

Muma, J. (1984). Clinical assessment. In K. Ruder & M. Smith (Eds.), *Developmental language intervention: Psycholinguistic applications* (pp. 57–80). Baltimore: University Park Press.

Muma, J. (1986). *Language acquisition: A functional perspective.* Austin, TX: Pro-Ed.

Muma, J., Lubinski, R., & Pierce, S. (1982). A new era in language assessment: Data or evidence. In N. Lass (Ed.), *Speech and language advances in basic research and practice* (Vol. 7) (pp. 135–147). New York: Academic Press.

Muma, J., & Pierce, S. (1981). Language intervention: Data or evidence? *Topics in Learning & Learning Disabilities, 1*(2), 1–12.

Muma, J., Pierce, D., & Muma, D. (1983). Language training in speech-language pathology. *ASHA, 26*(6), 35–42.

Mundell, C., & Lucas, E. (1978). *A parent conducted pragmatic language program for Down's Syndrome children.* An unpublished manuscript, Washington State University.

Musselwhite, C. (1983). Pluralistic assessment in speech-language pathology: Use of dual norms in the placement process. *Language, Speech, and Hearing Services in Schools, 14,* 29–37.

Musselwhite, C., & St. Louis, K. (1982). *Communication programming for the severely handicapped: Vocal and nonvocal strategies.* San Diego: College-Hill.

Nakamura, P., & Newhoff, M. (1982, November). Clinical speech adjustments to normal and language-disordered children. Paper presented at the American Speech-Language-Hearing Association annual convention, Toronto.

Nakayama, M. (1987). Performance factors in subject-auxiliary inversion in children. *Journal of Child Language, 14*, 113–127.

Narrol, H., & Giblon, S. (1984). *The fourth "R"—Uncovering hidden learning potential*. Baltimore: University Park Press.

National Council of Teachers of English Report. (1976). *Language development: Kindergarten through grade twelve*. Urbana, IL: National Council of Teachers of English.

Nelson, K. (1973). Structure and strategy in learning to talk. *Monographs of the Society for Research in Child Development, 38* (Serial No. 149).

Nelson, K. (1981a). Acquisition of words by first-language learners. *Annals of the New York Academy of Sciences, 379*, 148–159.

Nelson, K. (1981b). Social cognition in a script framework. In L. Ross & J. Flavell (Eds.), *The development of social cognition in children*. Cambridge: Cambridge University Press.

Nelson, K. (1981c). Toward a rare-event cognitive comparison theory of syntax acquisition. In P. Dale & D. Ingram (Eds.), *Child language—An international perspective* (pp.). Baltimore: University Park Press.

Nelson, K., & Denninger, M. (1977). The shadow technique in the investigation of children's acquisition of new syntactic forms. Unpublished manuscript, New School for Social Research, New York.

Nelson, K., & Gruendel, J. (1981). Generalized event representation: Basic building blocks of cognitive development. In A. Brown & M. Lamb (Eds.), *Advances in developmental psychology* (pp. 131–158). Hillsdale, NJ: Erlbaum.

Nelson, K., & Gruendel, J. (1979). At mornings its lunchtime: A scriptal view of children's stories. *Discourse Processes, 2*, 73–94.

Nelson, K., & Lucariello, J. (1983). The development of meaning in first words. In M. Barrett (Ed.), *Children's single-word speech* (pp. 59–86). New York: Wiley.

Nelson, L., & Weber-Olsen, M. (1980). The Elicited Language Inventory and the influence of contextual cues. *Journal of Speech and Hearing Disorders, 45*, 549–563.

Nelson, N. (1984). Beyond information processing: The language of teachers and textbooks. In

G. Wallach & K. Butler (Eds.), *Language learning disabilities in school-age children* (pp. 154–178). Baltimore: Williams & Wilkins.

Nelson, N. (1985). Teachers talk and children listen—Fostering a better match. In C. Simon (Ed.), *Communication skills and classroom success: Assessment of language-learning disabled students* (pp. 65–104). San Diego: College-Hill.

Nelson, N. (1986a). Individual processing in classroom settings. *Topics in Language Disorders, 6*(2), 13–27.

Nelson, N. (1986b). What is meant by meaning (and how can it be taught)? *Topics in Language Disorders, 6*(4), 1–14.

Nelson, N. (1988a). The consultant model. *ASHA Audioteleconference*. Rockville, MD: ASHA.

Nelson, N. (1988b). *Planning individualized speech and language intervention programs: Objectives for infants, children, and adolescents*. Tucson, AZ: Communication Skill Builders.

Nelson, N. (1989). Curriculum-based language assessment and intervention. *Language, Speech, and Hearing Services in Schools, 20*, 170–184.

Nestheide, C., & Culatta, B. (1980, November). Incorporating language training into daily activities. Paper presented at the American Speech-Language-Hearing Association annual convention, Detroit.

Newcomer, P., & Hammill, D. (1977). The Test of Language Development. Austin, TX: Empiric Press.

Newhoff, M., & Leonard, L. (1983). Diagnosis of developmental language disorders. In I. Meitus & B. Weinberg (Eds.), *Diagnosis in speech-language pathology* (pp. 71–112). Baltimore: University Park Press.

Newman, J., Lovett, M., & Dennis, M. (1986). The use of discourse analysis in neurolinguistics: Some findings from the narratives of hemidecorticate adolescents. *Topics in Language Disorders, 7*(1), 31–44.

Newport, E., Gleitman, H., & Gleitman, L. (1977). Mother, I'd rather do it myself: Some effects and non-effects of maternal speech style. In C. Snow & C. Ferguson (Eds.), *Talking to children: Language input and acquisition* (pp. 109–150). Cambridge: Cambridge University Press.

Newson, J. (1979). The growth of shared understandings between infant and caregiver. In N.

Bullowa (Ed.), *Before speech* (pp. 207–222). New York: Cambridge University Press.

Nietupski, J., Hamre-Nietupski, S., Clancy, P., & Veerhusen, K. (1986). Guidelines for making simulation an effective adjunct to in vivo community instruction. *The Journal of the Association for Persons with Severe Handicaps, 11*, 12–18.

Ninio, A., & Bruner, J. (1978). The achievements and antecedents of labeling. *Journal of Child Language, 5*, 1–15.

Noel, M. (1980). Referential communication abilities of learning disabled children. *Learning Disability Quarterly, 3*, 70–75.

Norris, J. (1989). Providing language remediation in the classroom: An integrated language-to-reading intervention model. *Language, Speech, and Hearing Services in Schools, 20*, 205–218.

Norris, J., & Bruning, R. (1988). Cohesion in the narratives of good and poor readers. *Journal of Speech and Hearing Disorders, 53*, 416–424.

Norris, J., and Hoffman, P. (1990). Comparison of adult-initiated vs. child-initiated interaction styles with handicapped prelanguage children. *Language, Speech, and Hearing Services in Schools, 21*, 28–36.

Norris, J., & Hoffman, P. (1990). Language intervention within naturalistic environments. *Language, Speech, and Hearing Services in Schools, 21*, 72–84.

Norris, M., Juarez, M., & Perkins, M. (1989). Adaptation of a screening test for bilingual and bidialectal populations. *Language, Speech, and Hearing Services in Schools, 20*, 381–390.

Nye, C., Foster, S., & Seaman, D. (1987). Effectiveness of language intervention with the language/learning disabled. *Journal of Speech and Hearing Disorders, 52*, 348–357.

Oakhill, J. (1984). Inferential and memory skills in children's comprehension of stories. *British Journal of Educational Psychology, 54*, 31–39.

O'Connor, L., & Schery, T. (1986). A comparison of microcomputer-aided and traditional language therapy for developing communication skills in nonoral toddlers. *Journal of Speech and Hearing Disorders, 51*, 356–361.

Odom, S. (1983). The development of social interchanges in infancy. In S. Garwood & R. Rewell (Eds.), *Educating handicapped infants: Issues in development and intervention*. Rockville, MD: Aspen.

O'Donnell, R., Griffin, W., & Norris, R. (1967). *Syntax of kindergarten and elementary school children: A transformational analysis* (Research Report No. 8). Champaign, IL: National Council of Teachers of English.

Oliver, C., & Halle, J. (1982). Language training in the everyday environment: Teaching functional sign use to a retarded child. *Journal of the Association for Persons with Severe Handicaps, 8*, 50–62.

Oller, D. (1974). Simplification as the goal of phonological processes in child speech. *Language Learning, 24*, 299–303.

Oller, J. (1983). *Issues in language testing research*. Rowley, MA: Newbury House.

Oller, J. (1979). *Language tests at school: A pragmatic approach*. London: Longman.

Olsen-Fulero, L. (1982). Style and stability in mother conversational behavior: A study of individual differences. *Journal of Child Language, 9*, 543–564.

Olson, D. (1970). Language and thought: Aspects of a cognitive theory of semantics. *Psychological Review, 77*, 257–273.

Olswang, L. (1978). The ontogenesis of agent: From cognitive notion to semantic expression. Unpublished doctoral dissertation, University of Washington.

Olswang, L., Kriegsmann, E., & Mastergeorge, A. (1982). Facilitating functional requesting in pragmatically impaired children. *Language, Speech, and Hearing Services in Schools, 13*, 202–222.

Orelove, F., & Sobsey, D. (1987). *Educating children with multiple disabilities: A transdisciplinary approach*. Baltimore: Brookes.

Owens, R. (1978). *Speech acts in the early language of non-delayed and retarded children: A taxonomy and distributional study*. Unpublished doctoral dissertation, The Ohio State University.

Owens, R. (1982a). Caregiver interview and environmental observation. *Program for the acquisition of language with the severely impaired*. San Antonio: Psychological Corporation.

Owens, R. (1982b). Developmental Assessment Tool. *Program for the acquisition of language with the severely impaired*. San Antonio: Psychological Corporation.

Owens, R. (1982c). *Program for the acquisition of*

language with the severely impaired (PALS). San Antonio: Psychological Corporation.

Owens, R., Haney, M., Giesow, V., Dooley, L., & Kelly, R. (1983). Language test content: A comparative study. *Language, Speech, and Hearing Services in Schools, 14,* 7–21.

Owens, R., & House, L. (1984). Decision-making processes in augmentative communication. *Journal of Speech and Hearing Disorders, 49,* 18–25.

Owens, R., McNerney, C., Bigler-Burke, L., & Lepre-Clark, C. (1987, June). Language facilitators with residential retarded populations. *Topics in Language Disorders, 7*(3), 47–63.

Owens, R., & Rogerson, B. (1988). Adults at the presymbolic level. In S. Calculator & J. Bedrosian (Eds.), *Communication assessment and intervention for adults with mental retardation* (pp. 189–230). Boston, MA: College-Hill.

Paccia-Cooper, J., & Curcio, F. (1982). Language processing and forms of immediate echolalia in autistic children. *Journal of Speech and Hearing Research, 25,* 42–47.

Paden, E., & Moss, S. (1985). Comparison of three phonological analysis procedures. *Language, Speech, and Hearing Services in Schools, 16,* 103–109.

Page, J. (1982, May). *The communication game: Pragmatics and early communication training for severely/profoundly retarded individuals.* Paper presented at the American Association on Mental Deficiency annual convention, Boston.

Page, J., & Horn, D. (1987). Comprehension in developmentally delayed children. *Language, Speech, and Hearing Services in Schools, 18,* 63–71.

Palermo, D. (1982). Theoretical issues in semantic development. In S. Kuczaj (Ed.), *Language development: Vol. 1. Syntax and semantics.* Hillsdale, NJ: Erlbaum.

Paluszek, S., & Feintuch, F. (1979). Comparing imitation and comprehension training in two language impaired children. *Working Papers in Experimental Speech-Language Pathology and Audiology, 8,* 72–91.

Panagos, J., Quine, H., & Klich, P. (1979). Syntactic and phonological influences in children's articulations. *Journal of Speech and Hearing Research, 22,* 841–848.

Parnell, M., & Amerman, J. (1983). Answers to wh- questions: Research and application. In T. Gallagher & C. Prutting (Eds.), *Pragmatic assessment and intervention issues in language* (pp. 129–150). San Diego: College-Hill.

Parnell, M., Amerman, J., & Harting, R. (1986). Responses of language-disordered children to wh- questions. *Language, Speech, and Hearing Services in Schools, 17,* 95–106.

Parnell, M., Patterson, S., & Harding, M. (1984). Answers to wh- questions: A developmental study. *Journal of Speech and Hearing Research, 27,* 297–305.

Paul, R., & Shriberg, L. (1982). Associations between phonology and syntax in speech-delayed children. *Journal of Speech and Hearing Research, 25,* 536–546.

Paynter, E., & Bumpas, T. (1977). Imitative and spontaneous articulatory assessment of 3-year-old children. *Journal of Speech and Hearing Disorders, 42,* 119–125.

Pearson, D. (1988). A group therapy idea for new clinicians in the school setting: Keep little hands busy. *Language, Speech, and Hearing Services in Schools, 19,* 432.

Pecyna, P. (1984). The use of nonspeech communication systems to facilitate language acquisition in severely handicapped preschool children. Unpublished doctoral dissertation, Kent State University, Ohio.

Pecyna, P. (1988). Rebus symbol communication training with a severely handicapped preschool child: A case study. *Language, Speech, and Hearing Services in Schools, 19,* 128–143.

Pecyna-Rhyner, P., Lehr, D., & Pudlas, K. (1990). An analysis of teacher responsiveness to communicative initiations of preschool children with handicaps. *Language, Speech, and Hearing Services in Schools, 21,* 91–97.

Peterson, C., & McCabe, A. (1983). Developmental psycholinguistics: Three ways of looking at a child's narrative. New York: Plenum.

Peterson, P., & Swing, S. (1985). Students' cognitions as mediators of the effectiveness of small-group learning. *Journal of Educational Psychology, 77,* 299–312.

Phillips, J., & Balthazar, E. (1979). Some correlates of language deterioration in severely and profoundly retarded long-term institutionalized residents. *American Journal of Mental Deficiency, 83,* 402–408.

Piaget, J. (1952). *Origins of intelligence in children.* New York: International Universities Press.

Piaget, J. (1954). *The construction of reality in the child.* New York; Basic Books.

Piche-Cragoe, L., Reichle, J., & Sigafoos, J. (1986). Requesting validity intervention. Unpublished manuscript, University of Minnesota, Minneapolis.

Pidek, C. (1987). *The assignment book.* Schaumburg, IL: Communication Concepts.

Polk, X., Schilmoeller, G., Emboy, L., Holman, J., & Baer, D. (1976, May). *Prompted generalization through experimenters' instructions: A parent training study.* Paper presented at the Midwestern Association of Behavior Analysis annual meeting, Chicago.

Prather, E., Breecher, S., Stafford, M., & Wallace, E. (1980). Screening Test of Adolescent Language. Seattle: University of Washington Press.

Prelock, P., Messick, C., Schwartz, R., & Terrell, B. (1981). Mother-child discourse during the one-word stage. *Proceedings from the Second Wisconsin Symposium on Research in Child Language Disorders.* Madison, WI: Department of Communicative Disorders, University of Wisconsin.

Prelock, P., & Panagos, J. (1980). Minicry versus imitative production in the speech of the retarded. *Journal of Psycholinguistic Research, 9,* 565–578.

Price, P. (1984). A study of mother-child interaction strategies with mothers of young developmentally delayed children. In J. Berg (Ed.), *Perspectives and progress in mental retardation.* Sixth Congress of the International Association for the Scientific Study of Mental Deficiency. Baltimore: University Park Press.

Prizant, B. (1983a). Echolalia in autism: Assessment and intervention. *Seminars in Speech and Language, 4,* 63–77.

Prizant, B. (1983b). Language acquisition and communicative behavior in autism: Toward an understanding of the ''whole'' of it. *Journal of Speech and Hearing Disorders, 48,* 296–307.

Prizant, B., & Duchan, J. (1981). The functions of immediate echolalia in autistic children. *Journal of Speech and Hearing Disorders, 46,* 241–249.

Prizant, B., & Rentschler, G. (1983). Language-impaired children's use of language across three conversational situations. *Australian Journal of Human Communication Disorders, 11,* 5–16.

Prutting, C. (1979). Process \prâ\,ses\n: The action of moving forward progressively from one point to another on the way to completion. *Journal of Speech and Language Disorders, 44,* 3–30.

Prutting, C. (1982). Pragmatic and social competence. *Journal of Speech and Hearing Disorders, 42,* 123–134.

Prutting, C. (1983). Scientific inquiry and communicative disorders: An emerging paradigm across six decades. In T. Gallagher & C. Prutting (Eds.), *Pragmatic assessment and intervention issues in language* (pp. 247–267). San Diego: College-Hill.

Prutting, C., Bagshaw, N., Goldstein, H., Juskowitz, S., & Umen, I. (1978). Clinician-child discourse: Some preliminary questions. *Journal of Speech and Hearing Disorders, 43,* 123–139.

Prutting, C., & Connolly, J. (1976). Imitation: A closer look. *Journal of Speech and Hearing Disorders, 41,* 412–422.

Prutting, C., & Kirchner, D. (1983). Applied pragmatics. In T. Gallagher & C. Prutting (Eds.), *Pragmatic assessment and intervention issues in language* (pp. 29–64). San Diego: College-Hill.

Quigley, S., Steinkamp, M., Power, D., & Jones, B. (1978). Test of Syntactic Abilities. Beaverton, OR: Dormac.

Quigley, S., Wilbur, R., & Montanelli, D. (1974). Question formation in the language of deaf students. *Journal of Speech and Hearing Research, 17,* 699–713.

Ratner, N., & Bruner, J. (1978). Games, social exchange and the acquisition of language. *Journal of Child Language, 5,* 391–402.

Ray, S. (1989). Context and psychoeducational assessment of hearing impaired children. *Topics in Language Disorders, 9*(4), 33–44.

Reason, J., & Mycielska, K. (1982). *Absent-minded? The psychology of mental lapses and everyday errors.* Englewood Cliffs, NJ: Prentice Hall.

Rees, N. (1978). Art and science of diagnosis in hearing, language, and speech. In S. Singh & J. Lynch (Eds.), *Diagnostic procedures in hearing, language, and speech* (pp. 3–22). Baltimore: University Park Press.

Rees, N., & Wollner, S. (1981, April). Paper presented at the New York State Speech-Language-Hearing Association annual convention, Liberty.

Reich, P. (1986). *Language Development.* Englewood Cliffs, NJ: Prentice Hall.

Reichle, J. (1990). *Intervention with presymbolic clients: Setting up an initial communication system.* Paper presented at the New York State Speech-Language-Hearing Association annual convention, Kiamesha Lake.

Reichle, J., Busch, C., & Doyle, S. (1986). The topical relationship among adjacent utterances in productively delayed children's language addressed to their mothers. *Journal of Communication Disorders, 19,* 63–74.

Reichle, J., & Karlan, G. (1985). The selection of an augmentative system in communication intervention: A critique of decision rules. *The Journal of the Association of Persons with Severe Handicaps, 10,* 146–156.

Reichle, J., Piche-Cragoe, L., Sigafoos, J., & Doss, S. (1988). Optimizing functional communication for persons with severe handicaps. In S. Calculator & J. Bedrosian (Eds.), *Communication assessment and intervention for adults with mental retardation* (pp. 239–264). San Diego: College-Hill.

Reichle, J., Rogers, N., & Barrett, C. (1984). Establishing pragmatic discriminations among the communicative functions of requesting, rejecting, and commenting in an adolescent. *Journal of the Association for Persons with Severe Handicaps, 9,* 31–36.

Reichle, J., & Yoder, D. (1985). Communication board use in severely handicapped learners. *Language, Speech, and Hearing Services in Schools, 16,* 58–63.

Rescorla, L. (1989). The language development survey: A screening tool for delayed language in toddlers. *Journal of Speech and Hearing Disorders, 54,* 587–599.

Rice, M. (1983). Contemporary accounts of the cognitive/language relationship: Implications for speech-language clinicians. *Journal of Speech and Hearing Disorders, 48,* 347–359.

Rice, M. (1984). Cognitive aspects of communication development. In R. Schiefelbusch & J. Pickar (Eds.), *The acquisition of communicative competence* (pp. 141–189). Baltimore: University Park Press.

Rice, M. (1986). Mismatched premises of the communicative competence model and language intervention. In R. Schiefelbusch (Ed.), *Language competence: Assessment and intervention* (pp. 261–281). San Diego: College-Hill.

Rice, M., Buhr, J., & Nemeth, M. (1990). Fast mapping word-learning abilities of language-delayed preschoolers. *Journal of Speech and Hearing Disorders, 55,* 33–42.

Richards, M. (1979). Sorting out what's in a word from what's not: Evaluating Clark's semantic feature acquisition theory. *Journal of Experimental Child Psychology, 27,* 1–47.

Rieke, J., & Lewis, J. (1984). Preschool intervention strategies: The communication base. *Topics in Language Disorders, 5*(1), 41–57.

Ripich, D., & Griffith, P. (1985, November). Story structure, cohesion, and propositions in learning disabled children. Paper presented at the American Speech-Language-Hearing Association annual convention, Washington, DC.

Ripich, D., & Panagos, J. (1985). Assessing children's knowledge of sociolinguistic rules for speech therapy lessons. *Journal of Speech and Hearing Disorders, 50,* 335–345.

Ripich, D., & Spinelli, F. (1985). *School discourse strategies.* San Diego: College-Hill.

Rizzo, J., & Stephens, M. (1981). Performance of children with normal and impaired oral language production on a set of auditory comprehension tests. *Journal of Speech and Hearing Disorders, 46,* 150–159.

Roberts, K., & Horowitz, F. (1986). Basic level categorization in seven- and nine-month-old infants. *Journal of Child Language, 13,* 191–208.

Robertson, S., & Suci, G. (1980). Event perception by children in the early stage of language production. *Child Development, 51,* 89–96.

Rodgon, M., Jankowski, W., & Alenskas, L. (1977). A multi-functional approach to single-word usage. *Journal of Child Language, 4,* 23–43.

Rogers, S., D'Eugenio, D., Brown, S., Donovan, C., & Lynch, E. (1978). Early Intervention Developmental Profile. Ann Arbor: University of Michigan Press.

Rogers-Warren, A., & Warren, S. (1980). Mands for verbalization: Facilitating the display of newly taught language. *Behavior Modification, 4,* 361–382.

Rogow, S. (1978). On the comprehension of questions by nonspeaking children. *Journal of Communication Disorders, 11,* 383–390.

Romski, M. (1987, August). Augmentative and alternative communication systems: Considerations for individuals with severe intellectual disabilities. Presentation at the think tank, Augmentative and Alternative Communication: State of the Art and Science, Purdue University, West Lafayette, IN.

Romski, M., & Sevcik, R. (1989). An analysis of visual-graphic symbol meanings for two nonspeaking adults with severe mental retardation. *Augmentative and Alternative Communication, 5,* 109–144.

Romski, M., Sevcik, R., & Joyner, S. (1984). Nonspeech communication systems: Implications for language intervention with mentally retarded children. *Topics in Language Disorders, 5,* 66–81.

Romski, M., Sevcik, R., & Pate, J. (1988). Establishment of symbolic communication in persons with severe retardation. *Journal of Speech and Hearing Disorders, 53,* 94–107.

Romski, M., Sevcik, R., & Washburn, D. (1987, May). Microcomputer communication system implementation in homes and classrooms of nonspeaking youngsters with retardation. Paper presented at the American Association on Mental Retardation annual meeting, Los Angeles.

Romski, M., White, R., Millen, C., & Rumbaugh, D. (1984). Effects of computer-keyboard teaching in symbolic communication of severely retarded persons: Five case studies. *The Psychological Record, 34,* 39–51.

Rondal, J., Ghiotto, M., Bredart, S., & Bachelet, J. (1987). Age-relation, reliability, and grammatical validity of measures of utterance length. *Journal of Child Language, 14,* 433–446.

Rosenfeld, H. (1987). Conversational control functions of nonverbal behavior. In A. Siegman & S. Feldman (Eds.), *Nonverbal behavior and communication* (pp. 563–601). Hillsdale, NJ: Erlbaum.

Rosinski-McClendon, M., & Newhoff, M. (1987). Conversational responsiveness and assertiveness in language-impaired children. *Language, Speech, and Hearing Services in Schools, 18,* 53–62.

Roth, F. (1986). Oral narrative abilities of learning-disabled students. *Topics in Language Disorders, 7*(1), 21–30.

Roth, F., & Spekman, N. (1984a). Assessing the pragmatic abilities of children: Part 1. Organizational framework and assessment parameters. *Journal of Speech and Hearing Disorders, 49,* 2–11.

Roth, F., & Spekman, N. (1984b). Assessing the pragmatic abilities of children: Part 2. Guidelines, considerations, and specific evaluation procedures. *Journal of Speech and Hearing Disorders, 49,* 12–17.

Roth, F., & Spekman, N. (1985, June). Story grammar analysis of narratives produced by learning disabled and normally achieving students. Paper presented at the Symposium on Research in Child Language Disorders, Madison, WI.

Roth, F., & Spekman, N. (1986). Narrative discourse: Spontaneously generated stories of learning-disabled and normally achieving students. *Journal of Speech and Hearing Disorders, 51,* 8–23.

Roth, F., & Spekman, N. (1989). The oral syntactic proficiency of learning disabled students: A spontaneous story sampling analysis. *Journal of Speech and Hearing Research, 32,* 67–77.

Rowland, C., & Schweigert, P. (1989a). Tangible symbols: Symbolic communication for individuals with multisensory impairments. *Augmentative and Alternative Communication, 5,* 226–234.

Rowland, C., & Schweigert, P. (1989b). Tangible symbol systems for individuals with multisensory impairments [Videotape and manual]. Tucson, AZ: Communication Skill Builders.

Ruder, K., Smith, M., & Hermann, P. (1974). Effect of verbal imitation and comprehension on verbal production of lexical items. *ASHA Monographs, 18,* 15–29.

Rummelhart, D. (1975). Notes on a schema for stories. In D. Bobrow & A. Collins (Eds.), *Representation and understanding: Studies in cognitive science* (pp. 211–236). New York: Academic Press.

Russo, J., & Owens, R. (1982). Development of an objective observation tool for parent-child interaction. *Journal of Speech and Hearing Disorders, 47,* 165–173.

Sacks, H., Schegloff, E., & Jefferson, G. (1974). A simplest systematics for the organization of turn-taking in conversation. *Language, 50,* 696–735.

Sacks, J., & Young, E. (1982). Infant Scale of Communication Intent. *Pediatrics Update, 7,* 1–5.

Salzberg, C., & Villani, T. (1983). Speech training by parents of Down syndrome toddlers: Generalization across settings and instructional contexts. *American Journal of Mental Deficiency, 87,* 403–413.

Samuels, S. (1983). Diagnosing reading problems. *Journal of Learning and Learning Disabilities, 2*(4), 1–11.

Saunders, R., & Sailor, W. (1979). A comparison of three strategies of reinforcement on two-choice learning problems with severely retarded children. *Journal of the Association for Persons with Severe Handicaps* (Formerly AAESPH Review), *4,* 323–333.

Sawyer, J. (1973). Social aspects of bilingualism in San Antonio, Texas. In R. Bailey & J. Robinson (Eds.), *Varieties of present-day English* (pp. 226–235). New York: Macmillan.

Scarborough, H., Wyckoff, J., & Davidson, R. (1986). A reconsideration of the relationship between age and mean utterance length. *Journal of Speech and Hearing Research, 29,* 394–399.

Scherer, N., & Olswang, L. (1989). Using structured discourse as a language intervention technique with autistic children. *Journal of Speech and Hearing Disorders, 54,* 383–394.

Scherer, N., & Owings, N. (1982, November). Mothers' role in conversational exchanges with retarded children. Paper presented at the American Speech-Language-Hearing Association annual convention, Toronto.

Schetz, K. (1989). Computer-aided language/concept enrichment in kindergarten: Consultation program model. *Language, Speech, and Hearing Services in Schools, 20,* 2–10.

Schmauch, V., Panagos, J., & Klich, P. (1978). Syntax influences and accuracy of consonant production in language-disordered children. *Journal of Communication Disorders, 11,* 315–323.

Schober-Peterson, D., & Johnson, C. (1989). Conversational topics of 4-year-olds. *Journal of Speech and Hearing Research, 32,* 857–870.

Schodorf, J. (1982). A comparative analysis of parent-child interactions of language-delayed and linguistically normal children. *Dissertation Abstracts International, 42*(5), 1838B.

Schreibman, L., & Carr, E. (1978). Elimination of echolalic responding to questions through the training of a generalized verbal response. *Journal of Applied Behavioral Analysis, 11,* 453–463.

Schuler, A., & Goetz, C. (1981). The assessment of severe language disabilities: Communicative and cognitive considerations. *Analysis and Intervention in Developmental Disabilities, 1,* 333–346.

Schumaker, J., & Deshler, D. (1984). Setting demand variables. *Topics in Language Disorders, 4*(2), 22–40.

Schwartz, L., & McKinley, N. (1984). *Daily communication: Strategies for the language disordered adolescent.* Eau Claire, WI: Thinking Publications.

Schwartz, R., Chapman, K., Terrell, B., Prelock, P., & Rowan, L. (1985). Facilitating word combination in language-impaired children in discourse structure. *Journal of Speech and Hearing Disorders, 50,* 31–39.

Scollon, R. (1979). A real early stage: An unzipped condensation of a dissertation on child language. In E. Ochs & V. Schiesselin (Eds.), *Developmental pragmatics* (pp. 215–227). New York: Academic Press.

Scollon, R., & Scollon, S. (1981). *Narrative, literacy and face in interethnic communication.* Norwood, NJ: Ablex.

Scott, C. (1984, November). *What happened in that: Structural characteristics of school children's narratives.* Paper presented at the American Speech-Language-Hearing Association annual convention, San Francisco.

Scott, C. (1987). *Summarizing text: Context effects in language disordered children.* Paper presented at the First International Symposium, Specific Language Disorders in Children, University of Reading, England.

Scott, C. (1988a). Producing complex sentences. *Topics in Language Disorders, 8*(2), 44–62.

Scott, C. (1988b). A perspective on the evaluation of school children's narratives. *Speech, Language, and Hearing Services in Schools, 19,* 67–82.

Scoville, R. (1983). Development of the intention to communicate: The eye of the beholder. In L. Feagans, C. Garvey, & R. Golinkoff (Eds.), *The origins and growth of communication* (pp. 109–122). Norwood, NJ: Ablex.

Seitz, S. (1975). Language intervention—Changing the language environment of the retarded child. In R. Koch, F. de la Cruz, & F. Menolascino (Eds.), *Down's syndrome: Research, prevention and management*. New York: Bruner/Mazel.

Semel, E. & Wiig, E. (1980). *Clinical evaluation of language functions*. San Antonio: Psychological Corporation.

Semmel, M., Peck, C., Haring, T., & Theimer, K. (1984, April). Assessment and training of social/communicative skills for children with autism and severe handicaps. Paper presented at the Council for Exceptional Children annual convention, Washington, DC.

Sevcik, R., & Romski, M. (1986). Representational matching skills of persons with severe retardation. *Augmentative and Alternative Communication, 2*, 160–164.

Seymour, H., Ashton, N., & Wheeler, L. (1986). The effect of race on language elicitation. *Language, Speech, and Hearing Services in Schools, 17*, 146–151.

Shane, H., & Bashir, A.(1980). Election criteria for the adoption of an augmentative communication system: Preliminary considerations. *Journal of Speech and Hearing Disorders, 45*, 408–414.

Shane, H., Lipshultz, R., & Shane, C. (1982). Facilitating the communicative interaction of nonspeaking persons in large residential settings. *Topics in Language Disorders, 2*, 73–84.

Shantz, C., & Wilson, K. (1972). Training communication skills in young children. *Child Development, 43*, 118–122.

Shatz, M. (1975). The relationship between cognitive processes and the development of communication skills. In B. Keasey (Ed.), *Nebraska Symposium on Motivation, 1977* (pp. 1–42). Lincoln: University of Nebraska Press.

Shevin, M., & Klein, M. (1984). The importance of choice-making skills for students with severe disabilities. *Journal of the Association for Persons with Severe Handicaps, 9*, 159–166.

Shriberg, L. (1983). Natural phonologic process approach. In W. Perkins (Ed.), *Current therapy of communication disorders: Phonologic-articulatory disorders* (pp. 3–10). New York: Thieme-Stratton.

Shriberg, L., & Kwiatkowski, J. (1980). *Natural process analysis: A procedure for phonological analysis of continuous speech samples*. New York: Wiley.

Shriberg, L., & Kwiatkowski, J. (1985). Continuous speech sampling for phonologic analysis of speech-delayed children. *Journal of Speech and Hearing Disorders, 50*, 323–334.

Shultz, J., Florio, S., & Erickson, F. (1982). Whers's the floor? Aspects of the cultural organization of social relationships in communication at home and at school. In P. Gilmore & A. Glatthorn (Eds.), *Children in and out of school* (pp. 88–123). Washington, DC: Center for Applied Linguistics.

Siegel, G. (1975). The use of language tests. *Language, Speech, and Hearing Services in Schools, 6*, 211–217.

Siegel, G. (1979). Appraisal of language development. In F. Darely (Ed.), *Evaluation of appraisal techniques in speech and language pathology*. Reading, MA: Addison-Wesley.

Siegel, G., & Broen, P. (1976). Language assessment. In L. Lloyd (Ed.), *Communication assessment and intervention strategies* (pp. 73–122). Baltimore: University Park Press.

Siegel, L., Cunningham, C., & van der Spuy, H. (1979, April). Interactions in language-delayed and normal preschool children and their mothers. Paper presented to the Conference of the Society for Research in Child Development, San Francisco.

Siegel, R., Winitz, H., & Conkey, H. (1963). The influence of testing instruments on articulatory responses of children. *Journal of Speech and Hearing Disorders, 28*, 67–76.

Siegel-Causey, E., & Downing, J. (1987). Nonsymbolic communication development: Theoretical concepts and educational strategies. In L. Goetz, D. Guess, & K. Stremel-Campbell (Eds.), *Innovative program design for individuals with sensory impairments* (pp. 15–48). Baltimore: Brookes.

Silliman, E. (1984). Interactional competencies in the instructional context: The role of teaching discourse in learning. In G. Wallach & K. Butler (Eds.), *Language learning disabilities in school-age children* (pp. 288–317). Baltimore: Williams & Wilkins.

Silverman, F. (1989). *Communication for the speechless* (2nd ed.). Englewood Cliffs, NJ: Prentice Hall.

Simmons-Miles, R. (1983, November). Assessment of phonological disorders and single-word picture naming. Paper presented at the American Speech-Language-Hearing Association annual convention, Cincinnati.

Simner, M. (1983). The warning signs of school failure: An updated profile of the at-risk kindergarten child. *Topics in Early Childhood Special Education, 3*(4), 17–28.

Simon, C. (1985). *Communication skills and classroom success: Therapy methodologies for language-learning disabled students.* San Diego: College-Hill.

Sininger, Y., Klatsky, R., & Kirchner, D. (1989). Memory scanning speed in language-disordered children. *Journal of Speech and Hearing Research, 32,* 289–297.

Sleight, C., & Prinz, P. (1985). Use of abstracts, orientations, and codes in narratives by language-disordered and nondisordered children. *Journal of Speech and Hearing Disorders, 50,* 361–371.

Sleight, M., & Niman, C. (1984). *Grossmotor & oral motor development in children with Down Syndrome: Birth through three years.* St. Louis, MO: St. Louis Association for Retarded Citizens.

Slobin, D. (1973). Cognitive prerequisites for the acquisition of grammar. In C. Ferguson & D. Slobin (Eds.), *Studies in child language development* (pp. 175–208). New York: Holt, Rinehart.

Smith, L., & vonTelzchner, S. (1986). Communicative, sensorimotor, and language skills of young children with Down syndrome. *American Journal of Mental Deficiency, 91,* 57–66.

Smitherman, G. (1985). What go round come round: Keep in perspective. In C. Brookes (Ed.), *Tapping potential: English and language arts for the Black learner* (pp. 41–62). Urbana, IL: Black Caucus of the National Council of Teachers of English.

Snell, M., & Gast, D. (1981). Applying time delay procedure to the instruction of the severely handicapped. *Journal of the Association for the Severely Handicapped, 6*(3), 3–14.

Snell, M., & Zirpoli, T. (1987). Intervention strategies. In M. Snell (Ed.), *Systematic instruction of persons with severe handicaps* (pp. 110–150). Columbus, OH: Merrill.

Snow, C. (1979). The role of social interaction in language acquisition. In A. Collins (Ed.), *Children's language and communication* (pp. 157–182). Hillsdale, NJ: Erlbaum.

Snow, C. (1977). Mothers' speech research: From input to interaction. In C. Snow & C. Ferguson (Eds.), *Talking to children: Language input and acquisition* (pp. 31–50). Cambridge: Cambridge University Press.

Snow, C., & Goldfield, B. (1983). Turn the page please: Situation-specific language learning. *Journal of Child Learning, 10,* 551–570.

Snow, C., Midkiff-Borunda, S., Small, A., & Proctor, A. (1984). Therapy as social interaction: Analyzing the contexts for language remediation. *Topics in Language Disorders, 4*(4), 72–85.

Snyder, L. (1975). Pragmatics in language disabled children: Their prelinguistic and early verbal performatives and presuppositions. Unpublished doctoral dissertation, University of Colorado.

Snyder, L., & Downey, D. (1983). Pragmatics and information processing. *Topics in Language Disorders, 4*(1), 75–86.

Snyder-McLean, L., Etter-Schroeder, R., & Rogers, N. (1986). Issues in Piagetian cognitive assessment of severely/profoundly retarded individuals. Paper presented at the American Speech-Language-Hearing Association annual convention, Detroit.

Sobsey, D., & Reichle, J. (1986). Components of reinforcement for attention signal switch activation. Unpublished manuscript, University of Minnesota, Minneapolis.

Song, A., Jones, S., Lippert, J., Metzger, K., Miller, J., & Borreca, C. (1980). Wisconsin Behavior Rating Scale, Revised. Madison, WI: Central Wisconsin Center for Developmental Disabilities.

Sonnenschein, S., & Whitehurst, G. (1984). Developing referential communication: A hierarchy of skills. *Child Development, 55,* 1936–1945.

Spekman, N. (1981). Dyadic verbal communication abilities of learning disabled and normally achieving fourth and fifth grade boys. *Learning Disability Quarterly, 4,* 139–151.

Spekman, N. (1983). Discourse and pragmatics. In C. Wren (Ed.), *Language learning disabilities: Diagnosis and remediation* (pp. 53–120). Rockville, MD: Aspen.

Spiegel, B. (1983). The effect of context on language learning by severely retarded young adults. *Language, Speech, and Hearing Services in Schools, 14,* 252–259.

Spinelli, F., & Terrell, B. (1984). Remediation in context. *Topics in Language Disorders, 5*(1), 29–40.

Spradlin, J., & Siegel, G. (1982). Language training in natural and clinical environments. *Journal of Speech and Hearing Disorders, 47,* 2–6.

Spragle, D., & Micucci, S. (1990). Signs of the week: A functional approach to manual sign training. *Augmentative and Alternative Communication, 6,* 29–37.

Staab, C. (1983). Language functions elicited by meaningful activities: A new dimension in language programs. *Language, Speech and Hearing Services in Schools, 14,* 164–170.

Stafford, M., Sundberg, M., & Braam, S. (1978, May). *An experimental analysis of mands and tacts.* Paper presented at the Fourth Annual Conference of the Midwestern Association of Behavior Analysis, Chicago.

Stallnaker, L., & Creaghead, N. (1982). An examination of language samples obtained under three experimental conditions. *Language, Speech, and Hearing Services in Schools, 13,* 121–128.

Stark, J. (1985, April). *Learning disabilities and reading: Myths and realities.* Paper presented at the New York State Speech-Language-Hearing Association annual convention, Kiamesha Lake.

Stein, N. (1982). What's in a story: Interpreting the interpretations of story grammars. *Discourse Processes, 5,* 319–335.

Stein, N., & Glenn, C. (1979). An analysis of story comprehension in elementary school children. In R. Freedle (Ed.), *New directions in discourse processing* (Vol. 2) (pp. 53–120). Norwood, NJ: Ablex.

Stein, N., & Policastro, M. (1984). The concept of story: A comparison between children's and teachers' viewpoints. In H. Mandl, N. Stein, & T. Trabasso (Eds.), *Learning and comprehension of text* (pp. 113–155). Hillsdale, NJ: Erlbaum.

Steinmann, M. (1982). Speech act theory and writing. In M. Nystrand (Ed.), *What writers know: The language, process, and structure of written discourse* (pp. 291–323). New York: Academic Press.

Stephens, M., & Montgomery, A. (1985). A critique of recent relevant standardized tests. *Topics in Language Disorders, 5*(3), 21–45.

Stern, D. (1971). A microanalysis of mother-infant interaction. *Journal of the American Academy of Child Psychiatry, 10,* 501–517.

Stern, D., Jaffee, J., Beebe, B., & Bennett, S. (1975). Vocalizing in unison and in alternation: Two modes of communication within the mother-infant dyad. *Annals of the New York Academy of Sciences, 263,* 89–100.

Sternat, J., Nietupski, J., Messina, R., Lyon, S., & Brown, L. (1977). Occupational and physical therapy services for severely handicapped students: Towards a naturalized public school service delivery model. In E. Sontag, J. Smith, & N. Certo (Eds.), *Educational programming for the severely and profoundly handicapped* (pp. 263–278). Reston, VA: Division on Mental Retardation. The Council for Exceptional Children.

Sternberg, L. (1984). *Prelanguage communication programming techniques.* Workshop at State University of New York, Geneseo.

Sternberg, L., McNerney, C., & Pegnatore, L. (1985). Developing co-active imitation behaviors with profoundly mentally handicapped students. *Education and Training of the Mentally Retarded, 20,* 260–267.

Sternberg, L., Pegnatore, L., & Hill, C. (1983). Establishing interactive communication behaviors with profoundly mentally handicapped students. *Journal of the Association for Persons with Severe Handicaps, 8,* 39–46.

Stillman, R. (1978). The Callier-Azusa Scale. Dallas: Callier Center for Communication Disorders, The University of Texas at Dallas.

Stillman, R., & Battle, C. (1984). Developing prelanguage communication in the severely handicapped: An interpretation of the VanDijk method. *Seminars in Speech and Language, 5,* 159–170.

Stockman, I., & Vaughn-Cooke, F. (1982). A re-examination of research on the language of black children: The need for a new framework. *Journal of Education, 164,* 157–172.

Stockman, I., & Vaughn-Cooke, F. (1986). Implications of semantic category research for the language assessment of nonstandard speakers. *Topics in Language Disorders, 6*(4), 15–25.

Stokes, T., & Baer, D. (1977). An implicit technology of generalization. *Journal of Applied Behavior Analysis, 10,* 349–367.

Stremel-Campbell, K., & Campbell, C. (1985). Training techniques that may facilitate generalization. In S. Warren & A. Rogers-Warren (Eds.), *Teaching functional language* (pp. 251–285). Baltimore: University Park Press.

Stremel-Campbell, K., Johnson-Dorn, N., Guida, J., & Udell, T. (1984). *Communication curriculum.* Teaching Research Integration Project for Children and Youth with Severe Handicaps, Monmouth, OR.

Sugarman, S. (1973). A description of communicative development in the prelanguage child. Unpublished thesis, Hunter College.

Sutton-Smith, B. (1981). *The folkstories of children.* Philadelphia: University of Pennsylvania Press.

Sutton-Smith, B. (1986). The development of fictional narrative performances. *Topics in Language Disorders, 7*(1), 1–10.

Sutton-Smith, B. & Heath, S. (1981). Paradigms of pretense. *Quarterly Newsletter of the Laboratory of Comparative Human Cognition, 3,* 41–45.

Switzy, H., Rotatori, A., Miller, T., & Freagon, S. (1979). The developmental model and its implications for assessment and instruction for the severely/profoundly handicapped. *Mental Retardation, 17,* 167–170.

Tager-Flusberg, H. (1981). Linguistic functioning in autism. *Journal of Autism and Developmental Disorders, 11,* 45–56.

Tallal, P., Ross, R., & Curtiss, S. (1989). Familial aggregation in specific language impairment. *Journal of Speech O. (1977). The autistic child: Language development through behavior modification.* New York: Wiley.

Tapajna, M., & Finn-Scardine, L. (1981, November). *Comprehensive program planning for nonspeech communication.* Paper presented at the American Speech-Language-Hearing Association annual convention, Los Angeles.

Tattershall, S. (1987). Mission impossible: Learning how a classroom works before it's too late. *Journal of Childhood Communication Disorders, 2*(1), 181–184.

Taylor, O. (1986). Language differences. In G. Shames & E. Wiig (Eds.), *Human Communication* (2nd ed.) (pp. 385–413). Columbus, OH: Merrill.

Templin, M. (1957). *Certain language skills in children.* Minneapolis: University of Minnesota Press.

Templin, M., & Darley, F. (1969). The Templin-Darley Tests of Articulation. Iowa City: Bureau of Educational Research and Services, University of Iowa.

Thal, D., & Bates, E. (1988). Language and gesture in late talkers. *Journal of Speech and Hearing Research, 31,* 115–123.

Thomas, J. (1989). A standardized method for collecting and analyzing language samples of preschool and primary children in the public schools. *Language, Speech, and Hearing Services in Schools, 20,* 85–92.

Thorndyke, P. (1977). Cognitive structures in comprehension and memory of narrative discourse. *Cognitive Psychology, 9,* 77–110.

Thorum, A. (1980). The Fullerton Language Test for Adolescents. Palo Alto, CA: Consulting Psychologists Press.

Tiegerman, E., & Siperstein, M. (1982). Communication training: Changing mother-child interaction. Paper presented at the New York State Speech and Hearing Association annual convention, Ellenville.

Tiegerman, E., & Siperstein, M. (1984). Individual patterns of interaction in the mother-child dyad: Implications for parent intervention. *Topics in Language Disorders, 4*(4), 50–61.

Tizard, B., Cooperman, D., Joseph, A., & Tizard, J. (1973). Environmental effects on language development: A study of young children in long stay residential nurseries. *Annual Progress in Child Psychiatry and Child Development,* 705–728.

Toler, S., & Bankson, N. (1976). Utilization of an interrogative model to evaluate mother's use and children's comprehension of question forms. *Journal of Speech and Hearing Disorders, 41,* 301–314.

Tomasello, M., Farrar, J., & Dines, J. (1984). Children's speech revisions for a familiar and an unfamiliar adult. *Journal of Speech and Hearing Research, 27,* 359–363.

Tomblin, J. (1989). Familial concentration of developmental language impairment. *Journal of Speech and Hearing Disorders, 54,* 287–295.

Tough, J. (1973). *Focus on meaning: Talking to some purpose with young children.* London: George Allen & Unwin.

Tough, J. (1979). *Talk for teaching and learning.* London: Ward Lock Educational.

Trantham, C., & Pedersen, J. (1976). *Normal lan-*

guage development. Baltimore: Williams & Wilkins.

Tronick, E., Als, H., & Adamson, L. (1979). Structure of early face-to-face communicative interactions. In M. Bullowa (Ed.), *Before Speech* (pp. 249–372). New York: Cambridge University Press.

Tucker, J. (1985). Curriculum-based assessment: An introduction. *Exceptional Children, 52,* 199–204.

Tyack, D. (1981). Teaching complex sentences. *Language, Speech, and Hearing Services in Schools, 12,* 49–56.

Tyack, D., & Gottsleben, R. (1977). *Language sampling, analysis, and training.* Palo Alto, CA: Consulting Psychologists Press.

Tyack, D., & Gottsleben, R. (1986). Acquisition of complex sentences. *Language, Speech, and Hearing Services in Schools, 17,* 160–174.

Tyack, D., & Ingram, D. (1977). Children's production and comprehension of questions. *Journal of Child Language, 4,* 211–224.

Tyler, A., Edwards, M., & Saxman, J. (1987). Clinical application of two phonologically based treatment procedures. *Journal of Speech and Hearing Disorders, 52,* 393–409.

Uzgiris, I., & Hunt, J. (1975). *Assessment in infancy: Ordinal scales of intellectual development.* Urbana: University of Illinois Press.

Vanderheiden, G., & Lloyd, L. (1986). Communication systems and their components. In S. Blackstone (Ed.), *Augmentative Communication* (pp. 49–162). Rockville, MD: American Speech-Language-Hearing Association.

van der Lely, H., & Harris, M. (1990). Comprehension of reversible sentences in specifically language-impaired children. *Journal of Speech and Hearing Disorders, 55,* 101–117.

VanDijk, J. (1985). An educational curriculum for deaf-blind multihandicapped persons. In D. Ellis (Ed.), *Sensory impairments in mentally handicapped people* (pp. 374–382). San Diego: College-Hill.

Vetter, D. (1982). Language disorders and schooling. *Topics in Language Disorders, 2*(4), 69–82.

Vicker, B. (1985). *Recognizing and enhancing the communication skills of your group home clients.* Bloomington: Indiana Developmental Training Center.

Wallach, G. (1980). So you want to know what to do with language disabled children above the age of six. *Topics in Language Disorders, 1*(1), 99–113.

Wallach, G., & Butler, K. (1984). *Language learning disabilities in school-age children.* Baltimore: Williams & Wilkins.

Wallach, G., & Liebergott, J. (1984). Who shall be called "Learning Disabled": Some new directions. In G. Wallach & K. Butler (Eds.), *Language learning disabilities in school-age children* (pp. 1–14). Baltimore: Williams & Wilkins.

Wallach, G., & Miller, L. (1988). *Language intervention and academic success.* San Diego: College-Hill.

Wanska, S., Bedrosian, J., & Pohlman, J. (1986). Effects of play materials on the topic performance of preschool children. *Language, Speech, and Hearing Services in Schools, 17,* 152–159.

Warren, S. (1985). Clinical strategies for the measurement of language generalization. In S. Warren & A. Rogers-Warren (Eds.), *Teaching functional language* (pp. 197–224). Baltimore: University Park Press.

Warren, S. (1988). A behavioral approach to language generalization. *Language, Speech, and Hearing Services in Schools, 19,* 292–303.

Warren, S., & Kaiser, A. (1986a). Generalization of treatment effects by young language-delayed children: A longitudinal analysis. *Journal of Speech and Language Disorders, 51,* 239–251.

Warren, S., & Kaiser, A. (1986b). Incidental language teaching: A critical review. *Journal of Speech and Hearing Disorders, 51,* 291–298.

Warren, S., McQuarter, R., & Rogers-Warren, A. (1984). The effects of mands and models on the speech of unresponsive socially isolated children. *Journal of Speech and Hearing Disorders, 47,* 42–52.

Warren, S., & Rogers-Warren, A. (1980). Current perspectives in language remediation: A special monograph. *Education and Treatment in Children, 5,* 133–153.

Warren, S., & Rogers-Warren, A. (1985). Teaching functional language: An introduction. In S. Warren & A. Rogers-Warren (Eds.), *Teaching functional language* (pp. 3–24). Baltimore: University Park Press.

Warren, S., Rogers-Warren, A., Baer, D., & Guess, D. (1980). Assessment and facilitation of generalization. In W. Sailor, B. Wilcox, & L.

Brown (Eds.), *Methods of instruction for severely handicapped students.* Baltimore: Paul H. Brookes.

Washington, D., & Naremore, R. (1978). Children's use of spatial prepositions in two- and three-dimensional tasks. *Journal of Speech and Hearing Research, 21,* 151–165.

Waterson, N. (1978). Growth of complexity in phonological development. In N. Waterson & C. Snow (Eds.), *The development of communication* (pp. 415–442). New York: Wiley.

Waterson, N., & Snow, C. (1978). *The development of communication.* New York: Wiley.

Watson, D., Omark, D., Gronell, S., & Heller, B. (1986). *Nondiscriminatory assessment: A practitioner's handbook.* Sacramento: California State Department of Education.

Watson, L. (1977, November). Conversational participation by language deficient and normal children. Paper presented at the American Speech and Hearing Association annual convention, Chicago.

Watson, L., & Bassinger, J. (1974). Parent training technology: A potential service delivery system. *Mental Retardation, 12,* 3–10.

Watzlawick, P., Beavin, J., & Jackson, D. (1967). *Pragmatics of human communication.* New York: W.W. Norton & Co.

Weaver, P., & Dickinson, D. (1982). Scratching below the surface structure: Exploring the usefulness of story grammars. *Discourse Processes, 5,* 225–243.

Weber-Olsen, M., Putnam-Sims, P., & Gannon, J. (1983). Elicited imitation and the Oral Language Sentence Imitation Screening Test (OLSIST): Content or context. *Journal of Speech and Hearing Disorders, 48,* 368–378.

Weeks, T. (1971). Speech registers in young children. *Child Development, 42,* 1119–1131.

Weiner, F. (1979). *Phonological process analysis.* Baltimore: University Park Press.

Weiner, F. (1981). Treatment of phonological disability using the method of meaningful minimal contrast: Two case studies. *Journal of Speech and Hearing Disorders, 46,* 97–103.

Weiner, F. (1984). A phonologic approach to assessment and treatment. In J. Costello (Ed.), *Speech disorders in children: Recent advances* (pp. 75–91). San Diego: College-Hill.

Weiner, P., & Hoock, W. (1973). The standardization of tests: Criteria and criticisms. *Journal of Speech and Hearing Research, 16,* 616–626.

Weiner, F., & Lewnau, L. (1979). *Nondiscriminatory speech and language testing of minority children: Linguistic interferences.* Paper presented at the American Speech-Language-Hearing Association annual convention, Atlanta.

Weinrich, B., Glaser, A., & Johnston, E. (1987). *A sourcebook of adolescent pragmatic activities.* Tucson, AZ: Communication Skill Builders.

Weisner, S., & Murray-Branch, J. (1989). Modeling versus modeling plus evoked production training: A comparison of two language intervention methods. *Journal of Speech and Hearing Disorders, 54,* 269–281.

Weistuch, L., & Lewis, M. (1986). Effect of maternal language intervention strategies on the language of delayed two to five year olds. Paper presented at the Eastern Psychological Association Conference, New York.

Welch, S. (1981). Teaching generative grammar to mentally retarded children: A review and analysis of a decade of behavioral research. *Mental Retardation, 19,* 277–284.

Wells, G. (1981). *Language through interaction.* New York: Cambridge University Press.

Wells, G. (1985). *Language development in the preschool years.* New York: Cambridge University Press.

Westby, C. (1984). Development of narrative abilities. In G. Wallach & K. Butler (Eds.), *Language learning disabilities in school-age children* (pp. 103–127). Baltimore: Williams & Wilkins.

Westby, C. (1985). Learning to talk—Talking to learn: Oral-literate language differences. In C. Simon (Ed.), *Communication skills and classroom success: Therapy methodologies for language-learning disabled students.* San Diego: College-Hill.

Wetherby, A., Yonclas, D., & Bryan, A. (1989). Communicative profiles of preschool children with handicaps: Implications for early identification. *Journal of Speech and Hearing Disorders, 54,* 148–158.

Wexler, K., Blau, A., Dore, J., & Leslie, S. (1982, April). *A pragmatic view of how nonverbal and vocal persons communicate.* Paper presented at the New York State Speech-Language-Hearing Association annual convention, West Liberty.

Whaley, J. (1981). Readers' expectation for story

structure. *Reading Research Quarterly, 17,* 90–114.

Wickstrom, S., Goldstein, H., & Johnson, L. (1985). On the subject of subjects: Suggestions for describing subjects in language intervention studies. *Journal of Speech and Hearing Disorders, 50,* 282–286.

Wiig, E. (1982). *Let's talk: Developing prosocial communication skills.* San Antonio: Psychological Corporation.

Wiig, E. (1982). *Let's talk inventory for adolescents.* San Antonio: Psychological Corporation.

Wiig, E., Becker-Redding, U., & Semel, E. (in press). A cross-cultural, cross-linguistic comparison of language abilities of 7-to-8- and 12-to-13-year-old children with learning disabilities. *Journal of Learning Disabilities,* in press.

Wiig, E., & Fleischmann, N. (1980, November). Knowledge of pronominalization, reflexivization and relativization by learning disabled college students. Paper presented at the American Speech-Language-Hearing Association annual convention, Los Angeles.

Wiig, E., & Semel, E. (1976). *Language disabilities in children and adolescents.* Columbus, OH: Merrill.

Wiig, E., & Semel, E. (1984). *Language assessment and intervention for the learning disabled* (2nd ed.). Columbus, OH: Merrill.

Wiig, E., Semel, E., & Abele, E. (1981). Perception and interpretation of ambiguous sentences by learning disabled twelve-year-olds. *Learning Disabilities Quarterly, 4,* 3–12.

Wilbur, R. (1983). Where do we go from here. In J. Miller, D. Yoder, & R. Schiefelbusch (Eds.), *Contemporary issues in language intervention* (pp. 137–143). Rockville, MD: American Speech-Language-Hearing Association.

Wilbur, R. (1987). *American Sign Language: Linguistic and applied dimensions* (2nd ed.). San Diego: College-Hill.

Wilcox, K., & McGuinn-Aasby, S. (1988). The performance of monolingual and bilingual Mexican children on the TACL. *Language, Speech, and Hearing Services in Schools, 19,* 34–40.

Wilcox, M., & Campbell, P. (1983, November). *Assessing communication in low-functioning multihandicapped children.* Paper presented at the American Speech-Language-Hearing annual convention, Cincinnati.

Wilcox, M., & Leonard, L. (1978). Experimental

acquisition of wh- questions in language-disordered children. *Journal of Speech and Hearing Research, 21,* 220–239.

Wilkinson, L., & Milosky, L. (1987). School-age children's metapragmatic knowledge of requests and responses in the classroom. *Topics in Language Disorders, 7*(2), 61–70.

Williams, F., Cairns, H., & Cairns, C. (1971). *An analysis of the variations from standard English pronunciation in the phonetic performance of two groups of nonstandard-English-speaking children.* Center for Communication Research, University of Texas.

Williams, R., & Wolfram, W. (1977). *Social dialects: Differences vs. disorders.* Washington, DC: American Speech-Language-Hearing Association.

Wimmer, H. (1979). Processing of script deviation by young children. *Discourse Processes, 2,* 301–310.

Winitz, H. (1973). Problem solving and the delay of speech as strategies in the teaching of language. *ASHA, 15,* 583–586.

Wolfram, W., & Christian, D. (1976). *Appalachian speech.* Arlington, VA: Center for Applied Linguistics.

Wong, B., & Jones, W. (1982). Increasing metacomprehension in learning disabled and normally achieving students through self-questioning training. *Learning Disability Quarterly, 5,* 228–240.

Wood, D. (1983). Teaching: Natural and contrived. *Child Development Society Newsletter, 32,* 2–8.

Woods, T. (1984). Generality on the verbal tacting of autistic children as a function of "naturalness" in antecedent control. *Journal of Behavior Therapy and Experimental Psychiatry, 15,* 27–32.

Wren, C. (1981). Identifying patterns of syntactic disorder in six-year-old children. *British Journal of Disorders of Communication, 16,* 101–109.

Wren, C. (1982). Identifying patterns of processing disorder in six-year-old children with syntax problems. *British Journal of Disorders of Communication, 17,* 83–92.

Wren, C. (1985). Collecting language samples from children with syntax problems. *Language, Speech, and Hearing Services in Schools, 16,* 83–102.

Wulz, S., Hall, M., & Klein, M. (1983). A home-centered instructional communication strategy for severely handicapped children. *Journal of Speech and Hearing Disorders, 48,* 2–10.

Yoder, D. (1985). *Communication and the severely-profoundly retarded.* Paper presented at the Conference on Communication and the Developmentally Disabled: The State of the Art in 1985, Buffalo.

Yorkston, K., & Dowden, P. (1984). Nonspeech language and communication systems. In A. Holland (Ed.), *Language disorders in adults.* San Diego: College-Hill.

Yorkston, K., Honsinger, M., Dowden, P., & Marriner, N. (1989). Vocabulary selection: A case report. *Augmentative and Alternative Communication, 5,* 101–108.

Yorkston, K., Smith, K., & Beukelman, D. (1990). Extended communication samples of augmented communicators I: A comparison of individualized versus standard single-word vocabularies. *Journal of Speech and Hearing Disorders, 55,* 217–224.

Young, E. (1983). A language approach to treatment of phonological process problems. *Language, Speech, and Hearing Services in Schools, 14,* 47–53.

Young, E. (1987). The effects of treatment on consonant cluster and weak syllable reduction processes in misarticulating children. *Language, Speech, and Hearing Services in Schools, 18,* 23–33.

Young, E., & Sacks, G. (1982, June). Remediation of developmental speech disorders with treatment of phonological processes. Paper presented at the American Speech-Language-Hearing Association regional convention, Philadelphia.

Youniss, J. (1980). *Parents and peers in social development.* Chicago: University of Chicago Press.

Zachman, L., Huisingh, R., Jorgensen, C., & Barrett, M. (1978a). Oral Language Sentence Imitation Diagnostic Inventory. Moline, IL: Lingui Systems.

Zachman, L., Huisingh, R., Jorgensen, C., & Barrett, M. (1978b). Oral Language Sentence Imitation Screening Test. Moline, IL: Lingui Systems.

Zimmerman, I., Steiner, V., & Pond, R. (1979). Preschool Language Scale—Revised. San Antonio: Psychological Corporation.

Zwitman, D., & Sonderman, J. (1979). A syntax program designed to present base linguistic structures to language-disordered children. *Journal of Communicative Disorders, 13,* 232–237.

Author Index

Subject Index

Adjectivals, 100–101
Adolescent Language Screening Test, 29, 46
Adverbs, 103
Adversive conjoining, 120
African-American children, 57–58
Agency, 154
American Speech-Language Hearing Association, 257
Analysis of the Language of Learning, 46
Anaphoric reference, 160
Anticipation shelves, 313
Antonyms, 230
Appropriateness:
  of illocutionary function, 88
  of topic initiation, 134–135
Articles, 100, 128
Asian English, 57–58, 336–340
Assessment of Phonological Processes, 46, 107
Assessment:
  classroom, 267–272
  criterion-referenced approach to, 26
  curriculum-based, 267–272
  descriptive
    advantages and disadvantages of, 35–36
    reliability and validity of, 36–39
  goals of, 25
  integrated functional

conversational language sampling, 58
description of, 39–41
formal testing stage, 45–58
observation stage, 42–45
questionnaire, interview, and referral stage, 41–42
neutralist approach to, 26
normalist approach to, 25–26
of presymbolic and minimally symbolic children, 283–305
process, 41–58
psychometric
  content, 29–30
  misuse of, 30–34
  test differences in, 28–29
  variables in selecting, 34
  use of tests in, 26–27
Assigning Structural Stage, 353–354
Assimilation, 110, 254, 387
Audiotaping, 78, 269
Auditory bombardment, 250–251, 255, 256
Augmentative communication, 88, 288, 300, 301, 310, 314–318, 387
Autism, 117, 128, 129, 132, 135, 141, 202, 230, 308
Auxiliary verbs, 104

Backing, 111
Bankson Language Screening Test, 28, 46
Behavior-chain interruption, 287, 312